WORLD HEALTH ORGANIZATION

INTERNATIONAL AGENCY FOR RESEARCH ON CANCER

SECOND CANCER IN RELATION TO RADIATION TREATMENT FOR CERVICAL CANCER

From the International Radiation Study Group on Cervical Cancer

EDITORS
N.E. DAY and J.D. BOICE, Jr

IARC SCIENTIFIC PUBLICATIONS No. 52

RC267
A1
I5
No. 52
1983

LYON 1983

The International Agency for Research on Cancer (IARC) was established in 1965 by the World Health Assembly, as an independently financed organization within the framework of the World Health Organization. The headquarters of the Agency are at Lyon, France.

The Agency conducts a programme of research concentrating particularly on the epidemiology of cancer and the study of potential carcinogens in the human environment. Its field studies are supplemented by biological and chemical research carried out in the Agency's laboratories in Lyon and, through collaborative research agreements, in national research institutions in many countries. The Agency also conducts a programme for the education and training of personnel for cancer research.

The publications of the Agency are intended to contribute to the dissemination of authoritative information on different aspects of cancer research.

OUP ISBN 0-19-723052-0

The authors alone are responsible for the views expressed in the signed articles in this publication.

PRINTED IN FRANCE

TABLE OF CONTENTS

FOREWORD

The risk of cancer following exposure to moderate or low levels of ionizing radiation cannot at present be estimated with precision. There is considerable public pressure for quantitative clarification of these hazards. The main source of additional information on radiation risks will be epidemiological studies on large populations exposed to doses of radiation which can be accurately assessed. Since, fortunately, the general population receives in the normal course of events levels of radiation lower than those at which any detectable effect might be expected, special situations have to be sought. The medical use of radiation presents such an opportunity, in particular the doses used for therapy.

The information collected by cancer registries represents an ideal source of this material. Many population-based cancer registries make great efforts to follow for life those patients they register, recording the appearance of subsequent malignancies. They cover large populations and have been in existence for many years. To develop the joint exploitation of these data, the International Agency for Research on Cancer and the National Cancer Institute of the United States invited those cancer registries which had been in existence for twenty or more years, and which practised lifelong follow-up, to examine the possibilities of collaborative studies. The enthusiastic response of those registries which were approached led to the elaboration of a large series of studies. This monograph represents the first fruits of this collaboration.

L. Tomatis, M.D.
Director, IARC

LIST OF PARTICIPANTS

THE INTERNATIONAL RADIATION STUDY ON CERVICAL CANCER

Those members of the group who participated in the work reported here are listed below, with their respective institutions.

CANADA

N.W. Choi	Manitoba Cancer Treatment and Research Foundation
E.A. Clarke	Ontario Cancer Treatment and Research Foundation
J.M. Elwood	Cancer Control Agency of British Columbia
G.R. Howe	National Cancer Institute of Canada
M. Koch	Alberta Cancer Board
A.B. Miller	National Cancer Institute of Canada
N.A. Nelson	Manitoba Cancer Treatment and Research Foundation
D. Robson	Saskatchewan Cancer Foundation
R.E. Spengler	Ontario Cancer Treatment and Research Foundation
C. Wall	National Cancer Institute of Canada

DENMARK

O.M. Jensen	Danish Cancer Registry
H.H. Storm	Danish Cancer Registry

FINLAND

M. Hakama	Finnish Cancer Registry
T. Hakulinen	Finnish Cancer Registry
K. Mäkelä	Finnish Cancer Registry
A. Rimpelä	Finnish Cancer Registry

NORWAY

A. Andersen	The Cancer Registry of Norway
K. Magnus	The Cancer Registry of Norway
J.E. Skjerven	The Cancer Registry of Norway

SWEDEN

B. Malker	The Cancer Registry of the National Board of Health and Welfare
F. Petterson	Radiumhemmet

UNITED KINGDOM

R. Brown	Birmingham Cancer Registry
M.P. Coleman	London School of Hygiene and Tropical Medicine
P. Fraser	London School of Hygiene and Tropical Medicine
C.C. Patterson	London School of Hygiene and Tropical Medicine
P. Prior	Birmingham Cancer Registry
R.G. Skeet	South Thames Cancer Registry
P.G. Smith	London School of Hygiene and Tropical Medicine
G.W.O. Tomkins	South Thames Cancer Registry

UNITED STATES OF AMERICA

J.D. Boice, Jr	National Cancer Institute
L.A. Brinton	National Cancer Institute
R.E. Curtis	National Cancer Institute
J.T. Flannery	Connecticut Tumor Registry
R. Kleinerman	National Cancer Institute

YUGOSLAVIA

V. Pompe-Kirn	Slovenia Cancer Registry
M. Primic-Žakelj	Slovenia Cancer Registry
B. Ravnihar	Slovenia Cancer Registry
M. Sok	Slovenia Cancer Registry

INTERNATIONAL AGENCY FOR
RESEARCH ON CANCER, LYON,
FRANCE
  N.E. Day
  G. Engholm
  J. Estève
  M. Liceaga de Gonzalez
  C.A. Linsell
  D. Magnin
  X. Nguyen-Dinh
  R. Saracci

PATHOLOGY REVIEW COMMITTEE
  H. Lisco   Harvard University, USA
  W. Moloney   Harvard University, USA
  H. Tulinius   Icelandic Cancer Registry, Reykjavik

DOSIMETRY SUB-COMMITTEE
  M. Rosenstein   Bureau of Radiological Health, Food and Drug Administration, USA
  M. Stovall   M.D. Anderson Hospital and Tumor Institute, USA
  G. Svensson   Harvard University, USA

The study group is deeply appreciative of the support and guidance it received from Professor Brian MacMahon, Dr George Hutchison and Dr Robin Mole. Professor MacMahon was chairman of all the meetings of the group, and his skilled helmsmanship was a major factor in the smooth progress of the study. Dr Hutchinson provided an invaluable link with the previous international study of cervical cancer patients, with which the present study is being merged, as well as contributing his gifts as a rapporteur. Dr Mole advised the group on the radiobiological aspects of the study, and the group benefited in high measure from his experience and knowledge.

The progress of the study was greatly aided by a series of working meetings at the IARC. The participants at these meetings were as follows:

FIRST MEETING - IARC, Lyon, 4-5 October 1979

F. Berrino	National Institute for the Study and Treatment of Tumours, via Venezian 1, 20133 Milan, Italy
J.D. Boice, Jr	Radiation Studies Section, Environmental Epidemiology Branch, National Cancer Institute, Landow Building, Room 3C07, Bethesda MD 20205, USA
R.R. Frentzel-Beyme	Department of Epidemiology, German Cancer Research Centre, Im Neuenheimer Feld 280, Postfach 101949, 6900 Heidelberg 1, Federal Republic of Germany
M. Hakama	Finnish Cancer Registry, Liisankatu 21B, 00170 Helsinki 17, Finland
G.B. Hutchison	Department of Epidemiology, Harvard School of Public Health, 677 Huntington Avenue, Boston MA 02115, USA
L.R. Karhausen	EURATOM-CEA Association, Nuclear Study Centre, 92260 Fontenay-aux-Roses, France
B. MacMahon	Department of Epidemiology, Harvard School of Public Health, 677 Huntington Avenue, Boston MA 02115, USA
K. Magnus	The Cancer Registry of Norway, The Norwegian Radium Hospital, Oslo 3, Norway
R. Mole	MRC Radiobiology Unit, Harwell, Didcot OX11 ORD, UK
P.G. Smith	Department of Medical Statistics and Epidemiology, London School of Hygiene and Tropical Medicine, Keppel Street (Gower Street), London WC1E 7HT, UK
G. Svensson	Division of Physics and Engineering, Harvard Medical School, Radiation Treatment Planning Center, Brookline MA 02146, USA

IARC Secretariat
N.E. Day
J.F. Duplan
J. Estève
O.M. Jensen
C.S. Muir
R. Saracci

SECOND MEETING - IARC, Lyon, 14-15 May 1980

J.D. Boice, Jr	Environmental Epidemiology Branch, National Cancer Institute, Landow Building, Room 3C07, Bethesda MD 20205, USA
L.A. Brinton	ICRF Cancer Epidemiology and Clinical Trials Unit, University of Oxford, 9 Keble Road, Oxford OX1 3OG, UK
M. Faber	Finsen Institute, Strandboulevarden 49, 2100 Copenhagen Ø, Denmark
R.R. Frentzel-Beym	Department of Epidemiology, German Cancer Research Centre, Postfach 101949, 6900 Heidelberg 1, Federal Republic of Germany
M. Hakama	Finnish Cancer Registry, Liisankatu 21B, 00170 Helsinki 17, Finland
O.M. Jensen	Danish Cancer Registry, Strandboulevarden 49, 2100 Copenhagen Ø, Denmark
L.R. Karhause	EURATOM-CEA Association, Nuclear Study Centre, 92260 Fontenay-aux-Roses, France
K.E. Kjørstad	Department of Gynaecology, Norwegian Radium Hospital, Oslo 3, Norway
H. Lisco	Harvard University, Division of Medical Sciences of the Faculty of Arts and Sciences, 25 Shattuck Street, Boston MA 02115, USA
B. MacMahon	Department of Epidemiology, Harvard University School of Public Health, 677 Huntington Avenue, Boston MA 02115, USA
K. Magnus	The Cancer Registry of Norway, Norwegian Radium Hospital, Oslo 3, Norway
B. Malker	The Cancer Registry of the National Board of Health and Welfare, 106 30 Stockholm, Sweden
A.B. Miller	Director, NCIC Epidemiology Unit, University of Toronto, Faculty of Medicine, McMurrich Building, Toronto, Ontario M5S 1A8, Canada
R. Mole	Visitor, MRC Radiobiology Unit, Harwell, Didcot OX11 0RD, UK
J.J. Nickson	Department of Radiation Oncology, The University of Tennessee Center for the Health Sciences, 800 Madison Avenue, Memphis, TN 38163, USA
F. Pettersson	Radiumhemmet, 104 01 Stockholm 60, Sweden
E. Pochin	National Radiological Protection Board, Harwell, Didcot OX11 0RD, UK
V. Pompe-Kirn	The Cancer Registry of Slovenia, Institute of Oncology, Zaloska 2, 61000 Ljubljana, Yugoslavia
P.G. Smith	Department of Medical Statistics and Epidemiology, London School of Hygiene and Tropical Medicine, Keppel Street (Gower Street), London WC1E 7HT, UK
M. Stovall	Physics Department, The University of Texas System Cancer Center, M.D. Anderson Hospital and Tumor Institute, Texas Medical Center, Houston, TX 77030, USA

IARC Secretariat
N.W. Choi
N.E. Day
J. Estève
D. Magnin
R. Saracci
J. Wahrendorf

THIRD MEETING - IARC, Lyon, 10-11 December 1980

F. Berrino	National Institute for the Study and Treatment of Tumours, via Venezian 1, 20133 Milan, Italy
J.D. Boice, Jr	Radiation Studies Section, Environmental Epidemiology Branch, National Cancer Institute, Landow Building, Room 3C07, Bethesda, MD 20205, USA
N.W. Choi	Epidemiology and Biostatistics, Manitoba Cancer Treatment and Research Foundation, University of Manitoba Faculty of Medicine, 700 Bannatyne Avenue, Winnipeg, Manitoba R3E OW3, Canada
J.M. Elwood	Chairman, Department of Community Health, University of Nottingham, Queen's Medical Centre, Nottingham NG7 2UH, UK
R.R. Frentzel-Beyme	Department of Epidemiology, German Cancer Research Centre, Postfach 101949, 6900 Heidelberg 1, Federal Republic of Germany
H. Hansen	Danish Cancer Registry, Strandboulevarden 49, 2100 Copenhagen Ø, Denmark

PARTICIPANTS

O.M. Jensen	Danish Cancer Registry, Strandboulevarden 49, 2100 Copenhagen Ø, Denmark
B. MacMahon	Department of Epidemiology, Harvard School of Public Health, 677 Huntington Avenue, Boston, MA 02115, USA
B. Malker	The Cancer Registry of the National Board of Health and Welfare, 106 30 Stockholm, Sweden
A.B. Miller	Director, NCIC Epidemiology Unit, University of Toronto, Faculty of Medicine, McMurrich Building, Toronto, Ontario M5S 1A8, Canada
R. Mole	MRC Radiobiology Unit, Harwell, Didcot OX11 ORD, UK
G. O'Conor	Director, Office of International Affairs, National Cancer Institute, Department of Health and Human Services, Washington, DC 20201, USA
F. Pettersson	Radiumhemmet, 104 01 Stockholm 60, Sweden
V. Pompe-Kirn	The Cancer Registry of Slovenia, Institute of Oncology, Zaloska 2, 61000 Ljubljana, Yugoslavia
P. Prior	Birmingham Cancer Registry, Queen Elizabeth Medical Centre, Birmingham B15 2TH, UK
P.G. Smith	Department of Medical Statistics and Epidemiology, London School of Hygiene and Tropical Medicine, Keppel Street (Gower Street), London WC1E 7HT, UK
R.F. Spengler	Division of Epidemiology and Statistics, The Ontario Cancer Treatment and Research Foundation, 7 Overlea Boulevard, Toronto, Ontario M4H 1A8, Canada
H.H. Storm	Danish Cancer Registry, Strandboulevarden 49, 2100 Copenhagen Ø, Denmark
M. Stovall	Physics Department, The University of Texas System Cancer Center, M.D. Andersen Hospital and Tumor Institute, Texas Medical Center, Houston, TX 77030, USA
H. Tulinius	Icelandic Cancer Registry, PO Box 523, Reykjavik, Iceland

IARC Secretariat
N.E. Day
J. Estève
A. Geser
Hu Meng-Xuan
C.A. Linsell
D. Magnin
C.S. Muir
R. Saracci
J. Wahrendorf
D. Zaridze

FOURTH MEETING - IARC, Lyon, 7-8 July 1981

J.D. Boice, Jr	Environmental Epidemiology Branch, National Cancer Institute, Landow Building, Room 3C07, Bethesda, MD 20205, USA
N.W. Choi	Epidemiology and Biostatistics, Manitoba Cancer Treatment and Research Foundation, University of Manitoba Faculty of Medicine, 700 Bannatyne Avenue, Winnipeg, Manitoba R3E OW3
M. Coleman	Department of Medical Statistics and Epidemiology, London School of Hygiene and Tropical Medicine, Keppel Street (Gower Street), London WC1E 7HT, UK
M. Hakama	Finnish Cancer Registry, Liisankatu 21B, 00170 Helsinki 17, Finland
G.R. Howe	NCIC Epidemiology Unit, University of Toronto Faculty of Medicine, McMurrich Building, Toronto, Ontario M5S 1A8, Canada
G.B. Hutchison	Department of Epidemiology, Harvard School of Public Health, 677 Huntington Avenue, Boston, MA 02115, USA
O.M. Jensen	Danish Cancer Registry, Strandboulevarden 49, 2100 Copenhagen Ø, Denmark
L.R. Karhausen	EURATOM-CEA, Nuclear Study Centre, 92260 Fontenay-aux-Roses, France
K.E. Kjørstad	Department of Gynaecology, Norwegian Radium Hospital, Oslo 3, Norway
B. MacMahon	Department of Epidemiology, Harvard School of Public Health, 677 Huntington Avenue, Boston, MA 02115, USA
K. Magnus	The Cancer Registry of Norway, The Norwegian Radium Hospital, Oslo 3, Norway

B. Malker	The Cancer Registry of the National Board of Health and Welfare, 106 30 Stockholm, Sweden
W.C. Moloney	Hematology Division, Brigham and Women's Hospital, 75 Francis Street, Boston, MA 02115, USA
F. Pettersson	Department of Gynaecology, Karolinska Hospital, 104 01 Stockholm 60, Sweden
P. Prior	Birmingham Cancer Registry, Queen Elizabeth Medical Centre, Birmingham B15 2TH, UK
N.T. Racoveanu	Radiation Health Unit, World Health Organization, avenue Appia, 1211 Geneva 27, Switzerland
P.G. Smith	Department of Medical Statistics and Epidemiology, London School of Hygiene and Tropical Medicine, Keppel Street (Gower Street), London WC1E 7TH, UK
R.F. Spengler	Division of Epidemiology and Statistics, The Ontario Cancer Treatment and Research Foundation, 7 Overlea Boulevard, Toronto, Ontario M4H 1A8, Canada
H.H. Storm	Danish Cancer Registry, Strandboulevarden 49, 2100 Copenhagen Ø, Denmark
H. Tulinius	Icelandic Cancer Registry, PO Box 523, Reykjavik, Iceland
M. Wilhelmsen	Department of Gynaecology, Haukeland Hospital, 5016 Haukeland, Norway

IARC Secretariat
N.E. Day
J. Estève
A. Geser
C.A. Linsell
D. Magnin
R. Saracci
J. Wahrendorf

FIFTH MEETING - IARC, Lyon, 5-7 January 1982

F. Berrino	National Institute for the Study and Treatment of Tumours, via Venezian 1, 20133 Milan, Italy
J.D. Boice, Jr	Radiation Studies Section, Environmental Epidemiology Branch, National Cancer Institute, Landow Building, Room 3C07, Bethesda, MA 20205, USA
N.W. Choi	Epidemiology and Biostatistics, Manitoba Cancer Treatment and Research Foundation, University of Manitoba Faculty of Medicine, 700 Bannatyne Avenue, Winnipeg, Manitoba R3E OW3, Canada
E.A. Clarke	Division of Epidemiology and Statistics, The Ontario Cancer Treatment and Research Foundation, 7 Overlea Boulevard, Toronto, Ontario M4H 1A8, Canada
M. Coleman	Epidemiological Monitoring Unit, London School of Hygiene and Tropical Medicine, Keppel Street (Gower Street), London WC1E 7HT, UK
V. Fournier	University Centre for Gynaecology and Obstetrics, Voss strasse 9, 6900 Heidelberg, Federal Republic of Germany
P. Fraser	Epidemiology Monitoring Unit, London School of Hygiene and Tropical Medicine, Keppel Street (Gower Street), London WC1E 7HT, UK
R.R. Frentzel-Beyme	Department of Epidemiology, German Cancer Research Centre, Postfach 101949, 6900 Heidelberg 1, Federal Republic of Germany
R. Frischkorn	Department of Gynaecological Radiation, University Women's Clinic, 3400 Gottingen, Federal Republic of Germany
M. Hakama	Finnish Cancer Registry, Liisankatu 21B, 00170 Helsinki 17, Finland
A. Hamburger	Department of Radiotherapy, M.D. Anderson Hospital and Tumor Institute, Texas Medical Center, Houston, TX 77030, USA
Z. Hlasivec	Radiotherapy Centre, Oncological Institute, Na Truhlarce 100, Prague 8, Czechoslovakia
G.R. Howe	NCIC Epidemiology Unit, University of Toronto Faculty of Medicine, McMurrich Building, Toronto, Ontario M5S 1A8, Canada
G.B. Hutchison	Department of Epidemiology, Harvard School of Public Health, 677 Huntington Avenue, Boston, MA 02115, USA
O.M. Jensen	Danish Cancer Registry, Strandboulevarden 49, 2100 Copenhagen Ø, Denmark

PARTICIPANTS

L.R. Karhausen	EURATOM-CEA, Nuclear Study Centre, 92260 Fontenay-aux-Roses, France
K.E. Kjorstad	Department of Gynaecology, Norwegian Radium Hospital, Oslo 3, Norway
H. Kucera	Radiation Department, University Women's Clinics I and II, Spitalgasse 23, 1090 Vienna, Austria
B. MacMahon	Department of Epidemiology, Harvard School of Public Health, 677 Huntington Avenue, Boston, MA 02115, USA
B. Malker	The Cancer Registry of the National Board of Health and Welfare, 106 30 Stockholm, Sweden
R. Mole	MRC Radiobiology Unit, Harwell, Didcot OX11 ORD, UK
W.C. Moloney	Hematology Division, Brigham and Women's Hospital, 75 Francis Street, Boston, MA 02115, USA
R.F. Mould	Physics Department - Statistics, Westminster Hospital, Page Street Wing, London SW1P 2AP, UK
F.E. Neal	Weston Park Hospital, Whitham Road, Sheffield SLO 2SJ, UK
M. Palmer	Christie Hospital and Holt Radium Institute, Withington, Manchester M20 9BX, UK
F. Pettersson	Department of Gynaecology, Karolinska Hospital, 104 01 Stockholm 60, Sweden
P. Pisani	National Institute for the Study and Treatment of Tumours, via Venezian 1, 20133 Milan, Italy
V. Pompe-Kirn	The Cancer Registry of Slovenia, Institute of Oncology, Zaloska 2, 61000 Ljubljana, Yugoslavia
P. Prior	Birmingham Cancer Registry, Queen Elizabeth Medical Centre, Birmingham B15 2TH, UK
N.T. Racoveanu	Radiation Health Unit, World Health Organization, avenue Appia, 1211 Geneva 27, Swizterland
A. Rimpelä	Finnish Cancer Registry, Liisankatu 21B, 00170 Helsinki 17, Finland
M.D. Schulz	Department of Radiation Medicine, Massachusetts General Hospital, Boston, MA 02114, USA
P.G. Smith	Department of Medical Statistics and Epidemiology, London School of Hygiene and Tropical Medicine, Keppel Street (Gower Street), London WC1E 7HT, UK
H.H. Storm	Danish Cancer Registry, Strandboulevarden 49, 2100 Copenhagen Ø, Denmark
M. Stovall	Physics Department, The University of Texas System Cancer Center, M.D. Anderson Hospital and Tumor Institute, Texas Medical Center, Houston, TX 77030, USA
H. Tulinius	Icelandic Cancer Registry, PO Box 523, Reykjavik, Iceland
J. Wolff	Clinical and Therapeutic Centre, Gustave Roussy Institute, Hautes Bruyères, rue Camille-Desmoulins, 94800 Villejuif, France

IARC Secretariat
N.E. Day
J. Estève
A. Geser
C.A. Linsell
D. Magnin
C.S. Muir
R. Saracci
L. Tomatis
J. Wahrendorf

PREFACE

B. MacMahon

Department of Epidemiology
Harvard University
School of Public Health
Boston, Massachusetts, USA

It is said that only a fool learns from his own experience. And yet much human experience that could prevent us from being fools is ignored. Millions suffer and die without the lessons learned from their suffering being transmitted to those who follow them. The antecedents and concomitants of their illnesses - what induced them, what relieved them, and what were their consequences - go largely unrecorded. This volume is the work of individuals who would have it otherwise.

By the late 1950s, the fact that large doses of radiation could cause leukaemia had been well established, but there was a great need for information on the relationship between level of exposure and level of risk - the so-called dose-response relationship. This information was needed to predict the risks of radiation, not at high doses such as those received by many of the atomic bomb survivors or patients treated with X-rays for ankylosing spondylitis, but at the relatively low doses to which millions of people are exposed in the course of their occupations - when undergoing medical diagnostic tests, or when watching television or climbing mountains. Any accurate point on a dose-response curve would be of value.

In 1957, Dr Hermann Lisco, then Secretary of the United Nations Scientific Committee on the Effects of Atomic Radiation, recognized one segment of human experience from which important information was being lost. This was experience of women treated with ionizing radiation for carcinoma of the cervix of the uterus. Patients with cervical cancer were of interest since there was presumably accurate measurement of their exposure and they had been irradiated by at least two distinct modalities - X-rays and radium.

With the invaluable support of Dr Lowry Dobson, then Chief of the Division of Radiological Health of the World Health Organization, a steering committee, consisting of Dr Lisco, Dr George Hutchison, Dr James Nickson and myself, organized an international collaborative effort, of which two reports have been published (Hutchison, 1968; Boice & Hutchison, 1980). The scientific conclusions of that first study are reviewed elsewhere in this volume.

In the last two decades, concern about the carcinogenic effects of ionizing radiation has expanded from its effects on the haematopoietic system to its potential effects on a wide variety of tissues, the most important of which from the practical point of view being, perhaps, the female breast. The editors of the present volume, one of whom (JDB) had participated in the earlier effort, recognized that organs other than the bone marrow receive varying doses

B. MACMAHON

of radiation as a consequence of X-ray or radium treatment of cervical cancer. The same population of patients with cervical cancer could, therefore, yield information much broader than that sought earlier and, for the breast, in a rather critical dose range. Accordingly, plans were initiated to follow up further the cervical cancer cohort in those clinical centres where it appeared feasible.

During the past two decades, a new data resource - the population-based cancer registry - has been greatly expanded. These too seemed capable of addressing the question of the risk of second tumours in patients irradiated for cervical cancer, although the number of patients required for a useful study was beyond the resources of any single registry. The International Agency for Research on Cancer, with financial support from the US National Cancer Institute, took on the task of coordinating the international collaborative effort, the results of which are reported here. For financial and administrative reasons, the studies based on cancer registries proceeded faster than the follow-up of the clinical series which prompted the programme of investigations. The latter, however, is under way and results will be reported in due course.

The data presented here are descriptive - they are intended to raise questions rather than to answer them. Interpretations are advanced for some of the findings, but many of the results are simply provocative. It is likely that many years of investigation will be needed to understand them or even to distinguish between alternative explanations of them. Some questions will be answered, others will not. But some components of this human experience have been preserved. They are offered to the future to make of them what it can.

REFERENCES

Hutchison, G.B. (1968) Leukemia in patients with cancer of the cervix uteri treated with radiation. A report covering the first 5 years of an international study. *J. natl Cancer Inst.*, *40*, 951-982

Boice, J.D. & Hutchison, G.B. (1980) Leukemia in women following radiotherapy for cervical cancer. Ten-year follow-up of an international study. *J. natl Cancer Inst.*, *65*, 115-129

INTRODUCTORY CHAPTER

The International Radiation Study of Cervical Cancer comprises a programme of individual studies on radiation carcinogenesis. The aim of the overall programme is to provide more precise quantitative information relating radiation dose to excess cancer risk for a number of organs, with an emphasis on moderate radiation dose levels. In addition, it is hoped that the study will help to increase understanding of the mechanisms of carcinogenesis. For this purpose, well-defined populations of women with a diagnosis of cancer of the uterine cervix are being followed up, and their subsequent cancer experience determined. For a variety of cancer sites, the treatment given for an initial cervical cancer in women who later developed a second primary cancer at a specific site will be compared with the treatment given to women who did not develop a second cancer at that site. The treatments will be defined in terms of radiation dose at the site in question. The investigations set in motion to achieve these ends include cohort studies of a large number of cancer registries and individual clinics, case-control studies within these cohorts, dosimetry studies, pathological evaluations and chromosomal studies. The design of the overall programme, showing the relationships between the different component investigations, is displayed in Figure 1.

The programme developed from a WHO-sponsored investigation of 30 000 women in nine countries who were treated for cancer of the cervix uteri and evaluated clinically in the period 1960-1970 (Hutchison, 1968; Boice & Hutchison, 1980). Follow-up of most of this population is being extended to the present day. However, to obtain a sample large enough to measure the effects of relatively low doses of radiation received by organs distant from the site of primary irradiation, the programme was expanded by including additional women treated for cancer of the cervix. This expansion was achieved through the collaboration of many population-based cancer registries. Registries were selected on the basis of completeness of registration, length of time in existence, availability of resources for epidemiological investigations, and willingness to participate in a collaborative study. The most important requirement, however, was that a registry should follow for life cancer patients who had been registered, so that the subsequent occurrence of second primary cancers and of death would be known. Results from the cohort studies conducted by the cancer registries and from preliminary dosimetry studies are presented in this monograph.

Data from the 15 collaborating population-based cancer registries were analysed individually in a standard fashion and also combined in a summary analysis. Participating countries and registries are those of: Canada (Alberta, British Columbia, Manitoba, New Brunswick, Nova Scotia, Ontario, Saskatchewan), Denmark, Finland, Norway, Sweden, the United Kingdom (Birmingham, South Thames), the United States of America (Connecticut) and Yugoslavia (Slovenia). As shown in Figure 1, these cohort studies are used as the basis for case-control studies of individual organ sites, in which radiation doses will be estimated for each woman from information available in her radiotherapy records. However, the present analysis is limited to the information available in the cancer registry records. Since few registries record extensive details of treatment, women with cervical cancer were distinguished simply by whether or not mention was made of any radiation treatment. It appears likely that most women not known to have received radiotherapy have been correctly classified as non-exposed, although some misclassification does occur (see Storm & Jensen, this volume, Table 1). Details of how

Figure 1. International Radiation Study of Cervical Cancer. Aim: To improve the precision of the quantitative estimates of risk for cancer induced by moderate doses of radiation, for a variety of body organs and tissues

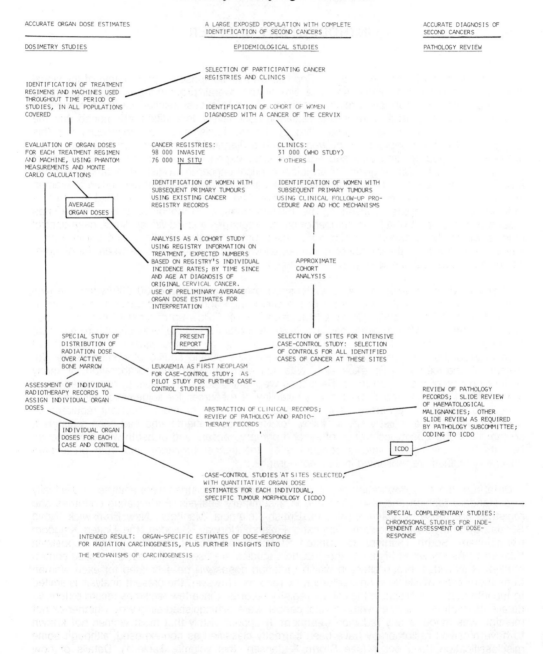

radiotherapy information was coded are given in the individual chapter for each registry, where appropriate. The information available on stage of disease varied among registries, and for the present purpose a distinction was made only between invasive and in-situ cancers of the cervix. The great majority of in-situ tumours did not receive radiotherapy. The radiation dose received by different organs and tissues of the body varies with the treatment regimen, which depends both on extent of disease, calendar year of treatment and treatment clinic. Most long-term survivors would have been in either Stage I or Stage II at the time of initial diagnosis. Approximate estimates of the average dose received by each organ have been made by consideration of generic type of treatment, without reference to individual radiotherapy records (see Stovall, this volume).

Information on second primary cancers was taken mainly from the records of the cancer registries, although, as noted in the individual chapters, a few registries chose to review histologically a number of organ sites. It is important to note that cancer registries participating in this study have made a routine practice of applying strict criteria before accepting a lesion as a second primary cancer.

The main purpose of this component of the programme is to examine the influence of radiation on cancer risk and to focus case-control studies upon sites of particular interest. It should be stressed that these studies cannot meaningfully be used to evaluate the therapeutic efficiency of different treatment regimens for cervical cancer. The possible occurrence of a low frequency of treatment-induced cancers is not likely to be a major criterion of the value of such treatment. The specific objectives of the cohort studies presented here are:

1. To determine the incidence of second cancers in women initially diagnosed as having invasive or in situ cervical cancer, by type of treatment (radiotherapy, no radiotherapy), and lapse of time since diagnosis of primary cervical cancer, with and without histological confirmation as recorded in the cancer registries;

2. To generate hypotheses regarding the possible influence of radiation dose on the development of second primary cancers; and

3. To provide the basis for case-control studies of specific cancers, to be undertaken in the future.

Eligibility of subjects for inclusion

All patients with invasive or in-situ cancer of the uterine cervix diagnosed between the first date of registry operation and the last year of complete registry follow-up were eligible for the study. Patients with in situ lesions recorded as having received radiation treatment were excluded. Patients with malignancies recorded either before the diagnosis of cervical cancer or during the subsequent month were also excluded. Other criteria for exclusion peculiar to particular cancer registries are specified in the chapters relating to the individual registries.

Methods

The period of observation for calculation of the risk of developing a second cancer began at the date of diagnosis of cervical cancer. Among women in whom no second cancer developed, the end of the period of risk was taken as the date of last contact, that is, the date of death for those who died or the date last known alive. For women who developed a second cancer, other than a non-melanoma skin cancer, the end of the period of risk was the date the second cancer was diagnosed. The total number of second cancers registered, with and without histological confirmation, is recorded for each site and for each time interval. For each cancer, five-year age and five-year calendar-year incidence rates from the relevant cancer registry were applied to the appropriate woman-years under observation to obtain the numbers of second primary cancers that would be expected had these patients experienced the same rates as prevailed in the corresponding general population. The information obtained from the 15 population-based cancer registries was combined and is evaluated in the summary chapter

Either the 7th or 8th revision of the International Classification of Diseases (ICD) was used by the various registries. Direct correspondences were made by following the guidelines given in Volume III of *Cancer Incidence in Five Continents* (Waterhouse *et al.*, 1976).

Table 1. Equivalence between ICD7 and ICD8 codes

7th Revision		8th Revision	
*140	Lip	*140	Lip
*141 (a)	Tongue	*141	Tongue
*142 (a)	Salivary gland	*142	Salivary gland
143 (b)	Floor of mouth	144	Floor of mouth
		143.1	*Lower gum*
144 (b)	Other parts of mouth and mouth unspecified	*145	Other and unspecified parts of mouth
		143.0	*Upper gum*
		143.9	*Gum unspecified*
*145 (a)	Oral mesopharynx	*146 (c)	Oropharynx
		(d)	
146	Nasopharynx	147	Nasopharynx
147	Hypopharynx	*148	Hypopharynx
148	Pharynx unspecified	149	Pharynx unspecified
150	Oesophagus	150	Oesophagus
151	Stomach	*151	Stomach
*152 (a)	Small intestine incl. duodenum	*152	Small intestine incl. duodenum
*153 (a)	Large intestine except rectum	*153	Large intestine except rectum
154	Rectum	*154	Rectum and rectosigmoid junction
*155 (a)	Biliary passages and liver (stated to be primary)	*155*	*Various*
		156	*Various*
155.0	*Liver*	*155	Liver and intrahepatic bile ducts specified primary
155.1	*Gallbladder and extrahepatic gall ducts, including ampulla of Vater*	*156	Gallbladder and bile ducts
155.8	*Multiple sites*		
156	Liver (secondary and unspecified)	*197.7*	*Liver secondary*
		197.8	*Liver unspecified*
157	Pancreas	*157	Pancreas
158	Peritoneum	*158	Peritoneum and retroperitoneal tissue
159	Unspecified digestive organs	159	Unspecified digestive organs
*160 (a)	Nose, nasal cavities, middle ear and accessory sinuses	*160	Nose, nasal cavities, middle ear and accessory sinuses
161 (d)	Larynx	*161	Larynx
*162 (a)	Bronchus and trachea and lung, primary	*162*	*Various*
		163 (part)	*Various*

7th Revision		8th Revision	
162.0	Trachea	162.0	Trachea
162.1	Bronchus and lung	162.1	Bronchus and lung
162.2	Pleura	163.0	Pleura
162.8	Multiple sites		
163	Lung unspecified whether primary or secondary	162 (part)	Various
		197 (part)	Various
164	Mediastinum	163.1	Mediastinum
		163.9	Site unspecified
165	Thoracic organs (secondary)	197.0	Lung secondary
		197.1	Mediastinum secondary
		197.2	Pleura secondary
		197.3	Other respiratory organs secondary
170	Breast	174	Breast
171 (h)	Cervix uteri	180	Cervix uteri
		234.0	Carcinoma in situ of cervix uteri
172	Corpus uteri	182.0	Corpus uteri
173	Other parts of uterus including chorione-pithelioma	181	Chorionepithelioma
		182.9 (part)	Uterus unspecified
174	Uterus unspecified	182.9 (part)	Uterus unspecified
*175 (a)	Ovary, fallopian tube and broad ligament	*183	Ovary, fallopian tube and broad ligament
*176 (a)	O and U female genital organs	*184	O and U female genital organs
177	Prostate	185	Prostate
178	Testis	186	Testis
*179 (a)	O and U male genital organs	*187	Various
		172 (part)	Various Various
		173 (part)	
179.0	Penis	187.0	Penis
179.1	Scrotum	172.5	Scrotum (melanoma)
		173.5	Scrotum (skin)
179.7	Other specified sites	187.8	Other specified sites
179.8	Multiple sites		
179.9	Site unspecified	187.9	Site unspecified
180	Kidney	*189 (part)	O and U urinary organs
		189.0	Kidney except pelvis
		189.1	Pelvis of kidney
		189.2	Ureter
*181 (a)	Bladder and other urinary organs	188	Various
		189 (part)	Various
181.0	Bladder	188	Bladder
181.7	Other urinary organs	189.9	Other and unspecified
181.8	Multiple sites		
*190 (a) (f)	Melanoma of skin	*172 (f) (part)	Melanoma of skin
*191 (a) (g)	Other skin (f)	*173 (f) (part)	Other skin (g)
192 (i)	Eye	190	Eye
*193 (a)	Brain and other parts of nervous system	191 *192	Brain
			Other parts of nervous system
193.0 (j)	Brain (continued)	191	Brain
		192.0	Cranial nerves including optic
193.1	Spinal cord	192.2	Spinal cord
193.2	Meninges	192.1	Cerebral meninges
		192.3	Spinal meninges
193.3	Peripheral nerves	192.4	Peripheral nerves
193.4	Sympathetic nervous system	192.5	Sympathetic nervous system
193.8	Multiple sites		
193.9	Site unspecified	192.9	Site unspecified

7th Revision		8th Revision	
194	Thyroid gland	193	Thyroid gland
*195 (a)	Other endocrine glands	*194	Other endocrine glands
*196 (e)	Bone	*170	Bone
*197	Connective tissue	*171	Connective tissue and other soft tissue
199 (c)	Other and unspecified sites	*195	Ill-defined sites
		197.4	*Small intestine including duodenum secondary*
		197.5	*secondary*
		197.6	*Large intestine and rectum secondary*
		198	*Peritoneum secondary*
		*199	Other secondary
			Without specification of site
*200	Lymphosarcoma and reticulosarcoma	*200*	*Various*
		202 (part)	*Various*
200.0	*Reticulum-cell sarcoma*	*200	Lymphosarcoma and reticulum-cell sarcoma
200.1	*Lymphosarcoma*		
200.2	*Other primary lymphoid tissue*	*202.2*	*Other primary lymphoid tissue*
201	Hodgkin's disease	201	Hodgkin's disease
*202	Other forms of lymphoma (reticulosis)	*202 (part)	Other lymphoid tissue
203	Multiple myeloma (plasmocytoma)	203	Multiple myeloma
*204	Leukaemia and aleukaemia	*204-207*	*Various*
204.0	*Lymphatic leukaemia*	*204.1*	*Chronic lymphatic leukaemia*
		204.9	*Unspecified lymphatic leukaemia*
204.1	*Myeloid leukaemia*	*205.1*	*Chronic myeloid leukaemia*
		205.9	*Unspecified myeloid leukaemia*
204.2	*Monocytic leukaemia*	*206	Monocytic leukaemia
204.3	Acute leukaemia	*204.0*	*Acute lymphatic leukaemia*
		205.0	*Acute myeloid leukaemia*
		207.0	*Acute leukaemia unspecified*
204.4	*O and U leukaemia*	*207.1*	*Leukaemia chronic (O and U)*
		207.2	*Acute erythraemia*
		207.9	*Leukaemia unspecified (O and U)*
205	Mycosis fungoides	*202.1*	*Mycosis fungoides*

(a) In ICD7 this number includes a sub-rubric for 'multiple sites'. There is no equivalent in ICD8 for this sub-rubric, secondary neoplasms of multiple lymph nodes (ICD8 196.8) excepted (see note (e) below)

(b) 'Gum' (ICD8 143) is distributed between 'floor of mouth' (ICD7 143) and 'other parts of mouth and mouth unspecified' (ICD7 144), there being no separate rubric or sub-rubric for gum in ICD7

(c) 'Branchial cleft or vestiges' included as an inclusion term (ICD8 146.8) in 'oropharynx' is coded to 'other and unspecified sites' (ICD7 199)

(d) 'Epiglottis, anterior surface' included as an inclusion term (ICD8 146.8) in 'oropharynx' was probably coded to larynx (ICD7 161)

(e) 'Multiple sites' of bone (ICD7 196.9) is merged with 'bones of site unspecified' in ICD7 whereas the comparable rubric of the 8th Revision (ICD8 170.9) is entitled 'site unspecified'

(f) 'Melanoma of skin' (ICD7 190) and 'other skin' (ICD7 191) exclude 'scrotum' which is coded to 'male genital organs' (ICD7 179.1) whereas the scrotum is included in skin in ICD8

(g) 'Other skin' in both Revisions (ICD8 173, ICD7 191) has the same 4th digit breakdown as 'melanoma of skin' (ICD8 172, ICD7 190)

(h) 'Cervix uteri' (ICD7 171) probably includes 'carcinoma *in situ* of cervix' since this specification term appears neither in the list of histological terms preceeding the Tabular List itself nor in the Index of ICD7. It was therefore likely to have been coded as 'carcinoma, any type'

(i) 'Optic nerve' is included with 'eye' in the 7th Revision (ICD7 192)

(j) 'Cranial nerves', except the 'optic nerve', are included in 'brain' (ICD7 193.0) in ICD7

* Fourth digit sub-rubrics exist for this site in the classification

Format

The collected material has been presented in five tables in a standard format, registry by registry. The stage of the initial cervical cancer was classified as either 'invasive' or 'in situ'. The treatment regimens were grouped into two categories, those in which radiotherapy was specifically mentioned, and others. At least five tables are provided by each registry as follows:

Characteristics of the population under study

Observed and expected numbers of second cancers among patients with invasive disease treated by radiotherapy

Observed and expected numbers of second cancers among patients with invasive disease not treated by radiotherapy

Observed and expected numbers of second cancers among patients with in-situ disease

Observed and expected numbers of breast cancers by age at diagnosis of cervical cancer and by period of observation

Each participating registry provided a description of its material to precede the tables. This includes a brief account of the registry, exceptions to the general guidelines, special difficulties, and observations that warrant special consideration. Although all second cancers were evaluated by age at treatment, the individual registry chapters provide this information only for the breast: the breast is given special emphasis because the risk of radiogenic breast cancer is known to vary appreciably by age at exposure (Boice et al., 1979) and because the protective effect of an artificial menopause also varies according to the age at which it is induced (Trichopoulos et al., 1972). The distributions of other cancers by age at diagnosis of cervical cancer and by period of observation are given for the combined registry material in the appendices.

Registries were also asked to list the numbers of women with three or more primary cancers. A total of 238 third and subsequent tumours were identified, but no analysis has been made of this material.

Radiation treatment

Radiation treatment was usually either by external beam, intracavitary radium, or a combination of both. The type of external beams commonly used included orthovoltage (200-400 kVp), cobalt-60, and megavoltage (2-33 MV photons) from betatrons, van de Graaff generators and linear accelerators.

Although exposure or tissue dose for individual subjects is usually not found in registry records, organs have been roughly classified according to their location with respect to the cervix and thus to the level of exposure likely to be received (see Stovall, this volume). The bladder, rectum, uterine corpus, large intestine, ovaries, bone, and lymphatic and haematopoietic systems are close to the cervix and therefore considered to be heavily irradiated sites. The stomach, pancreas, kidney and liver would be less heavily irradiated and are classed as sites of intermediate irradiation. The buccal cavity, lung, breast, brain and thyroid are sites remote from the cervix and will have received much lower doses of radiation.

Doses of radiation are given in rads, and not in Grays, the SI unit, by common preference among the majority of authors.

Cautions in interpretation

The material presented in this monograph should be interpreted with caution, since observations derived from the 15 different registries in eight different countries are not likely to be entirely comparable. There may be specific differences in cancer registration, in the practice of radiation therapy, in host and environmental factors, and in the comparison of cervical cancer patients with the general population. Such factors are considered in detail in the summary chapter (Day & Boice).

The records of many cancer registries undergo minor modifications as further information becomes available. Since the same sets of data were not used in all of the tabulations presented in this monograph, minor inconsistencies may be noticed, for example, between Appendix A and Appendix B. Such differences are, however, of no quantitative importance.

The specific value of this study

Despite the cautions listed above, factors that give special value to the current investigation are the exceptionally large numbers of subjects studied, the long follow-up available in many registries (over 30 years in some instances), the existence of two comparison populations of women with cervical cancer not known to have been treated by radiation, the stringent criteria normally used by cancer registries to record second primary cancers, and the ability to estimate accurately radiation doses to specific organs in individuals. Because this is a study of cancer incidence, a wider view of radiation risk can be expected than that of investigations of mortality. The two major epidemiological surveys of irradiated populations to date, i.e., the Japanese atomic bomb survivors (Kato & Schull, 1982) and the British patients with ankylosing spondylitis treated by radiotherapy (Smith & Doll, 1982), are both in large part studies of mortality. Thus, this current survey of cervical cancer patients treated or not treated by radiation can potentially substantially increase our knowledge of the carcinogenic effects of ionizing radiation in women.

REFERENCES

Boice, J. D. & Hutchison, G. B. (1980) Leukemia in women following radiotherapy for cervical cancer. Ten-year follow-up of an international study. *J. natl Cancer Inst.*, *65*, 115-129

Boice, J. D., Land, C. E., Shore, R. E., Norman, J. E. & Tokunaga, M. (1979) Risk of breast cancer following low-dose radiation exposure. *Radiology*, *131*, 589-597

Hutchison, G. B. (1968) Leukemia in patients with cancer of the cervix uteri treated with radiation. A report covering the first 5 years of an international study. *J. natl Cancer Inst.*, *40*, 951-982

Kato, H. & Schull, W. J. (1982) Studies of the mortality of A-bomb survivors. 7. Mortality, 1950-1978: Part I. Cancer mortality. *Radiat. Res.*, *90*, 395-432

Smith, P. G. & Doll, R. (1982) Mortality among patients with ankylosing spondylitis after a single treatment course with X rays. *Br. med. J.*, *284*, 449-460

Trichopoulos, D., MacMahon, B. & Cole, P. (1972) Menopause and breast cancer risk. *J. natl Cancer Inst.*, *48*, 605-613

Waterhouse, J., Muir, C., Correa, P. & Powell, J., eds (1976) *Cancer Incidence in Five Continents*, Vol. III (*IARC Scientific Publications No.15*), Lyon, International Agency for Research on Cancer

ALBERTA CANCER REGISTRY

G.B. Hill, G.R. Howe, M. Koch, A.B. Miller & C. Wall

Records have been kept on cancer patients in Alberta since 1941 when the Alberta cancer programme was initiated to provide a radiotherapy service and financial assistance for cancer patients. Since 1951, these records have been used to form the basis of a population based cancer registry. The Cancer Registry was computerized in the mid-1970s and now contains detailed information on all patients diagnosed within the province since 1941.

Data are supplied primarily by physicians within the province, who register either by referring patients to one of the three provincial cancer clinics or by submitting a report form. Pathology and autopsy reports on all malignancies are sent to the Registry, and the Division of Vital Statistics of the Alberta provincial government supplies information on those deaths of which cancer was the primary or secondary cause.

In the past, collection was voluntary and was considered to be complete for the majority of patients in the province who were referred for treatment to provincial cancer clinics. Cancer has been a reportable disease, by law, since 1976.

Follow-up of registered patients is carried out by a treating physician, a cancer clinic or both. Patients treated at clinics are contacted by mail and telephone for follow-up, while letters of inquiry are sent on a regular basis to doctors who are following up patients outside the clinics.

Data are coded from registration forms and patient files and checked for valid codes, missing information and for registration from multiple sources. Files are updated as new information is received. Subsequent primary neoplasms occurring in a given patient are recorded separately from the first, and are noted as such.

In 1976, the population of the registry area comprised 1 838 200, of whom 932 500 were males and 905 700 females.

The Registry covers the province of Alberta, which lies between Saskatchewan on the east, British Columbia on the west, the Northwest Territories to the north and the United States to the south. It lies between latitudes 49° and 60° north and longitudes 110° and 120° west and covers an area of 661,688 km^2.

Table 1. Alberta Cancer Registry: Characteristics of the population under study

	Invasive tumours			*In situ* (no radiotherapy)	Total
	Radiotherapy	No Radiotherapy	Total invasive		
Number of women	2 096	411	2 507		
Woman-years at risk by time since diagnosis					
<1 year	2 096	411	2 507		
1-4 years	6 082	1 015	7 097		
5-9 years	4 593	690	5 283		
10-14 years	2 801	343	3 144		
15-19 years	1 406	155	1 561		
20-24 years	519	53	572		
25-29 years	72	7	79		
30+ years	0	0	0		
All years	17 569	2 674	20 243		
Number of women by age at diagnosis:					
<35	94	51	145		
35-44	376	117	493		
45-54	560	87	647		
55-64	475	68	543		
65-74	335	43	378		
75+	256	45	301		
Number of women excluded because of:					
- second cancer (excluding non-melanoma skin) diagnosed simultaneously with cervical cancer	11	4	15		

Table 2. Observed and expected numbers of second primary cancers in women diagnosed with primary cervical cancer in Alberta

A. Cases of invasive cervical cancer treated by radiotherapy

TIME SINCE DIAGNOSIS OF PRIMARY CERVICAL CANCER (IN YEARS)

Number of women starting intervals		<1 2096			1-4 1903			5-9 1102			10-14 708			15-19 403			20-24 173			25-29 46			30+ 0			Total (excl. <1)		
ICD7	ICD8	O	O'	E	O	O'	E	O	O'	E	O	O'	E	O	O'	E	O	O'	E	O	O'	E	O	O'	E	O	O'	E
140	140			0.05			0.13			0.12			0.09			0.05			0.02			0.00			0.00			0.41
141	141			0.02			0.06			0.06			0.05			0.03			0.01			0.00			0.00	1	1	0.21
142	142			0.03			0.08			0.07			0.05	1		0.03			0.01			0.00			0.00	1		0.24
143-4	143-5			0.03			0.09			0.09			0.07			0.04			0.01			0.00			0.00			0.30
145,7-8	146,8-9			0.02			0.05			0.05			0.03			0.02			0.00			0.00			0.00			0.16
146	147			0.02			0.04			0.04			0.02			0.01			0.02			0.00			0.00			0.11
150	150			0.04			0.12			0.11			0.09			0.05			0.14			0.00			0.00			0.39
151	151			0.28	3	3	0.75	1	1	0.73	1	1	0.57	2	2	0.33			0.01			0.01			0.00	7	7	2.53
152	152			0.02			0.06			0.06			0.05			0.02			0.01			0.00			0.00	1	1	0.20
153	153			0.87	4	4	2.33	3	3	2.26	1	1	1.73	3	3	0.98	1	1	0.40	2	2	0.04			0.00	14	14	7.74
154	154			0.37	3	3	1.00	2	2	0.97	2	2	0.73	2	2	0.42	1	1	0.17			0.01			0.00	10	10	3.30
155.0	155			0.03			0.09			0.08			0.06			0.04			0.01			0.00			0.00			0.28
155.1	156			0.11			0.30			0.29			0.23			0.13			0.06			0.00			0.00			1.01
157	157	1	1	0.22	1	1	0.59			0.59	1	1	0.46			0.27			0.12			0.01			0.00			2.04
160	160			0.02			0.04			0.04			0.03			0.02			0.01			0.00			0.00	2	2	0.14
161	161			0.01			0.04			0.04			0.03			0.01			0.01			0.00			0.00			0.13
162-3	162-3			0.40	3	3	1.09	2	2	1.05	4	4	0.77	2	2	0.42			0.16			0.01			0.00	10	10	3.50
170	174			2.86	4	4	7.95	5	5	7.25	3	3	4.90	2	2	2.56	1	1	0.92	1	1	0.07			0.00	15	15	23.65
172	182.0			0.83			2.36			2.24	2	2	1.62			0.88			0.31			0.02			0.00	2	2	7.43
173-4	181,2.9			0.01			0.03			0.03			0.02			0.01			0.00			0.00			0.00			0.09
175	183	1	1	0.45	1	1	1.26	2	2	1.17	2	2	0.81	2	2	0.43			0.16			0.01			0.00	4	4	3.84
176	184			0.08			0.20			0.19			0.14			0.08			0.03			0.00			0.00	3	3	0.64
180	189.0-.1	1	1	0.16			0.45	2	2	0.43			0.31	2	2	0.17	2	2	0.07			0.01			0.00	10	10	1.44
181	188			0.20	3	3	0.52	1	1	0.51	1	1	0.40	2	1	0.22			0.09			0.01			0.00	10	10	1.75
190	172	1	1	0.14	1	1	0.37	2	2	0.32	1	1	0.21			0.11			0.04			0.00			0.00	2	2	1.05
191	173	1	1	2.30	3	3	6.18	5	5	5.81	7	7	4.20	3	3	2.29	3	3	0.94			0.07			0.00	18	18	19.49
192	190			0.03			0.09			0.08			0.06			0.03	1	1	0.03			0.00			0.00	1	1	0.27
193	191-2			0.13			0.37			0.33			0.22			0.11	1	1	0.11			0.00			0.00	1	1	1.07
194	193			0.12			0.31			0.25			0.16			0.08	1	1	0.04			0.00			0.00	1	1	0.83
195	194			0.01			0.03			0.02			0.02			0.01			0.03			0.00			0.00			0.08
196	170			0.01			0.04			0.03			0.02			0.01			0.00			0.00			0.00			0.10
197	171	1	1	0.05			0.13			0.11			0.08			0.04			0.00			0.01			0.00			0.38
200,202	200,202			0.20			0.54	1	1	0.50			0.37			0.21			0.09			0.02			0.00	1	1	1.72
201	201			0.06			0.17	1	1	0.14			0.09			0.09			0.02			0.01			0.00	1	1	0.46
203	203			0.11	1	1	0.30			0.29	1	1	0.22			0.04			0.05			0.00			0.00	2	2	0.99
204.0	204.1,.9			0.07	1	1	0.19			0.19			0.15			0.13			0.04			0.00			0.00	1	1	0.66
204.1-4	204.0,5-7			0.12	1	1	0.31			0.29			0.20			0.09			0.05			0.00			0.00	1	1	0.96
204	204-207			0.19			0.51			0.48	1	1	0.36			0.20			0.08			0.00			0.00	1	1	1.63
TOTAL		5	5	10.48	28	28	28.67	25	25	26.83	26	26	19.27	15	15	10.48	11	11	4.07	3	3	0.28	0	0	0.00	108	108	89.60

O : All tumours
O': Histologically confirmed
E : Expected

B. Cases of invasive cervical cancer not treated by radiotherapy

TIME SINCE DIAGNOSIS OF PRIMARY CERVICAL CANCER (IN YEARS)

Number of women starting intervals: <1 = 411, 1–4 = 322, 5–9 = 177, 10–14 = 87, 15–19 = 49, 20–24 = 17, 25–29 = 3, 30+ = 0

ICD7	ICD8	<1 E	1–4 O	1–4 O'	1–4 E	5–9 O	5–9 O'	5–9 E	10–14 O	10–14 O'	10–14 E	15–19 O	15–19 O'	15–19 E	20–24 E	25–29 O	25–29 O'	25–29 E	30+ E	Total O	Total O'	Total E
140	140	0.01			0.01			0.01			0.01			0.01	0.00			0.00	0.00			0.04
141	141	0.00			0.01			0.00			0.00			0.00	0.00			0.00	0.00			0.02
142	142	0.00			0.01			0.01			0.01			0.00	0.00			0.00	0.00			0.03
143–4	143–5	0.00			0.01			0.00			0.00			0.00	0.00			0.00	0.00			0.03
145,7–8	146,8–9	0.01			0.01			0.00			0.00			0.00	0.00			0.00	0.00			0.01
146	147	0.03			0.01			0.01			0.01			0.03	0.02			0.00	0.00			0.03
150	150	0.00			0.07			0.06			0.06			0.00	0.05			0.00	0.00			0.26
151	151	0.11			0.01			0.00			0.00			0.03	0.02			0.01	0.00			0.02
152	152	0.05			0.01			0.18			0.00			0.00	0.05			0.00	0.00			0.02
153	153	0.00			0.22			0.08	1	1	0.10			0.10	0.02			0.00	0.00	1	1	0.82
154	154	0.01			0.10			0.01			0.08	1	1	0.04	0.01			0.00	0.00	1	1	0.35
155.0	155	0.03			0.01			0.01			0.01			0.00	0.00			0.00	0.00			0.03
155.1	156	0.00			0.03			0.02			0.03			0.01	0.00			0.00	0.00			0.10
157	157	0.00			0.06			0.04			0.06			0.03	0.03			0.00	0.00			0.20
160	160	0.00			0.00			0.00			0.00			0.00	0.00			0.00	0.00			0.00
161	161	0.05			0.00			0.00			0.00			0.00	0.00			0.00	0.00			0.00
162–3	162–3	0.38	1	1	0.11			0.09			0.11			0.05	0.09	1	1	0.02	0.00	1	1	0.40
170	174	0.10	1	1	0.87	1	1	0.56	1	1	0.87			0.25	0.25			0.09	0.00	3	3	2.78
172	182.0	0.01			0.25			0.19			0.25			0.10	0.10			0.03	0.00			0.84
173–4	181,2.9	0.06			0.01			0.00			0.00			0.00	0.00			0.00	0.00			0.01
175	183	0.01			0.14			0.10			0.14			0.05	0.05			0.00	0.00			0.47
176	184	0.02			0.02			0.01			0.02			0.01	0.01			0.00	0.00			0.06
180	189,0–.1	0.02			0.05			0.03			0.05			0.02	0.02			0.00	0.00			0.16
181	188	0.02			0.05			0.04			0.05			0.02	0.02			0.01	0.00			0.18
190	172	0.30			0.04			0.02			0.04			0.01	0.01			0.00	0.00			0.12
191	173	0.00			0.62			0.46			0.62			0.24	0.10	1	1	0.10	0.00	1	1	2.15
192	190	0.02			0.01			0.01			0.01			0.01	0.00			0.00	0.00			0.03
193	191–2	0.02			0.04			0.03			0.04			0.01	0.01			0.00	0.00			0.13
194	193	0.00			0.03			0.02			0.03			0.01	0.01			0.00	0.00			0.11
196	194	0.00			0.00			0.00			0.00			0.00	0.00			0.00	0.00			0.00
197	170	0.01			0.01			0.01			0.01			0.00	0.00			0.00	0.00			0.00
200,202	171	0.03			0.05			0.04			0.05			0.02	0.02			0.00	0.00			0.03
201	200,202	0.01			0.02			0.01			0.02			0.01	0.00			0.00	0.00			0.18
203	201	0.01			0.03			0.02			0.03			0.02	0.01			0.00	0.00			0.06
204.0	203	0.02			0.02			0.01			0.02			0.01	0.01			0.00	0.00			0.10
204.1–4	204,1.9	0.03			0.03			0.02			0.03			0.01	0.00			0.00	0.00			0.06
204	204,0.5–7				0.02			0.03			0.03			0.01	0.01			0.00	0.00			0.10
	204–207				0.05			0.05			0.05			0.02	0.02			0.01	0.00			0.18
TOTAL		1.34	2	2	3.41	1	1	2.94	2	2	2.10	1	1	1.04	0.42	1	1	0.03	0.00	7	7	9.94

O : All tumours
O' : Histologically confirmed
E : Expected

Table 3. Breast cancer in women in Alberta by age at diagnosis of cervical cancer, stage and treatment

TIME SINCE DIAGNOSIS OF PRIMARY CERVICAL CANCER (IN YEARS)

INVASIVE / RADIOTHERAPY

RADIOTHERAPY	<1 O'	<1 E	1-4 O'	1-4 E	5-9 O'	5-9 E	10-14 O'	10-14 E	15-19 O'	15-19 E	20-24 E	25-29 E	30+ E	Total O'	Total E
<30		0.01		0.03		0.05		0.07		0.09	0.06	0.00	0.00		0.30
30-39		0.13		0.52		0.81		0.76	1	0.46	0.15	0.01	0.00	1	2.72
40-49	3	0.64	1	2.19	2	2.31	2	1.70	1	0.01	0.35	0.02	0.00	8	7.58
50-59	1	0.81	1	2.42	1	2.18	1	1.34		0.63	0.26	0.03	0.00	3	6.89
60-69		0.69	1	1.66	1	1.25		0.76		0.31	0.08	0.01	0.00	1	4.08
70+		0.59	2	1.13		0.63		0.26		0.06	0.01	0.00	0.00	2	2.09

INVASIVE / NO THERAPY

NO THERAPY	<1 E	1-4 O'	1-4 E	5-9 O'	5-9 E	10-14 E	15-19 E	20-24 E	25-29 E	30+ E	Total O'	Total E
<30	0.00		0.01		0.01	0.01	0.00	0.00	0.00	0.00		0.03
30-39	0.04		0.13		0.18	0.13	0.06	0.02	0.00	0.00	1	0.53
40-49	0.09	1	0.29	1	0.28	0.18	0.08	0.03	0.01	0.00	1	0.88
50-59	0.10		0.26		0.21	0.13	0.06	0.02	0.00	0.00		0.67
60-69	0.08		0.20		0.15	0.11	0.05	0.02	0.00	0.00		0.52
70+	0.08		0.11		0.04	0.00	0.00	0.00	0.00	0.00		0.15

IN SITU / RADIOTHERAPY

RADIOTHERAPY	<1	1-4	5-9	10-14	15-19	20-24	25-29	30+	Total
<30									
30-39									
40-49									
50-59									
60-69									
70+									

O : All tumours
O': Histologically confirmed
E : Expected

BRITISH COLUMBIA CANCER REGISTRY

J.M. Elwood, G.R. Howe, A.B. Miller & C. Wall

Cancer was added to the list of diseases notifiable to the Provincial Department of Health in 1932 at the request of the British Columbia Medical Association. The reporting system went into effect in 1935, utilizing direct notifications from physicians. However, a cancer register was not established until 1966, when the notifications from private physicians were supplemented by reports from the British Columbia Cancer Institute and from the medical records departments of several of the larger hospitals. This still did not achieve complete ascertainment, since, by the end of 1968, about 30% of the neoplasms recorded by the cancer register were ascertained only through death registrations.

In 1966, arrangements were made with pathologists throughout the province that duplicates of all pathology reports mentioning cancer should be submitted. By 1970, such reports were being received from nearly every regional hospital pathology laboratory in the province. By 1976, death registrations accounted for only 9% of new reports. However, because complete registration is dependent on pathology reports, it seems likely that a number of cases of disease were being registered as newly diagnosed whereas they were recurrences from previous years with incomplete registration. Duplication is eliminated as far as possible by checking with an alphabetical patient index.

In 1979, arrangements were made to transfer the Registry from the jurisdiction of the Division of Vital Statistics of the British Columbia provincial government to the government-supported British Columbia Cancer Control Agency. Following this transfer, the Registry was computerized and the records available from the provincial cancer clinics were more directly incorporated within the registry reporting system. However, until that time, the Registry was an incidence reporting registry only and no follow-up was conducted.

Nevertheless, for the purposes of this monograph, reporting of cancer of the cervix can be regarded as complete, as the records used for the present purpose have come not from the Provincial Cancer Registry but from the Cancer Control Agency of British Columbia. The Cancer Control Agency runs the Provincial Cervical Cytology Register, which has been in place since a screening programme for cancer of the cervix was initiated in 1949. As part of the documentation for this register, complete, independent ascertainment of all invasive and non-invasive cases of cancer of the cervix has been maintained by the Provincial Cytology Register since 1955. Follow-up has been carried out through the mechanisms of the Cancer Control Agency. Not only are individuals followed through records of cancer clinics and physicians but deaths are ascertained both through this active follow-up and through receipt of copies of death certificates and causes of death, then methodically and accurately ascertained and confirmed. Thus, for cancer of the cervix, complete registration, elimination of duplication and follow-up with identification of second primary tumours has been determined through a mechanism independent of the Provincial Cancer Registry.

The population of the province of British Columbia in 1976 was 2 466 500, of whom 1 232 500 were males and 1 234 000 females. The two registries referred to here have covered all of British Columbia, the most westerly province of Canada, bordered on the east by Alberta, on the west by the Pacific Ocean. The province lies between latitudes 49° and 60° north and longitudes 120° and 130° west. A considerable portion is mountainous; most of the population lives within 100 meters of sea level, particularly in the valley and delta of the Frazer River. The registration area is 948 600 km².

Table 1. British Columbia Cancer Registry: Characteristics of the population under study

	Invasive tumours			*In situ* (no radiotherapy)	Total
	Radiotherapy	No radiotherapy	Total invasive		
Number of women	2 232	81	2 313	230	2 543
Woman-years at risk by time since diagnosis:					
<1 year	2 232	81	2 313	230	2 543
1-4 years	6 558	200	6 758	835	7 593
5-9 years	4 752	134	4 886	789	5 675
10-14 years	2 911	76	2 987	565	3 552
15-19 years	1 624	43	1 667	348	2 015
20-24 years	746	18	764	21	785
25-29 years	247	2	249	6	255
30+ years	4	0	4	0	4
All years	19 074	554	19 628	2 794	22 422
Number of women by age at diagnosis:					
<35	79	13	92	50	142
35-44	327	21	348	74	422
45-54	553	13	566	47	613
55-64	537	18	555	32	587
65-74	432	8	440	9	449
75+	304	8	312	18	330
Number of women excluded because of:					
- second cancer (excluding non-melanoma skin) diagnosed simultaneously with cervical cancer	32	6	38	12	50

Table 2. Observed and expected numbers of second primary cancers in women diagnosed with primary cervical cancer in British Columbia

A. Cases of invasive cervical cancer treated by radiotherapy

TIME SINCE DIAGNOSIS OF PRIMARY CERVICAL CANCER (IN YEARS)

Number of women starting intervals		<1 2232			1-4 2087			5-9 1191			10-14 718			15-19 428			20-24 208			25-29 83			30+ 4			Total (excl. <1)		
ICD7	ICD8	O	O'	E	O	O'	E	O	O'	E	O	O'	E	O	O'	E	O	O'	E	O	O'	E	O	O'	E	O	O'	E
140	140			0.03			0.08			0.07			0.05			0.03			0.02			0.00			0.00			0.25
141	141			0.06			0.17			0.15			0.11			0.07			0.03			0.00			0.00			0.54
142	142			0.03			0.08			0.07			0.05			0.03			0.01			0.00			0.00			0.24
143-4	143-5			0.05			0.15			0.13			0.09			0.05			0.02			0.01			0.00			0.45
145,7-8	146,8-9			0.04	1	1	0.10			0.09			0.06			0.04			0.02			0.00			0.00	1	1	0.31
146	147			0.02			0.05			0.04			0.03			0.02			0.01			0.00			0.00			0.15
150	150			0.10			0.29			0.27			0.20			0.13			0.07			0.02			0.00			0.98
150	151			0.37	1	1	1.07	2	2	1.00			0.77			0.48			0.27	1	1	0.09			0.00	6	6	3.68
151	152	1	1	0.04			0.10			0.09	2	2	0.06			0.04	1	1	0.02			0.01			0.00			0.32
152	153			1.26	6	6	3.60	2	2	3.28	2	2	2.45	2	2	1.52			0.81	1	1	0.25			0.00	14	14	11.91
153	154			0.56	1	1	1.58			1.43	1	1	1.06			0.66	2	2	0.35	1	1	0.11			0.00	5	5	5.19
154	155			0.06			0.16			0.15			0.21			0.07			0.04			0.01			0.00			0.54
155.0	156			0.14	2	2	0.41			0.38			0.29			0.18			0.10			0.03			0.00	3	3	1.39
155.1	157			0.33	4	3	0.96			0.88	1	1	0.67			0.42			0.23	1	1	0.07			0.00	5	3	3.23
157	160			0.02			0.06			0.05	1	1	0.04			0.02			0.01			0.00			0.00			0.18
160	161			0.05			0.15			0.13			0.09			0.05			0.02			0.01			0.00	3	3	0.45
161	162-3	1	1	0.75	4	3	2.12	8	8	1.82	6	6	1.28	2	2	0.76	1	1	0.37			0.10			0.00	18	17	6.45
162-3	174			3.88	4	4	10.86	7	7	9.16	2	2	6.19	2	1	3.53	2	2	1.65			0.45			0.00	16	16	31.84
170	182.0			1.05	1	1	2.96	4	4	2.49	2	2	1.75	1	1	1.03			0.47			0.12			0.00	8	8	8.82
172	181,2.9			0.03			0.10			0.08			0.05			0.03			0.01			0.00			0.00			0.27
173-4	183			0.66	2	2	1.87	1	1	1.59			1.09			0.63	1	1	0.30			0.08			0.00	5	5	5.56
175	184			0.20	3	3	0.57	3	3	0.50			0.36			0.22			0.11			0.03			0.00	8	8	1.79
176	189.0-.1	1	1	0.15			0.44	1	1	0.39	1	1	0.27			0.17			0.09			0.03			0.00	8	7	1.39
180	188	1	1	0.33	3	3	0.95	1	1	0.87			0.65	2		0.41	2	2	0.22			0.07			0.00	7	1	3.17
181	172			0.20	3	3	0.56	1	1	0.45			0.28	1		0.15			0.07			0.02			0.00	1		1.53
190	173	7	7	3.66	6	6	10.31	4	4	9.07	2	2	6.57			4.02	1	1	2.08			0.63			0.00	13	13	32.68
191	190			0.03			0.07			0.06	1	1	0.04			0.03			0.01			0.00			0.00			0.21
192	191-2			0.17	1		0.47	1	1	0.38	1	1	0.26			0.15			0.07			0.02			0.00	1	1	1.35
193	193			0.12			0.31			0.24			0.15			0.08	1	1	0.04	1	1	0.01			0.00	3	3	0.83
194	194			0.01			0.04	1		0.03			0.03			0.01			0.01	1	1	0.00			0.00	1	1	0.11
195	170			0.02			0.05			0.05			0.03			0.02			0.01			0.00			0.00			0.16
196	171			0.04	1		0.11			0.09	1	1	0.06			0.04			0.02			0.01			0.00	1	1	0.33
197	200,202			0.28	1	1	0.78	1	1	0.69	1	1	0.49			0.29			0.15			0.04			0.00	2	2	2.44
200,202	201			0.06			0.16			0.13			0.08			0.05			0.02			0.01			0.00			0.45
201	203			0.10	1	1	0.28			0.25			0.18	1	1	0.11			0.06			0.02			0.00	1	1	0.90
203	204.1,.9			0.06			0.16			0.15			0.12			0.07			0.04			0.01			0.00			0.55
204.0	204.0,5-7			0.14			0.40	1		0.35	1	1	0.26	1	1	0.16			0.08			0.03			0.00	1	1	1.28
204.1-4	204-207			0.20			0.57			0.51	1	1	0.37	1	1	0.23	1	1	0.12			0.04			0.00	1	1	1.84
TOTAL		11	11	15.10	42	39	42.59	35	34	37.06	23	23	26.30	9	7	15.77	10	10	7.91	6	6	2.30	0	0	0.00	125	119	131.93

O : All tumours
O' : Histologically confirmed
E : Expected

B. Cases of invasive cervical cancer not treated by radiotherapy

TIME SINCE DIAGNOSIS OF PRIMARY CERVICAL CANCER (IN YEARS)

ICD7	ICD8	<1 O	<1 O'	<1 E	1-4 O	1-4 O'	1-4 E	5-9 O	5-9 O'	5-9 E	10-14 O	10-14 O'	10-14 E	15-19 O	15-19 O'	15-19 E	20-24 O	20-24 O'	20-24 E	25-29 O	25-29 O'	25-29 E	30+ O	30+ O'	30+ E	Total O	Total O'	Total E
Number of women starting intervals		81			63			36			18			11			6			1			0			1		
140	140			0.00			0.00			0.00			0.00			0.00			0.00			0.00			0.00			0.00
141	141			0.00			0.00			0.00			0.00			0.00			0.00			0.00			0.00			0.00
142	142			0.00			0.00			0.00			0.00			0.00			0.00			0.00			0.00			0.00
143-4	143-5			0.00			0.00			0.00			0.00			0.00			0.00			0.00			0.00			0.00
145,7-8	146,8-9			0.00			0.00			0.00			0.00			0.00			0.00			0.00			0.00			0.00
146	147			0.00			0.00			0.01			0.01			0.00			0.00			0.00			0.00			0.00
150	150			0.01			0.02			0.00			0.00			0.00			0.00			0.00			0.00			0.04
151	151			0.00			0.00			0.02			0.00			0.00			0.00			0.00			0.00			0.00
152	152			0.02			0.06			0.04			0.03			0.02			0.01			0.00			0.00			0.16
153	153			0.01			0.03			0.02			0.01			0.01			0.00			0.00			0.00			0.07
154	154			0.00			0.00			0.00			0.01			0.00			0.00			0.00			0.00			0.00
155.0	155			0.00			0.01			0.01			0.00			0.00			0.00			0.00			0.00			0.04
155.1	156			0.01			0.02			0.01			0.01			0.00			0.00			0.00			0.00			0.00
157	157			0.00			0.00			0.01			0.00			0.00			0.00			0.00			0.00			0.00
160	160			0.00			0.00			0.00			0.00			0.00			0.00			0.00			0.00			0.00
161	161			0.01			0.04			0.03			0.02			0.01			0.01			0.00			0.00			0.11
162-3	162-3			0.08			0.21			0.17			0.12			0.08			0.03			0.01			0.00			0.61
170	174			0.02			0.05			0.04			0.03			0.02			0.01			0.00			0.00			0.15
172	182.0			0.00			0.00			0.00			0.00			0.00			0.00			0.00			0.00			0.00
173-4	181,2.9			0.01	1	1	0.03			0.03			0.02			0.01			0.01			0.00			0.00	1	1	0.10
175	183			0.00			0.01			0.01			0.00			0.00			0.00			0.00			0.00			0.02
176	184			0.00			0.01			0.01			0.00			0.00			0.00			0.00			0.00			0.01
180	189.0-.1			0.00			0.02			0.01			0.01			0.00			0.00			0.00			0.00			0.04
181	188			0.02			0.01			0.01			0.01			0.01			0.00			0.00			0.00			0.03
190	172			0.00			0.19			0.13			0.09			0.06			0.03			0.00			0.00			0.50
191	173			0.08			0.00			0.00			0.00			0.00			0.00			0.00			0.00			0.00
192	190			0.00			0.01			0.01			0.00			0.00			0.00			0.00			0.00			0.02
193	191-2			0.00			0.00			0.01			0.00			0.00			0.00			0.00			0.00			0.02
194	193			0.00			0.00			0.00			0.00			0.00			0.00			0.00			0.00			0.00
195	194			0.00			0.00			0.01			0.00			0.00			0.00			0.00			0.00			0.00
196	170			0.00			0.01			0.00			0.00			0.00			0.00			0.00			0.00			0.00
197	171			0.00			0.00			0.00			0.01			0.00			0.00			0.00			0.00			0.00
200,202	200,202			0.01			0.01			0.01			0.00			0.00			0.00			0.00			0.00			0.03
201	201			0.00			0.00			0.00			0.00			0.00			0.00			0.00			0.00			0.00
203	203			0.00			0.00			0.00			0.00			0.00			0.00			0.00			0.00			0.00
204.0	204.1,.9			0.00			0.00			0.00			0.00			0.00			0.00			0.00			0.00			0.00
204.1-4	204.0,5-7			0.00			0.00			0.01			0.00			0.00			0.00			0.00			0.00			0.01
204	204-207			0.00			0.01						0.00			0.00			0.00			0.00			0.00			0.02
TOTAL				0.27	1	1	0.75			0.55			0.37			0.21			0.10			0.00			0.00	1	1	1.98

O : All tumours
O': Histologically confirmed
E : Expected

C. Cases of carcinoma in situ not treated by radiotherapy

TIME SINCE DIAGNOSIS OF PRIMARY CERVICAL CANCER (IN YEARS)

Number of women starting intervals		<1 (230)			1-4 (221)			5-9 (182)			10-14 (131)			15-19 (95)			20-24 (42)			25-29 (8)			30+ (0)			Total (excl. <1) (13, 11, 14.43)		
ICD7	ICD8	O	O'	E	O	O'	E	O	O'	E	O	O'	E	O	O'	E	O	O'	E	O	O'	E	O	O'	E	O	O'	E
140	140			0.00			0.01			0.01			0.01			0.00			0.00			0.00			0.00			0.03
141	141			0.00			0.01			0.01			0.01			0.01			0.00			0.00			0.00			0.04
142	142			0.00			0.01			0.01			0.01	1	1	0.00			0.00			0.00			0.00	1	1	0.03
143-4	143-5			0.00			0.01			0.02			0.01			0.01			0.00			0.00			0.00			0.06
145,7-8	146,8-9			0.00			0.00			0.01			0.00			0.00			0.00			0.00			0.00			0.04
146	147			0.00			0.00			0.00			0.00			0.00			0.00			0.00			0.00			0.00
150	150			0.02			0.02			0.02			0.02			0.01			0.01			0.00			0.00			0.09
151	151			0.02			0.07			0.09			0.09			0.06			0.02			0.01			0.00			0.33
152	152			0.06			0.01			0.01			0.01			0.01			0.00			0.00			0.00			0.04
153	153			0.03			0.22			0.28	1	1	0.29			0.21			0.08			0.01			0.00	1	1	1.09
154	154			0.00			0.10			0.13			0.13			0.10			0.04			0.00			0.00			0.50
155.0	155			0.01			0.01			0.01			0.01			0.01			0.01			0.00			0.00			0.04
155.1	156			0.02			0.02			0.03			0.03			0.02			0.01			0.00			0.00			0.11
157	157			0.00			0.06			0.07			0.07			0.05			0.02			0.00			0.00			0.27
160	160			0.00			0.00			0.00			0.00			0.00			0.00			0.00			0.00			0.00
161	161			0.01			0.01			0.01			0.02	1	1	0.01			0.01			0.00			0.00	1	1	0.05
162-3	162-3			0.04	1	1	0.14	2	2	0.18	1		0.20			0.14			0.05			0.00			0.00			0.71
170	174			0.23			0.90	2	2	1.14	1	1	1.07	1		0.67			0.23			0.05			0.00	4	3	4.03
172	182.0			0.05			0.21			0.28			0.29			0.22			0.08			0.02			0.00			1.09
173-4	181,2,9			0.00			0.01			0.01			0.01			0.01			0.00			0.01			0.00			0.04
175	183			0.04			0.14			0.18			0.18			0.12			0.04			0.00			0.00	1	1	0.66
176	184			0.01			0.04			0.05			0.05			0.03			0.01		1	0.01			0.00	1	1	0.18
180	189.0-.1			0.02			0.03			0.04			0.04			0.02			0.01			0.00			0.00			0.14
181	188			0.02			0.06			0.07	2	2	0.07			0.05			0.05			0.00			0.00			0.27
190	172			0.20			0.06			0.07			0.06			0.03			0.03			0.00			0.00			0.23
191	173			0.00			0.74			0.92			0.90			0.61	1	1	0.22			0.00			0.00	3	3	3.41
192	190			0.01			0.20			0.05			0.04			0.00			0.00			0.00			0.00			0.03
193	191-2			0.01			0.04	1		0.04			0.03			0.03			0.01			0.00			0.00			0.17
194	193			0.00			0.04			0.00			0.03			0.01			0.00			0.00			0.00			0.12
195	194			0.00			0.00			0.00			0.00			0.00			0.00			0.00			0.00			0.00
196	170			0.00			0.00			0.00			0.00			0.00			0.00			0.00			0.00			0.00
197	171			0.02			0.01			0.01			0.01			0.01			0.01			0.00			0.00			0.04
200,202	200,202			0.01			0.06			0.07			0.07			0.05			0.02			0.02			0.00	1		0.27
201	201			0.00			0.02			0.02			0.01			0.01			0.00			0.00			0.00			0.06
203	203			0.00			0.01			0.01			0.01			0.02			0.01			0.00			0.00			0.08
204.0	204.1,.9			0.01			0.01			0.01			0.01			0.01			0.01			0.00			0.00			0.04
204.1-4	204.0,5-7			0.01			0.03			0.04			0.03			0.02			0.02			0.00			0.00			0.13
204	204-207						0.04			0.05			0.05			0.03			0.03			0.00			0.00			0.18
TOTAL				0.82	1	1	3.13	3	2	3.92	5	4	3.84	2	2	2.58	1	1	0.90	1	1	0.06	0	0	0.00	13	11	14.43

O : All tumours
O': Histologically confirmed
E : Expected

Table 3. Breast cancer in women in British Columbia by age at diagnosis of cervical cancer, stage and treatment

TIME SINCE DIAGNOSIS OF PRIMARY CERVICAL CANCER (IN YEARS)

Stage	Treatment	Age	<1 O	<1 O'	<1 E	1-4 O	1-4 O'	1-4 E	5-9 O	5-9 O'	5-9 E	10-14 O	10-14 O'	10-14 E	15-19 O	15-19 O'	15-19 E	20-24 O	20-24 O'	20-24 E	25-29 O	25-29 O'	25-29 E	30+ O	30+ O'	30+ E	Total (excl. <1) O	Total (excl. <1) O'	Total (excl. <1) E
INVASIVE	RADIOTHERAPY	<30			0.01			0.03			0.05			0.07			0.06			0.04			0.02			0.00			0.27
		30-39	1		0.11			0.53			0.89			0.96			0.70			0.38			0.10			0.00			3.55
		40-49			0.72			2.36		2	2.49		1	1.90		1	1.17			0.55			0.15			0.00	4		8.63
		50-59		2	1.14		4	3.30			2.57			0.54			0.88			0.47			0.15			0.00	6		8.90
		60-69		2	1.06		3	2.80			2.01			1.25			0.66			0.21			0.04			0.00	6		6.96
		70+			0.82			1.83			1.12			0.47			0.05			0.00			0.00			0.00			3.47
IN SITU	NO THERAPY	<30			0.00			0.00			0.00			0.01			0.01			0.01			0.00			0.00			0.03
		30-39			0.01			0.02			0.04			0.04			0.03			0.00			0.00			0.00			0.14
		40-49			0.01			0.05			0.06			0.04			0.02			0.01			0.00			0.00			0.18
		50-59			0.02			0.06			0.04			0.01			0.01			0.01			0.00			0.00			0.14
		60-69			0.02			0.05			0.03			0.01			0.00			0.00			0.00			0.00			0.09
		70+			0.02			0.03			0.00			0.00			0.00			0.00			0.00			0.00			0.03
IN SITU	SURGERY	<30			0.00			0.02			0.02			0.02			0.02			0.01			0.00			0.00			0.09
		30-39			0.03			0.16		1	0.31		1	0.39			0.22			0.08			0.01			0.00	2		1.18
		40-49			0.06			0.27		1	0.38			0.35		1	0.27			0.11			0.00			0.00	2		1.39
		50-59			0.07			0.26			0.29			0.22			0.13			0.03			0.00			0.00			0.92
		60-69			0.02			0.05			0.04			0.04			0.02			0.00			0.00			0.00			0.16
		70+			0.05			0.13			0.10			0.05			0.00			0.00			0.00			0.00			0.28

O : All tumours
O': Histologically confirmed
E : Expected

MANITOBA CANCER REGISTRY

N.W. Choi & N.A. Nelson

Epidemiology and Biostatistics
Manitoba Cancer Treatment and Research Foundation
University of Manitoba Faculty of Medicine
Winnipeg, Manitoba R3E OW3
Canada

In 1937, the province of Manitoba created a central registry to enumerate cancer cases. In 1950, the Registry was reorganized on a population basis, and further reorganization in 1956, 1969 and again in 1974 enabled compilation of more detailed data. The Registry is situated in and administered by the Manitoba Cancer Treatment and Research Foundation. Registry personnel comprise a director in charge, medical records technologists, computer personnel and support staff.

Virtually all cancer cases diagnosed in the province are reported to the Cancer Registry. The sources of data are hospital admission and discharge records from the Manitoba Health Services Commission - which operates the governmental compulsory health insurance scheme - physicians' claims to that Commission for treatment of out-patients and for office visits, pathology and autopsy reports on malignancies, hospital charts from the two university-affiliated hospitals, vital statistics records of deaths in Manitoba and cancer report forms from rural physicians. With computer assistance, follow-up is based on a combination of passive and active procedures; patients treated by radiation and chemotherapy are followed the most actively. These follow-up procedures are considered to assure relatively complete registration of second primaries, particularly in patients who received radiation therapy.

Data are maintained on computer tape files, giving registration number, name and address, date of birth, SNOP topography and morphology, method and date of diagnosis, stage, treatment modality, hospital chart number and date of death. All data received are checked against the computerized alphabetical index for previous registration. The information is then codified for computer entry and update. Although each patient is assigned one number, multiple primaries are identified by a sub-number, so that the unit of registration is the primary tumour rather than the patient. In 1974, computer software was developed to store linked files of patient identification data and primary cancer data. Other files are being developed that include treatment details and follow-up information. When fully implemented, the files will be cross-linked to provide computerized patient profiles on request.

Incidence and mortality rates are published annually in the annual report of the Manitoba Cancer Foundation. Data are provided to medical staff, epidemiologists and other registries. The number of requests for information has increased steadily each year.

All hospitals and most physicians in Manitoba function under the Manitoba Health Services Commission. On 31 December 1975, there were 110 hospitals comprising 9642 beds, and 1732 active physicians in the province, i.e., about 9.5 beds and some 1.7 active physicians per 1 000 population.

The Registry covers all of Manitoba, the most central province of Canada, bordered on the east by Ontario and Hudson Bay, on the west by Saskatchewan, on the north by the Northwest Territories and on the south by the United States, between latitudes 49° and 60° north and longitudes 90° and 102° west. The altitude varies from sea level to 823 metres, and the province covers an area of 650 000 km².

The population in 1975 was 504 700 males and 508 900 females. Of these, 37% of the males and 36% of the females were under 20 years of age. The population includes approximately 42% of British extraction; 12.5% German; 12% Ukrainian; 9% French; 4% Dutch, 4% Polish; 3% Scandinavian; 2% Jewish and 4% native Indian Eskimo. Manitoba's population is stable, with an immigrant population of 15.5%. Some 60% of the population are Protestant, 33% Catholic and 7% other religions.

Predominant occupations include clerical and service occupations, construction and production work and farming.

Table 1. Manitoba Cancer Registry: Characteristics of the population under study

	Invasive tumours			*In situ* (no radiotherapy)	Total
	Radiotherapy	No radiotherapy	Total invasive		
Number of women	1 337	1 035	2 372	4 832	7 204
Woman-years at risk by time since diagnosis:					
<1 year	1 225.92	930.92	2 156.84	4 672.00	6 828.84
1-4 years	3 160.25	2 889.25	6 049.50	15 453.92	21 503.42
5-9 years	2 708.33	2 542.67	5 251.00	13 535.58	18 786.58
10-14 years	1 958.83	1 439.67	3 398.50	7 015.17	10 413.67
15-19 years	1 215.92	461.58	1 677.50	1 839.00	3 516.50
20-24 years	616.50	127.33	743.83	326.33	1 070.16
25-29 years	174.25	16.50	190.75	45.67	236.42
All years	11 060.00	8 407.92	19 467.92	42 887.67	62 355.59
Number of women by age at diagnosis:					
<30	47	150	197	1 482	1 679
30-39	221	218	439	1 756	2 195
40-49	347	280	627	1 017	1 644
50-59	303	159	462	369	831
60-69	267	116	383	159	541
70+	152	112	265	50	314

Table 2. Observed and expected numbers of second primary cancers in women diagnosed with primary cervical cancer in Manitoba

A. Cases of invasive cervical cancer treated by radiotherapy

TIME SINCE DIAGNOSIS OF PRIMARY CERVICAL CANCER (IN YEARS)

Number of women starting intervals		<1 1337			1-4 1090			5-9 629			10-14 465			15-19 326			20-24 167			25-29 79			30+			Total (excl. <1)		
ICD7	ICD8	O	O'	E	O	O'	E	O	O'	E	O	O'	E	O	O'	E	O	O'	E	O	O'	E	O	O'	E	O	O'	E
140	140			0.00			0.07			0.06			0.06			0.00			0.00			0.00			0.00			0.19
141	141			0.00			0.06			0.07			0.07			0.05			0.00			0.00			0.00			0.25
142	142			0.00			0.12			0.09			0.06			0.00			0.00			0.00			0.00			0.27
143-4	143-5			0.00			0.07			0.07			0.06			0.00			0.00			0.00			0.00			0.20
145,7-8	146,8-9																											
146	147																											
150	150			0.00			0.12	2		0.12			0.10			0.07			0.00			0.00			0.00	2		0.41
151	151	1	1	0.35			0.95	1		0.90			0.74			0.51			0.31			0.09			0.00	1		3.50
152	152			0.07			0.07			0.06			0.05			0.00			0.00			0.00			0.00			0.18
153	153	1	1	0.71			1.96			1.91	1		1.64			1.17			0.72			0.21			0.00	1		7.61
154	154			0.29			0.79			0.78	1		0.65			0.47			0.29			0.09			0.00	1		3.07
155.0	155			0.00			0.10			0.10			0.08			0.06			0.00			0.00			0.00			0.34
155.1	156			0.11			0.30			0.29			0.24			0.17			0.11			0.00			0.00			1.11
157	157			0.21			0.58	1	1	0.57	1	1	0.50	1	1	0.37			0.24			0.07			0.00	3	3	2.33
160	160																											
161	161																											
162-3	162-3	2	2	0.22	4	3	0.63	3	1	0.64	5	4	0.56			0.40			0.23			0.07			0.00	12	8	2.53
170	174	2	1	1.83	5	5	4.99	4	4	4.73			3.81	1	1	2.55			1.36			0.39			0.00	10	10	17.83
172	182.0	1	1	0.47			1.29	2	1	1.21	1	1	0.99	1	1	0.66			0.35			0.10			0.00	4	3	4.60
173-4	181,2.9																											
175	183			0.42	1	1	1.14	1	1	1.02	1		0.77	2	1	0.51			0.27			0.08			0.00	5	3	3.79
176	184			0.06	1	2	0.18	1		0.17	1	1	0.13	1	1	0.09			0.06			0.00			0.00	4	4	0.63
180	189.0-.1	1	1	0.11	1	1	0.32	1	1	0.32	1	1	0.27			0.18	1	1	0.10	1	1	0.00			0.00	5	5	1.19
181	188	2	2	0.11			0.30	1	1	0.33	1	1	0.31	1		0.23			0.14			0.00			0.00	3	2	1.31
190	172	2	1	0.06	1	1	0.16	1	1	0.16	1	2	0.14	2	1	0.09			0.00			0.00			0.00	5	5	0.55
191	173	1	1	1.02	4	4	2.81	5	5	2.84	2	2	2.50	2	2	1.93	1	1	1.20	1	1	0.36			0.00	15	15	11.64
192	190																											
191-2	191-2			0.15	1		0.39			0.33			0.24			0.15			0.08			0.00			0.00	1		1.19
193	193			0.08			0.20			0.17			0.13			0.08			0.00			0.00			0.00			0.58
195	194																											
196	170																											
197	171			0.00			0.08			0.09			0.07			0.00			0.00			0.00			0.00			0.24
200,202	200,202			0.10	1		0.37			0.37			0.31			0.23			0.08			0.00			0.00	1		1.36
201	201			0.08			0.13			0.11			0.08			0.05			0.00			0.00			0.00			0.37
203	203			0.08			0.22			0.23			0.21			0.16			0.10			0.00			0.00			0.92
204.0	204.1,.9			0.13			0.33			0.29			0.22			0.13			0.07			0.00			0.00			1.04
204.1-4	204.0,5-7			0.00			0.07			0.09			0.10			0.09			0.06			0.00			0.00			0.41
204	204-207			0.13			0.40			0.38			0.32			0.22			0.13			0.00			0.00			1.45
TOTAL		13	11	6.51	19	17	18.80	23	16	18.12	16	13	15.09	11	8	10.40	2	2	5.77	2	2	1.46			0.00	73	58	69.64

O : All tumours
O' : Histologically confirmed
E : Expected

B. Cases of invasive cervical cancer not treated by radiotherapy

TIME SINCE DIAGNOSIS OF PRIMARY CERVICAL CANCER (IN YEARS)

		<1 (1035)			1–4 (872)			5–9 (605)			10–14 (425)			15–19 (159)			20–24 (50)			25–29 (11)			30+			Total (excl. <1)		
ICD7	ICD8	O	O'	E	O	O'	E	O	O'	E	O	O'	E	O	O'	E	O	O'	E	O	O'	E	O	O'	E	O	O'	E
140	140																											
141	141			0.00			0.00			0.06			0.00			0.00			0.00			0.00			0.00			0.06
142	142			0.00			0.08			0.06			0.00			0.00			0.00			0.00			0.00			0.14
143-4	143-5			0.00			0.00			0.05			0.00			0.00			0.00			0.00			0.00			0.05
145,7-8	146,8-9																											
146	147																											
150	150			0.00			0.07			0.08			0.06			0.00			0.00			0.00			0.00			0.21
151	151			0.15	1	1	0.45	1	1	0.47			0.33			0.13			0.05			0.00			0.00			1.43
152	152	1	1	0.35			1.10	1	1	1.20			0.89			0.36			0.13			0.00			0.00	2	2	3.68
153	153			0.14			0.47			0.53	1		0.39	2	2	0.16			0.06			0.00			0.00	3	2	1.61
154	154			0.00			0.06			0.07			0.05			0.00			0.00			0.00			0.00			0.18
155.0	155			0.00			0.14			0.15			0.11			0.00			0.00			0.00			0.00			0.40
155.1	156			0.10			0.29			0.35			0.27			0.12			0.00			0.00			0.00			1.03
157	157																											
160	160																											
161	161			0.00			0.00			0.00	1	1	0.00			0.00			0.00			0.00			0.00	1	1	0.00
162-3	162-3	2	2	0.12	1	1	0.41	1	1	0.48	2		0.37	1	1	0.15			0.00			0.00			0.00	5	3	1.41
170	174			1.10	3	3	3.70	4	4	4.00	3	3	2.65			0.93	1	1	0.27			0.00			0.00	11	11	11.55
172	182.0			0.25			0.82			0.92			0.67			0.26			0.07			0.00			0.00			2.74
173-4	181,2.9						0.72			0.73			0.48			0.18			0.05			0.00			0.00			2.16
175	183	1	1	0.22	1	1	0.10	1	1	0.11			0.08			0.00	1	1	0.05			0.00			0.00	3	3	0.29
176	184	2	2	0.00			0.20			0.22	1	1	0.16			0.06	1	1	0.00			0.00			0.00	2	2	0.64
180	189.0-.1	1	1	0.06			0.20			0.24			0.19			0.07			0.00			0.00			0.00			0.70
181	188			0.06			0.16			0.16			0.10			0.00			0.00			0.00			0.00			0.42
190	172			0.00			0.00			0.00			0.00			0.00			0.00			0.00			0.00			0.00
191	173			0.55	2	2	1.83	4	3	2.10	2	2	1.57	2	2	0.65			0.23			0.00			0.00	10	9	6.38
192	190																											
193	191-2			0.08			0.24			0.23			0.15			0.06			0.00			0.00			0.00			0.68
194	193			0.00			0.15			0.14			0.09			0.00			0.00			0.00			0.00			0.38
195	194																											
196	170																											
197	171																											
200,202	200,202	1	1	0.00	1	1	0.08			0.08			0.05			0.05			0.00			0.00			0.00	1	1	0.21
201	201			0.05			0.28			0.32			0.20			0.05			0.00			0.00			0.00			0.85
203	203			0.00			0.12			0.09			0.00			0.00			0.00			0.00			0.00			0.21
204.0	204.1,.9			0.06			0.13			0.15			0.12			0.00			0.00			0.00			0.00			0.40
204.1-4	204.0,5-7			0.00			0.17			0.15			0.11			0.00			0.00			0.00			0.00			0.43
204	204-207			0.06			0.26			0.28			0.20			0.00			0.00			0.00			0.00			0.74
TOTAL		8	8	3.29	9	9	12.06	11	10	13.27	10	7	9.18	5	5	3.18	3	3	0.86			0.00			0.00	38	34	38.55

O : All tumours
O' : Histologically confirmed
E : Expected

C. Cases of carcinoma in situ not treated by radiotherapy

TIME SINCE DIAGNOSIS OF PRIMARY CERVICAL CANCER (IN YEARS)

ICD7	ICD8	<1 O	<1 O'	<1 E	1-4 O	1-4 O'	1-4 E	5-9 O	5-9 O'	5-9 E	10-14 O	10-14 O'	10-14 E	15-19 O	15-19 O'	15-19 E	20-24 O	20-24 O'	20-24 E	25-29 O	25-29 O'	25-29 E	30+ O	30+ O'	30+ E	Total O	Total O'	Total E
	Number of women starting intervals			4832			4513			3309			2085			798			127			26						(excl. <1)
140	140			0.00			0.10			0.14			0.10			0.00			0.00			0.00			0.00			0.34
141	141			0.00			0.10			0.15			0.14			0.06			0.06			0.00			0.00			0.45
142	142			0.11			0.34			0.23			0.11			0.00			0.00			0.00			0.00			0.68
143-4	143-5			0.00			0.15			0.18			0.14			0.00			0.00			0.07			0.00			0.47
145,7-8	146,8-9			0.00			0.06			0.06			0.00			0.00			0.00			0.00			0.00			0.12
146	147																											
150	150			0.00	1		0.15			0.21	1	1	0.19			0.07			0.12			0.00			0.00	2	2	0.62
151	151	2	1	0.24	1	1	0.97	1	1	1.12	1		0.91			0.37			0.37			0.00			0.00	1	1	3.49
152	152	1	1	0.00	1	1	0.13			0.14	2	2	0.09			0.00			0.00			0.00			0.00	5	4	0.36
153	153	1	1	0.70	2	2	2.85	2	2	3.47			2.73	1		1.04			0.29			0.07			0.00	1	1	10.45
154	154	1	1	0.28	2	2	1.19			1.60			1.31			0.49			0.13			0.00			0.00	2	2	4.72
155.0	155			0.06			0.14			0.19			0.15			0.06			0.00			0.00			0.00			0.54
155.1	156			0.13			0.26	1		0.33			0.30			0.13			0.09	1		0.00			0.00			1.02
157	157				1		0.57	1	1	0.81	2	2	0.76			0.32			0.00			0.00			0.00	5	3	2.55
160	160			0.00			0.09			0.10			0.07			0.00			0.00			0.00			0.00			0.26
161	161			0.00			0.09			0.11			0.08			0.00			0.00			0.00			0.00			0.28
162-3	162-3	1		0.00	3	3	1.14	18	17	1.56	4	4	1.29	1	1	0.48			0.11			0.00			0.00	9	8	4.58
170	174	2	2	3.10	11	10	12.95			16.10	7	7	11.13	3	2	3.46	1	1	0.68			0.11			0.00	40	37	44.43
172	182.0	3	3	0.59			2.46	17		3.14	1	1	2.52			0.91			0.19			0.00			0.00	1	1	9.22
173-4	181,2,9																											
175	183			0.60	2	2	2.31	4	4	2.59	1	1	1.84	1		0.63			0.13			0.00			0.00	7	7	7.50
176	184			0.08	3	3	0.30	8	8	0.35			0.26			0.09			0.00			0.00			0.00	11	11	1.00
180	189.0-.1			0.14	1	1	0.58			0.71			0.56			0.21			0.00			0.00			0.00	2	2	2.06
181	188			0.13			0.54	1	1	0.72			0.59			0.22			0.06			0.00			0.00	1	1	2.13
190	172			0.20	1	1	0.77			0.80			0.45			0.12			0.00			0.00			0.00	1	1	2.14
191	173			1.25	2	2	5.27	5	5	6.91	4	4	5.29			1.91			0.52			0.12			0.00	11	11	20.02
192	190	1	1	0.00			0.10			0.12			0.10			0.00			0.00			0.00			0.00			0.32
193	191-2			0.25	1		0.89			0.91			0.60			0.19			0.19			0.00			0.00	1		2.59
194	193			0.20			0.70			0.66			0.37			0.10			0.10			0.00			0.00			1.83
195	194			0.05			0.17			0.14			0.09			0.00			0.00			0.00			0.00			0.40
196	170			0.00			0.13			0.13			0.09			0.00			0.00			0.00			0.00			0.35
197	171			0.10			0.37			0.37			0.20	1		0.06			0.00			0.00			0.00	1	1	1.00
200,202	200,202	1		0.26	2	2	1.08	3	3	1.24	1	1	0.85			0.27			0.00			0.00			0.00	6	6	3.44
201	201			0.20	2	2	0.67	1		0.53	1	1	0.22			0.05			0.00			0.00			0.00	2	2	1.47
203	203			0.08	1	1	0.31	1	1	0.40			0.35			0.15			0.00			0.00			0.00	2	2	1.21
204.0	204.1,.9			0.13	1		0.47			0.45			0.32			0.12			0.00			0.00			0.00	2	2	1.36
204.1-4	204.0,5-7			0.07			0.34			0.53			0.38			0.12			0.00			0.00			0.00			1.37
204	204-207			0.20	1	1	0.81	1	1	0.98			0.70			0.24			0.00			0.00			0.00	2	2	2.73
TOTAL		12	9	8.95	35	33	38.74	45	43	47.20	24	23	34.58	7	5	11.63	1	1	2.32	1		0.30			0.00	113	105	134.77

O : All tumours
O' : Histologically confirmed
E : Expected

Table 3. Breast cancer in women in Manitoba by age at diagnosis of cervical cancer, stage and treatment

TIME SINCE DIAGNOSIS OF PRIMARY CERVICAL CANCER (IN YEARS)

	<1 :O	<1 O'	<1 E	1-4 :O	1-4 O'	1-4 E	5-9 :O	5-9 O'	5-9 E	10-14 :O	10-14 O'	10-14 E	15-19 :O	15-19 O'	15-19 E	20-24 :O	20-24 O'	20-24 E	25-29 :O	25-29 O'	25-29 E	30+ :O	30+ O'	30+ E	Total (excl. <1) :O	Total O'	Total E
INVASIVE — RADIOTHERAPY																											
<30						0.01			0.03			0.06			0.07			0.08			0.04						0.29
30-39			0.09			0.39			0.66			0.79			0.69			0.38			0.13						3.04
40-49	1		0.43	1		1.28			1.33			1.08			0.75			0.43			0.12				2		4.99
50-59	2		0.48	1		1.27			1.19			0.91			0.56			0.31			0.08				2		4.32
60-69	1		0.49	1		1.32			1.11			0.84			0.44			0.18			0.02				3		3.91
70+	1		0.33	2		0.72			0.40			0.13			0.04			0.00			0.00				3		1.29
INVASIVE — NO RADIOTHERAPY																											
<30						0.03			0.08			0.09			0.03			0.01			0.00						0.24
30-39			0.10	1		0.50	2		0.77			0.65			0.29			0.08			0.01				4		2.30
40-49			0.37	1		1.40			1.67			1.09			0.38			0.12			0.01				4		4.67
50-59	1		0.26			0.81	1		0.78			0.48	1		0.15			0.02			0.00				2		2.24
60-69	1		0.21			0.64			0.48			0.21			0.06			0.02			0.00						1.41
70+	1		0.16	1		0.32	1		0.22			0.13			0.03			0.01			0.00				1		0.71
IN-SITU — NO RADIOTHERAPY																											
<30			0.07			0.35			0.91			0.92			0.31			0.08			0.00						2.57
30-39			0.67	6		3.63	3		5.68			4.32			1.46			0.24			0.02				11		15.35
40-49	6		1.29	7		5.36	2		6.33	1		3.98	1		1.11			0.22			0.04				17		17.04
50-59	1		0.63	4		2.18	2		2.15			1.38			0.43			0.10			0.02				7		6.26
60-69	1		0.32	1		1.10			0.84			0.45			0.13			0.04			0.02				2		2.58
70+	3		0.11			0.33			0.19			0.08			0.00			0.00			0.00				3		0.60

O : All tumours
O' : Histologically confirmed
E : Expected

NEW BRUNSWICK CANCER REGISTRY

G.R. Howe, A.B. Miller, D. Smith & C. Wall

A provincial tumour registry was established in the main cancer treatment clinic in Saint John, New Brunswick in 1955. Registration is sought by Registry staff from hospital in-patients and out-patients and from the Radiotherapy Department. Pathologists report cases with a mention of cancer from pathology departments, and data on deaths with a mention of cancer are obtained from the Provincial Registrar of Vital Statistics. Physicians treating cases at home are also urged to register them. Cancer is not a reportable disease by law in New Brunswick, but the collection of data on patients with cancer is accepted as policy by the Department of Health of New Brunswick, which has also given approval for the follow-up of patients with cancer. Follow-up is active, being conducted through the cancer clinic and through contact with individual physicians.

The Registry is not computerized, but registered cases are entered on punch cards for mechanical sorting. Quality control is assured by linking manual records pertaining to the same individual, primarily through an alphabetical card index.

In 1976, the total population of the registration area was 677 200, of whom 339 300 were males and 337 900 females. The Registry covers the entire province of New Brunswick, which is bordered on the west by Quebec and on the est by Nova Scotia. It lies between latitudes 45° and 48° north and longitude 69° and 65° west. The total registration area is 73 437 km².

HOWE *et al.*

Table 1. New Brunswick Cancer Registry: Characteristics of the population under study

	Invasive tumours			*In situ* (no radiotherapy)	Total
	Radiotherapy	No radiotherapy	Total invasive		
Number of women	1 449				
Woman-years at risk by time since diagnosis:					
<1 year	1 449				
1-4 years	4 359				
5-9 years	3 491				
10-14 years	2 264				
15-19 years	1 238				
20-24 years	517				
25-29 years	89				
30+ years	0				
All years					
Number of women by age at diagnosis:					
<35	78				
35-44	290				
45-54	389				
55-64	327				
65-74	226				
75+	139				
Number of women excluded because of:					
- malignancy prior to diagnosis of cervical cancer	37				
- second cancer (excluding non-melanoma skin) diagnosed simultaneously with cervical cancer	3				

Table 2. Observed and expected numbers of second primary cancers in women diagnosed with primary cervical cancer in New Brunswick

A. Cases of invasive cervical cancer treated by radiotherapy

TIME SINCE DIAGNOSIS OF PRIMARY CERVICAL CANCER (IN YEARS)

ICD7	ICD8	<1 (1449) O	O'	E	1-4 (1349) O	O'	E	5-9 (826) O	O'	E	10-14 (541) O	O'	E	15-19 (338) O	O'	E	20-24 (163) O	O'	E	25-29 (46) O	O'	E	30+ O	O'	E	Total (excl. <1) O	O'	E
140	140			0.01			0.03			0.03			0.03			0.02			0.01			0.00			0.00			0.12
141	141			0.01			0.04			0.04			0.03	1		0.02			0.01			0.00			0.00	1		0.14
142	142			0.02			0.06			0.06			0.05			0.03			0.01			0.00			0.00			0.21
143-4	143-5			0.03			0.08			0.08			0.06			0.04			0.02			0.00			0.00			0.28
145,7-8	146,8-9			0.02	1		0.05			0.04			0.04			0.02			0.01			0.00			0.00	1		0.16
146	147			0.00			0.01			0.01			0.01			0.00			0.00			0.00			0.00			0.03
150	150	1		0.03			0.09			0.09			0.07			0.05			0.03			0.03			0.00	1		0.33
151	151			0.26	3		0.69			0.69			0.54			0.37			0.20			0.00			0.00	3		2.52
152	152			0.02			0.05			0.05			0.04			0.02			0.01			0.03			0.00			0.17
153	153			0.70			1.94			1.89	4		1.47	2		0.99			0.50	1		0.07			0.00	8		6.86
154	154			0.30			0.85	1		0.82			0.64			0.41			0.20			0.03			0.00	1		2.95
155.0	155			0.02			0.07			0.07			0.05			0.03			0.02			0.00			0.00			0.24
155.1	156			0.06			0.17			0.17			0.13			0.10			0.05			0.01			0.00			0.63
157	157			0.16	3		0.43			0.43	1		0.33	1		0.23			0.12	1		0.02			0.00	6		1.56
160	160			0.01			0.02			0.02			0.01			0.01			0.01			0.00			0.00			0.07
161	161			0.02	1		0.05	1		0.04			0.03			0.02			0.01			0.00			0.00	2		0.15
162-3	162-3			0.27	3		0.77	5		0.74			0.56	1		0.34			0.15			0.02			0.00	12		2.58
170	174	1		1.84	7		5.29	5		5.00	3		3.64	1		2.12			0.90			0.11			0.00	16		17.06
172	182.0			0.44			1.28			1.20	2		0.93	2		0.58			0.26			0.03			0.00			4.28
173-4	181,2.9			0.00			0.00			0.00			0.00			0.00			0.00			0.00			0.00			0.00
175	183			0.29	1		0.82	1		0.78	1		0.58			0.35			0.16			0.02			0.00	3		2.71
176	184			0.07			0.20	1		0.20			0.15			0.10			0.05			0.01			0.00	1		0.71
180	189.0-.1			0.10	1		0.30	2		0.28			0.22			0.13			0.07			0.01			0.00	3		1.01
181	188			0.14	1		0.39	1		0.39	1		0.29			0.20			0.11			0.02			0.00	3		1.40
190	172			0.10			0.30			0.27			0.19			0.11			0.04			0.01			0.00			0.92
191	173			1.61	4		4.47	3		4.32	3		3.23	2		2.08			1.04			0.15			0.00	12		15.29
192	190			0.01			0.03			0.03			0.02			0.02			0.01			0.00			0.00			0.11
193	191-2			0.09			0.25			0.22			0.16			0.10			0.04			0.01			0.00	1		0.78
194	193			0.09			0.03			0.22			0.02			0.08			0.03			0.00			0.00			0.73
195	194			0.01			0.01			0.02			0.01			0.01			0.00			0.00			0.00			0.08
196	170			0.00			0.00			0.01			0.01			0.00			0.00			0.00			0.00			0.03
197	171			0.04	1		0.11	1		0.10	1		0.07	1		0.04			0.02			0.00			0.00			0.34
200,202	200,202			0.14			0.39			0.37			0.29			0.19			0.09			0.02			0.00	1		1.34
201	201			0.03			0.08			0.07			0.05			0.03			0.01			0.09			0.00	3		0.24
203	203			0.07			0.19			0.18			0.15			0.09			0.04			0.01			0.00			0.66
204.0	204.1,.9			0.02			0.06			0.06			0.05			0.04			0.02			0.04			0.00	1		0.23
204.1-4	204.0,5-7			0.08			0.22			0.21	1		0.15			0.09			0.05			0.00			0.00			0.73
204	204-207			0.10			0.28			0.27	1		0.20			0.13			0.07			0.01			0.00	1		0.96
TOTAL		2		7.11	27		20.07	22		19.20	18		14.44	11		9.06			4.30	2		0.58			0.00	80		67.65

O : All tumours
O' : Histologically confirmed
E : Expected

Table 3. Breast cancer in women in New Brunswick by age at diagnosis of cervical cancer, stage and treatment

TIME SINCE DIAGNOSIS OF PRIMARY CERVICAL CANCER (IN YEARS)

INVASIVE — RADIOTHERAPY

Age	<1 O'	<1 Ex	1–4 O'	1–4 Ex	5–9 O'	5–9 Ex	10–14 O'	10–14 Ex	15–19 O'	15–19 Ex	20–24 O'	20–24 Ex	25–29 O'	25–29 Ex	30+ O'	30+ Ex	Total (excl. <1) O	Total (excl. <1) Ex
<30		0.00		0.03		0.05		0.08		0.08		0.04		0.01		0.00		0.29
30–39	1	0.10	1	0.46		0.73		0.80		0.59		0.24		0.03		0.00	1	2.85
40–49	1	0.40	1	1.46	3	1.66	1	1.30		0.73		0.35		0.03		0.00	6	5.53
50–59	3	0.55	3	1.51	1	1.31	1	0.85		0.43		0.20		0.03		0.00	5	4.33
60–69	1	0.44	1	1.14	1	0.84		0.51		0.25		0.06		0.01		0.00	2	2.81
70+	1	0.35	1	0.70	1	0.40		0.11		0.03		0.00		0.00		0.00	2	1.24

INVASIVE — SURGERY

Age
<30
30–39
40–49
50–59
60–69
70+

IN-SITU

Age
<30
30–39
40–49
50–59
60–69
70+

O : All tumours
O' : Histologically confirmed
Ex : Expected

NOVA SCOTIA CANCER REGISTRY

G.R. Howe, A.B. Miller, J.A. Myrden & C. Wall

The Nova Scotia Cancer Registry was established in 1964, is supported by the National Health Grants Fund under the Cancer Control Programme and is administered jointly by the Department of Public Health and the Medical Society of Nova Scotia. Cancer is a reportable disease by law in Nova Scotia, and cancer patients diagnosed in hospitals, clinics and physicians' offices are reported; in addition, the Registry maintains a systematic search for all potential patients, aided by regular submission of pathology reports of cases with a diagnosis of cancer. Vital statistics records of deaths are supplied routinely to the Cancer Registry and are perused for those with a mention of cancer, although patients with no other record of cancer than a mention on a death certificate are not registered.

Follow-up is largely passive, although approximately half the patients registered are followed up actively through the Nova Scotia Tumour Clinic, which is adjacent. For the remainder, information on deaths is obtained from vital statistics records and from other sources, and requests for follow-up are sent periodically to physicians. Between 1964 and the end of 1979, more than 40 000 patients with cancer had been registered.

The Registry is not computerized, but details of registered cases are entered on punch cards. Quality control is dependent largely on clerical checking, and multiple records for the same individual are linked through an alphabetical card index.

In 1976, the total population of the registration area was 826 600, of whom 414 100 were males and 414 500 females. The Registry covers the province of Nova Scotia, which lies to the south of the Gulf of St Lawrence and the province of New Brunswick, between the Gulf of Maine and the Atlantic Ocean. The province lies between longitudes 59° and 67° west and latitudes 43° and 47° north. It covers an area of 55 491 km².

Table 1. Nova Scotia Cancer Registry: Characteristics of the population under study

	Invasive tumours			*In situ* (no radiotherapy)	Total
	Radiotherapy	No radiotherapy	Total invasive		
Number of women	695	84	779		
Woman-years at risk by time since diagnosis:					
<1 year	695	84	779		
1-4 years	2 180	277	2 457		
5-9 years	1 888	290	2 178		
10-14 years	750	122	872		
15-19 years	27	8	35		
20-24 years	0	0	0		
25-29 years	0	0	0		
30+ years	0	0	0		
All years	5 540	781	6 321		
Number of women by age at diagnosis:					
<35	23	9	32		
35-44	126	20	146		
45-54	199	22	221		
55-64	179	14	193		
65-74	93	7	100		
75+	75	12	87		
Number of women excluded because of:					
- second cancer (excluding non-melanoma skin) diagnosed simultaneously with cervical cancer	1	2	3		

Table 2. Observed and expected numbers of second primary cancers in women diagnosed with primary cervical cancer in Nova Scotia

A. Cases of invasive cervical cancer treated by radiotherapy

TIME SINCE DIAGNOSIS OF PRIMARY CERVICAL CANCER (IN YEARS)

Number of women starting intervals — <1: 695; 1-4: 657; 5-9: 446; 10-14: 246; 15-19: 27; 20-24: 0; 25-29: 0; 30+: 0

ICD7	ICD8	<1 O	<1 O'	<1 E	1-4 O	1-4 O'	1-4 E	5-9 O	5-9 O'	5-9 E	10-14 O	10-14 O'	10-14 E	15-19 O	15-19 O'	15-19 E	20-24 O	20-24 O'	20-24 E	25-29 O	25-29 O'	25-29 E	30+ O	30+ O'	30+ E	Total O	Total O'	Total E
140	140			0.00			0.01			0.01			0.01			0.00			0.00			0.00			0.00			0.03
141	141			0.01			0.02			0.02			0.01			0.00			0.00			0.00			0.00			0.05
142	142			0.01			0.02			0.02			0.01			0.00			0.00			0.00			0.00			0.05
143-4	143-5			0.01	1		0.03	1		0.03			0.01			0.00			0.00			0.00			0.00	2		0.07
145,7-8	146,8-9			0.01			0.02			0.02			0.01			0.00			0.00			0.00			0.00			0.05
146	147			0.00			0.00			0.00			0.00			0.00			0.00			0.00			0.00			0.00
150	150			0.01			0.04			0.04			0.02			0.00			0.00			0.00			0.00			0.10
151	151			0.10			0.32	1		0.33			0.13			0.00			0.00			0.00			0.00	1		0.78
152	152			0.01			0.02			0.02			0.01			0.00			0.00			0.00			0.00			0.05
153	153			0.37	2		1.17			1.23			0.49			0.00			0.00			0.00			0.00	2		2.89
154	154			0.12	1		0.40			0.42			0.16			0.00			0.00			0.00			0.00	1		0.98
155.0	155			0.01			0.03			0.03			0.01			0.00			0.00			0.00			0.00			0.07
155.1	156			0.03			0.10			0.11			0.04			0.00			0.00			0.00			0.00			0.25
157	157			0.06			0.17			0.19	1		0.08			0.00			0.00			0.00			0.00	1		0.44
160	160			0.01			0.01			0.01			0.00			0.00			0.00			0.00			0.00			0.02
161	161			0.01			0.02			0.02			0.01			0.00			0.00			0.00			0.00			0.05
162-3	162-3	1		0.13			0.42	2		0.42	1		0.16			0.00			0.00			0.00			0.00	3		1.00
170	174			0.89	5		2.80	2		2.71	2		0.97			0.00			0.00			0.00			0.00	9		6.48
172	182.0			0.19			0.61	1		0.61	2		0.23			0.00			0.00			0.00			0.00	3		1.45
173-4	181,2.9			0.01			0.04	1		0.03			0.01			0.00			0.00			0.00			0.00	1		0.08
175	183			0.16			0.52			0.51	1		0.18			0.00			0.00			0.00			0.00	1		1.21
176	184			0.03	1		0.10	1		0.10	1		0.04			0.00			0.00			0.00			0.00	3		0.24
180	189.0-.1			0.04			0.12			0.13			0.05			0.00			0.00			0.00			0.00			0.30
181	188			0.06			0.18			0.20			0.08			0.00			0.00			0.00			0.00			0.46
190	172			0.03			0.10			0.09			0.03			0.00			0.00			0.00			0.00			0.22
191	173	1		0.41			1.29	1		1.32	1		0.51			0.00			0.00			0.00			0.00	2		3.12
192	190			0.01			0.02			0.02			0.01			0.00			0.00			0.00			0.00			0.05
193	191-2			0.04			0.11			0.10			0.03			0.00			0.00			0.00			0.00			0.24
194	193	1		0.04			0.11	1		0.10			0.03			0.00			0.00			0.00			0.00	1		0.24
195	194			0.00			0.01			0.01			0.00			0.00			0.00			0.00			0.00			0.02
196	170			0.00			0.01			0.01			0.00			0.00			0.00			0.00			0.00			0.02
197	171			0.01			0.03			0.03			0.01			0.00			0.00			0.00			0.00			0.07
200,202	200,202			0.06			0.20			0.21			0.08			0.00			0.00			0.00			0.00			0.49
201	201			0.02			0.05			0.05			0.02			0.00			0.00			0.00			0.00			0.12
203	203			0.02			0.07			0.07			0.03			0.00			0.00			0.00			0.00			0.17
204.0	204.1,.9			0.00			0.02			0.02			0.01			0.00			0.00			0.00			0.00			0.05
204.1-4	204.0,5-7			0.03			0.11			0.11			0.04			0.00			0.00			0.00			0.00			0.26
204	204-207			0.04			0.13			0.12			0.05			0.00			0.00			0.00			0.00			0.30
TOTAL		3		2.95	10		9.30	11		9.34	9		3.52			0.00			0.00			0.00			0.00	30		22.16

O : All tumours
O' : Histologically confirmed
E : Expected

B. Cases of invasive cervical cancer not treated by radiotherapy

TIME SINCE DIAGNOSIS OF PRIMARY CERVICAL CANCER (IN YEARS)

ICD7	ICD8	<1 (84) O	O'	E	1–4 (72) O	O'	E	5–9 (66) O	O'	E	10–14 (45) O	O'	E	15–19 (9) O	O'	E	20–24 (0) O	O'	E	25–29 (0) O	O'	E	30+ (0) O	O'	E	Total (exel. <1) O	O'	E
140	140			0.00			0.00			0.00						0.00												0.00
141	141			0.00			0.00			0.00						0.00												0.00
142	142			0.00			0.00			0.00						0.00												0.00
143–4	143–5			0.00			0.00			0.00						0.00												0.00
145,7–8	146,8–9			0.00			0.00			0.00						0.00												0.00
146	147			0.00			0.00			0.00						0.00												0.00
150	150			0.00			0.00			0.00						0.00												0.00
151	151			0.01			0.01			0.04						0.00												0.09
152	152			0.03			0.03			0.14			0.02			0.02												0.31
153	153			0.03			0.11			0.05			0.06			0.06												0.11
154	154			0.01			0.04			0.01			0.02			0.02												0.00
155.0	155			0.00			0.01			0.02			0.01			0.01												0.03
155.1	156			0.00			0.02			0.00			0.01			0.00												0.05
157	157			0.00			0.00			0.00			0.00			0.00												0.00
160	160			0.00			0.00			0.00			0.00			0.00												0.00
161	161			0.01			0.04			0.05			0.02			0.02												0.11
162–3	162–3			0.08			0.29			0.34			0.14			0.14												0.77
170	174			0.01			0.05			0.07			0.03			0.03												0.15
172	182.0			0.00			0.00			0.01	1		0.00			0.00									1		0.01
173–4	181,2.9			0.01			0.05			0.07			0.03			0.03												0.15
175	183			0.01			0.01			0.01			0.00			0.00												0.02
176	184			0.01			0.01			0.01			0.01			0.01												0.03
180	189.0–.1			0.00			0.02			0.01			0.01			0.01												0.05
181	188			0.04			0.00			0.02			0.01			0.01												0.02
190	172			0.00			0.13			0.01			0.07			0.07												0.36
191	173			0.00			0.00			0.16			0.00			0.00												0.00
192	190			0.00			0.01			0.00			0.00			0.00												0.02
193	191–2			0.00			0.01			0.01			0.01			0.01												0.02
194	193			0.00			0.00			0.01			0.00			0.00												0.00
195	194			0.00			0.00			0.00			0.00			0.00												0.00
196	170			0.00			0.00			0.00			0.00			0.00												0.05
197	171			0.00			0.02			0.02			0.01			0.01												0.01
200,202	200,202			0.00			0.00			0.01			0.00			0.00												0.02
201	201			0.00			0.01			0.01			0.00			0.00												0.00
203	203			0.00			0.00			0.00			0.00			0.00												0.01
204.0	204.1,.9			0.00			0.01			0.00			0.00			0.00												0.02
204.1–4	204.0,5–7			0.00			0.01			0.01			0.01			0.01												0.03
204	204–207			0.00			0.01			0.02			0.01			0.01												0.04
TOTAL				0.20			0.88			1.09	1		0.45		9	0.00		0			0			0	1		2.42

0 : All tumours
0': Histologically confirmed
E : Expected

Table 3. Breast cancer in women in Nova Scotia by age at diagnosis of cervical cancer, stage and treatment

TIME SINCE DIAGNOSIS OF PRIMARY CERVICAL CANCER (IN YEARS)

		<1			1-4			5-9			10-14			15-19			20-24			25-29			30+			Total (excl. <1)		
	Age	O'	:O	E	O'	:O	E	O'	:O	E	O'	:O	E	O'	:O	E	O'	:O	E	O'	:O	E	O'	:O	E	O'	:O	E
INVASIVE / RADIOTHERAPY	<30			0.00			0.00			0.01			0.02			0.01			0.00			0.00			0.00			0.04
	30-39			0.04			0.21			0.36			0.16			0.00			0.00			0.00			0.00			0.73
	40-49			0.23	1		0.80			0.84	1		0.31			0.00			0.00			0.00			0.00	2		1.95
	50-59	1		0.29	1		0.86			0.79			0.28			0.00			0.00			0.00			0.00	1		1.94
	60-69			0.19	2		0.56			0.48	1		0.15			0.00			0.00			0.00			0.00	3		1.18
	70+			0.15	1		0.36	2		0.22			0.06			0.00			0.00			0.00			0.00	3		0.64
INVASIVE / NOT RADIOTHERAPY	<30			0.00			0.00			0.01			0.00			0.00			0.00			0.00			0.00			0.01
	30-39			0.01			0.03			0.06			0.03			0.00			0.00			0.00			0.00			0.13
	40-49			0.02			0.11			0.13			0.04			0.00			0.00			0.00			0.00			0.28
	50-59			0.02			0.07			0.07			0.04			0.00			0.00			0.00			0.00			0.19
	60-69			0.01			0.05			0.03			0.02			0.00			0.00			0.00			0.00			0.10
	70+			0.01			0.04			0.04			0.01			0.00			0.00			0.00			0.00			0.09
IN SITU / NOT RADIOTHERAPY	<30																											
	30-39																											
	40-49																											
	50-59																											
	60-69																											
	70+																											

O : All tumours
O': Histologically confirmed
E : Expected

ONTARIO CANCER REGISTRY

E.A. Clarke & R.F. Spengler

Division of Epidemiology and Statistics
The Ontario Cancer Treatment and Research Foundation
Toronto, Ontario M5S 1A8, Canada

The Ontario Cancer Registry was established in 1964 to collect information on all cancer cases diagnosed in the province, which in 1981 included a population of approximately 8.5 million people in an area of more than 1 million square kilometres. Cancer is not a reportable disease in Ontario, and the Registry uses information collected for other purposes to generate incidence data. The sources of this information are all hospital discharge records with a mention of cancer, patient registrations from seven treatment centres (including the Princess Margaret Hospital) associated with the Ontario Cancer Treatment and Research Foundation, and death certificates on which cancer is given as the primary or secondary cause of death. Since 1972, pathology reports on cancer specimens have been forwarded to the Registry. Originally, the records from these multiple sources were linked manually to produce a single record on each new case of cancer diagnosed in the province. Recently, the Registry has been developing computerized record linkage techniques to produce more timely incidence data. Such computer processing is necessary in view of the large volume of incoming data (375 000 records per year) and the fact that no unique personal identifying number is available on health records. There are approximately 25 000 incident cases each year in the province.

A cohort study was undertaken, which included 8 039 incident cases of cervical cancer admitted to the treatment centres associated with the Ontario Cancer Treatment and Research Foundation from 1960 to 1975 and followed to the end of 1979. The cohort was selected from the treatment centres because (i) these centres have registered and actively followed every cervical cancer patient referred for radiotherapy in the province since 1930, (ii) over 80% of all incident cervical cancer cases in the province are referred to these centres, and (iii) 70% of the 'incident' cases reported in the province that were not referred to these centres were found to have diagnoses other than cervical cancer. Thus, the non-referred incident cases reported to the Ontario Cancer Registry without radiotherapy would not have been a suitable cohort, and the 717 cervical cancer cases not given radiotherapy (see Table 1) at the centres are the only valid internal comparison group. Excluded from the cohort analysis were women who were found to have a second primary tumour within 30 days after the date of diagnosis of cervical cancer, women with third primary tumours or with prior malignancies (with the exception of non-melanotic skin cancer, ICD8 173), and women with in-situ carcinoma of the cervix. In addition, the records of patients with second primary tumours with the same histology as the cervical cancer were reviewed by a physician who had been a pathology resident to determine which were true second primaries (included in the study) and which were metastases.

Table 1. Ontario Cancer Registry: Characteristics of the population under study

	Invasive tumours			*In situ* (no radiotherapy)	Total
	Radiotherapy	No radiotherapy	Total invasive		
Number of women	7 322	717	8 039		
Woman-years at risk by time since diagnosis:					
<1 year	7 322	717	8 039		
1-4 years	22 472	2 215	24 687		
5-9 years	16 735	1 795	18 530		
10-14 years	8 293	740	9 033		
15-19 years	1 983	130	2 113		
20-24 years	0	0	0		
25-29 years	0	0	0		
30+ years	0	0	0		
All years	56 805	5 597	62 402		
Number of women by age at diagnosis:					
<35	571	138	709		
35-44	1 677	211	1 888		
45-54	1 981	173	2 154		
55-64	1 662	95	1 757		
65-74	986	56	1 042		
75+	445	44	489		
Number of women excluded because of:					
- malignancy prior to diagnosis of cervical cancer	99	13	112		
- second cancer (excluding non-melanoma skin) diagnosed simultaneously with cervical cancer	25	6	31		

Incidence rates for the years 1966 and 1971 were used in the person-year analysis. The National Cancer Institute of Canada provided the computer program used for the analysis, which included only calendar year, rather than day, month and year, for estimation of time intervals. The dates used in the analysis are the dates of *registration* (admission) at the treatment centres and not the dates of diagnosis of cervical cancer. As the median time interval between date of diagnosis and date of registration (admission) was one month, the use of date of registration should not affect the findings.

Our results may be different from those of other cancer registries. We believe that the low observed/expected ratios for second primary cancers of the stomach, large intestine and rectum reflect underreporting of these sites among treatment-centre patients because such surgically-treated tumours may not be identified at the centres, where major surgery is not performed. We also see an excess in the observed/expected ratio for cancers of the liver and small intestine, possibly because these tumours are rare and because the use of incidence data from 1966 to estimate the expected cases for the time period 1960 to 1968 and from 1971 for the time period 1969 to 1979, does not allow a parallel to be drawn with the year-to-year variation of the observed numbers. Apart from these exceptions, our reported excesses and deficits of cancer at other sites seem to be comparable with those of other cancer registries.

We would like to thank the directors of all the treatment centres for their collaboration in this study.

Table 2. Observed and expected numbers of second primary cancers in women diagnosed with primary cervical cancer in Ontario

A. Cases of invasive cervical cancer treated by radiotherapy

TIME SINCE REGISTRATION OF PRIMARY CERVICAL CANCER (IN YEARS) [a]

ICD7	ICD8	<1 (7322) O	O'	E	1-4 (6835) O	O'	E	5-9 (4209) O	O'	E	10-14 (2355) O	O'	E	15-19 (802) O	O'	E	20-24 O	O'	E	25-29 O	O'	E	30+ O	O'	E	Total (excl. <1) O	O'	E
140	140			0.08			0.28			0.25			0.13			0.03												0.69
141	141			0.16			0.53			0.46			0.24			0.05												1.28
142	142			0.08			0.27			0.23			0.12			0.03												0.65
143-4	143-5			0.20	1		0.68			0.62	1		0.35			0.07									2		1.72
145,7-8	146,8-9			0.16	1		0.55	2		0.52			0.28			0.06									2	1	1.41
146	147			0.04	1		0.12	1		0.09			0.04			0.01									1		0.26
150	150			0.28	1		0.89	2	1	0.76	2	2	0.41			0.09									5	4	2.15
151	151	2		1.61	7	3	5.08	1		4.22	2		2.34			0.51									8	3	12.15
152	152			0.11	1		0.38			0.35			0.20			0.04									5	4	0.97
153	153			4.65	10	7	14.68	10	6	12.21	4	2	6.59			1.40									24	15	34.88
154	154			1.96	2	1	6.09	6	3	4.94	4	3	2.58			0.55									12	7	14.16
155.0	155			0.11	1		0.37	2	1	0.31			0.17			0.04									3	2	0.89
155.1	156			0.47			0.49			1.25			0.68			0.15											3.57
157	157			1.08	4		3.48	1		2.99	3		1.63			0.35									8	2	8.45
160	160			0.06			0.19			0.15	1		0.08			0.02											0.44
161	161			0.12			0.39			0.34	1		0.18			0.04									1	1	0.95
162-3	162-3	6		1.56	21	13	5.19	30	23	4.62	9	1	2.49	1	1	0.51									61	46	12.81
170	174	3	3	11.73	16	15	36.64	23	19	29.81	5	5	14.88	3	3	2.93									47	42	84.26
172	182.0			2.60			8.23	4	3	6.87	10	9	3.50			0.72									15	13	19.32
173-4	181,2.9			0.27			0.91	1		0.82			0.43	1		0.09									1		2.25
175	183			1.99	3	1	6.17	6	6	4.95	2	2	2.44			0.48									12	9	14.04
176	184			0.44	2	2	1.38	2	2	1.12	2	2	0.57			0.12									6	6	3.19
180	189.0-.1	1	1	0.54	2		1.74			1.48			0.78			0.16									2	1	4.16
181	188,9.2,.9	1	1	1.05	4	3	3.33	7	7	2.81	2	2	1.56	3	1	0.33									16	13	8.03
190	172			0.57			1.71	2	2	1.28			0.57			0.10									2	2	3.66
191	173																										
192	190			0.08			0.27			0.23			0.12			0.02									2	1	0.64
193	191-2	1		0.50	1		1.59	2	1	1.30	2		0.63			0.12									3	2	3.64
194	193			0.40			1.21			0.96			0.46			0.09											2.72
195	194			0.04			0.12			0.08			0.03			0.01											0.24
196	195			0.06			0.22			0.20			0.11			0.02											0.55
197	170	1	1	0.16	1		0.53			0.46			0.25	1		0.05									1	1	1.29
200,202	171		1	0.81			2.61	3	2	2.20	1		1.16			0.24									5	4	6.21
201	200,202			0.26			0.77			0.57			0.27			0.05											1.66
203	201			0.35			1.17	2		1.06			0.61			0.13									2		2.97
204.0	203	2		0.29			0.93	1		0.77			0.41			0.09									1		2.20
204.1-4	204.0,.9			0.56	3	1	1.70	3		1.33	1		0.70			0.15									5	2	3.88
204	204.0,5-7			0.86	3		2.62	1		2.10	1		1.11			0.24									6	2	6.07
	204-207																										
TOTAL [b]	:	14	7	35.44	82	55	111.88	113	82	92.61	48	40	47.99	9	6	9.85									252	183	262.33

O : All tumours
O' : Histologically confirmed
E : Expected

[a] Calendar year (see text)
[b] Excludes non-melanoma skin cancer (ICD8 173)

B. Cases of invasive cervical cancer not treated by radiotherapy

TIME SINCE REGISTRATION OF PRIMARY CERVICAL CANCER (IN YEARS) [a]

ICD7	ICD8	<1 (717) O	O'	E	1-4 (612) O	O'	E	5-9 (463) O	O'	E	10-14 (213) O	O'	E	15-19 (59) O	O'	E	20-24 O	O'	E	25-29 O	O'	E	30+ O	O'	E	Total (excl. <1) O	O'	E
140	140			0.00			0.02			0.02			0.01			0.00										0.05
141	141			0.01			0.03			0.03			0.02			0.00										0.08
142	142			0.01			0.02			0.02			0.01			0.00										0.05
143-5	143-5			0.01			0.05			0.05			0.02			0.00										0.12
145,7-8	146,8-9			0.01			0.03			0.03			0.02			0.00										0.08
146	147			0.00			0.01			0.00			0.00			0.00										0.01
150	150			0.02			0.05	1		0.05			0.02			0.00										0.12
151	151			0.10			0.31			0.26			0.12			0.02										0.71
152	152			0.01			0.02			0.02			0.01			0.00										0.05
153	153			0.30			0.92			0.80			0.38			0.06									1		2.16
154	154			0.12			0.39			0.32			0.15			0.02										0.88
155.0	155			0.01			0.02			0.02			0.01			0.00										0.05
155.1	156			0.03			0.09			0.07			0.04			0.01										0.21
157	157			0.07			0.21			0.20			0.10			0.02										0.53
160	160			0.00			0.01			0.01			0.00			0.00										0.02
161	161			0.01			0.03			0.02			0.01			0.00										0.06
162-3	162-3			0.10			0.35	2	2	0.34	1	1	0.17			0.03								3	3	0.89
170	174			0.84	1	1	2.89	1	1	2.50			1.09			0.17								2	2	6.65
182.0	182.0			0.16			0.57			0.51			0.24			0.04										1.36
173-4	181,2.9			0.02			0.07			0.07			0.03			0.00										0.17
175	183			0.14			0.47			0.40			0.18			0.03										1.08
176	184	1	1	0.03			0.10			0.08			0.04			0.00										0.22
180	189.0-1			0.04			0.12			0.10			0.05			0.01										0.28
181	188,9,2,.9			0.06			0.20			0.18			0.08			0.01										0.47
190	172			0.05			0.16			0.12			0.05			0.01										0.34
191	173																										
192	190			0.01			0.02			0.02			0.01			0.00										0.05
193	191-2			0.04			0.13			0.12			0.05			0.01										0.31
194	193	1	1	0.03			0.10			0.08			0.03			0.00										0.21
195	194			0.00			0.01			0.01			0.00			0.00										0.02
196	170			0.00			0.02			0.02			0.01			0.00										0.05
197	171			0.01			0.04			0.03			0.02			0.01										0.09
200,202	200,202			0.06			0.18			0.16			0.07			0.01										0.42
201	201			0.02			0.07			0.05			0.04			0.00										0.14
203	203			0.02			0.07			0.07			0.04			0.01										0.19
204.0	204.1,.9			0.02			0.05			0.05			0.02			0.00										0.12
204.1-4	204.0.5-7			0.04			0.12			0.09			0.04			0.00										0.26
204	204-207			0.06			0.17			0.14			0.06			0.01										0.38
TOTAL [b]		2	2	2.40	1	1	7.95	4	3	6.92	1	1	3.16			0.47								6	5	18.50

O : All tumours
O': Histologically confirmed
E : Expected

[a] Calendar year (see text)
[b] Excludes non-melanoma skin cancer (ICD8 173)

Table 3. Breast cancer in women in Ontario by age at diagnosis of cervical cancer, stage and treatment

TIME SINCE REGISTRATION OF PRIMARY CERVICAL CANCER (IN YEARS) [a]

Group	Treatment	Age	<1 O	<1 O'	<1 E	1-4 O	1-4 O'	1-4 E	5-9 O	5-9 O'	5-9 E	10-14 O	10-14 O'	10-14 E	15-19 O	15-19 O'	15-19 E	20-24 O	20-24 O'	20-24 E	25-29 O	25-29 O'	25-29 E	30+ O	30+ O'	30+ E	Total O	Total O'	Total E
INVASIVE	RADIOTHERAPY	<30			0.02			0.10			0.17			0.17			0.05												0.49
INVASIVE	RADIOTHERAPY	30-39			0.47	1	1	2.31	2	2	3.32	1	1	2.46			0.63										4	4	8.72
INVASIVE	RADIOTHERAPY	40-49	1	1	2.71	4	4	9.26	5	5	8.99	1	1	4.95	1	1	1.04										11	11	24.23
INVASIVE	RADIOTHERAPY	50-59	1	1	3.41	6	6	10.81	5	5	8.74	3	3	4.00	1	1	0.78										15	15	24.32
INVASIVE	RADIOTHERAPY	60-69	1	1	2.74	3	3	8.30	6	5	5.76			2.52			0.40										9	8	16.99
INVASIVE	RADIOTHERAPY	70+	3		2.39	2	1	5.86	5	2	2.83	1	1	0.79			0.03										8	4	9.51
INVASIVE	NO RADIOTHERAPY	<30			0.00			0.03			0.06			0.03			0.01												0.13
INVASIVE	NO RADIOTHERAPY	30-39			0.07			0.42	1	1	0.57			0.30			0.06										1	1	1.35
INVASIVE	NO RADIOTHERAPY	40-49			0.25			0.98	1	1	0.89			0.38			0.07										1	1	2.33
INVASIVE	NO RADIOTHERAPY	50-59			0.21			0.73			0.53			0.24			0.03												1.53
INVASIVE	NO RADIOTHERAPY	60-69			0.14			0.38			0.27			0.09			0.01												0.74
INVASIVE	NO RADIOTHERAPY	70+			0.16			0.34			0.18			0.04			0.00												0.56
IN SITU	UNTREATED	<30																											
IN SITU	UNTREATED	30-39																											
IN SITU	UNTREATED	40-49																											
IN SITU	UNTREATED	50-59																											
IN SITU	UNTREATED	60-69																											
IN SITU	UNTREATED	70+																											

O : All tumours
O': Histologically confirmed
E : Expected
[a] Calendar year (see text)

SASKATCHEWAN CANCER REGISTRY

G.R. Howe, A.B. Miller, D. Robson & C. Wall

Records of cancer cases have been available in Saskatchewan since two major cancer clinics were opened in Regina and Saskatoon by the provincial government in 1932. Since 1944, all Saskatchewan residents have been provided with free diagnosis and treatment of cancer, and cancer registration is regarded as almost complete from that date. Cancer is a reportable disease by law in Saskatchewan, and no physician is paid for services to cancer patients unless the patient was first reviewed at one of the two treatment clinics. By 1948, 85% of all cancer patients were seen at the cancer clinics, and the percentage rose to over 90% by the early 1950s. Since the early 1970s, 4% or less of registrations are first discovered from death certificates, and 95% are based on histological information. Registration therefore results from referrals to a clinic from physicians and surgeons, from records of hospital in-patients and out-patients, from copies of pathology report forms from pathology departments, from reports submitted by physicians attending patients at home and from copies of death certificates provided by the Provincial Registrar of Vital Statistics.

All patients with cancer are followed clinically by the cancer clinics from the date of diagnosis for the duration of their lives. Those who do not attend a cancer clinic are followed either directly or by their physicians.

For many years, records were kept in the two separate cancer clinics; however, since the end of the 1970s a computerized provincial cancer registry has been in operation in the offices of the Saskatchewan Cancer Foundation. Duplication of registration is avoided by cross-filing through an alphabetical patient index. Multiple primary sites in the same patient are recorded.

In 1976, the population of the registration area was 921 300, of whom 464 700 were males and 456 600 females. The Registry covers the province of Saskatchewan, which lies between Alberta on the west and Manitoba on the east, between latitudes 49° and 60° north and longitudes 110° and 102° west. The total registration area is 651 903 km^2.

HOWE *et al.*

Table 1. Saskatchewan Cancer Registry: Characteristics of the population under study

	Invasive tumours			*In situ* (no radiotherapy)	Total
	Radiotherapy	No radiotherapy	Total invasive		
Number of women	1 277	232	1 509		
Woman-years at risk by time since diagnosis:					
<1 year	1 277	232	1 509		
1-4 years	3 771	665	4 436		
5-9 years	3 144	628	3 772		
10-14 years	2 224	370	2 594		
15-19 years	1 311	198	1 509		
20-24 years	772	96	868		
25-29 years	240	24	264		
30+ years	0	0	0		
All years	12 739	2 213	14 952		
Number of women by age at diagnosis:					
<35	47	22	69		
35-44	225	44	269		
45-54	332	51	383		
55-64	294	47	341		
65-74	216	31	247		
75+	163	37	200		
Number of women excluded because of:					
- malignancy prior to diagnosis of cervical cancer	24	5	29		
- second cancer (excluding non-melanoma skin) diagnosed simultaneously with cervical cancer	22	9	31		

Table 2. Observed and expected numbers of second primary cancers in women diagnosed with primary cervical cancer in Saskatchewan

A. Cases of invasive cervical cancer treated by radiotherapy

TIME SINCE DIAGNOSIS OF PRIMARY CERVICAL CANCER (IN YEARS)

		<1			1–4			5–9			10–14			15–19			20–24			25–29			30+			Total (excl. <1)		
Number of women starting intervals		1277			1177			731			534			349			207			93			0					
ICD7	ICD8	O	O'	E	O	O'	E	O	O'	E	O	O'	E	O	O'	E	O	O'	E	O	O'	E	O	O'	E	O	O'	E
140	140			0.02			0.06			0.06			0.06			0.05			0.04			0.01			0.00			0.28
141	141			0.01			0.03			0.04			0.03			0.03			0.02			0.01			0.00			0.16
142	142			0.03			0.08			0.07			0.06			0.04			0.03			0.01			0.00			0.29
143–4	143–5			0.02			0.04			0.04			0.04			0.02			0.02			0.00			0.00			0.16
145,7–8	146,8–9			0.01			0.04			0.05	1		0.04			0.03			0.02			0.00			0.00	1		0.18
146	147			0.01			0.02			0.02			0.01			0.01			0.00			0.00			0.00			0.06
150	150			0.02			0.06			0.06			0.06			0.06			0.03			0.01			0.00			0.27
151	151			0.20			0.54			0.58			0.54	1		0.42			0.31			0.08			0.00			2.47
152	152			0.02			0.07	1		0.07			0.07			0.05			0.03			0.01			0.00	1		0.30
153	153			0.55	3		1.51			1.61	2		1.46	2		1.09	1		0.76			0.20			0.00	8		6.63
154	154			0.27	2		0.75	1		0.80			0.70			0.50			0.34			0.09			0.00	6		3.18
155.0	155			0.02			0.05			0.06			0.05			0.04			0.01			0.01			0.00			0.24
155.1	156			0.09			0.23			0.25			0.24			0.18	1		0.14			0.04			0.00			1.08
157	157			0.14	3		0.39			0.43			0.39	1		0.32	1		0.22			0.06			0.00	5		1.81
160	160			0.01			0.02			0.03			0.02			0.01			0.01			0.00			0.00			0.09
161	161			0.01			0.03			0.03			0.03			0.02			0.01			0.00			0.00			0.12
162–3	162–3			0.26	2		0.74	2		0.78	1		0.65			0.44			0.27			0.06			0.00	5		2.94
170	174			1.78			5.16	2		5.26	2		4.16			2.73			1.65			0.40			0.00	5		19.36
172	182.0			0.54			1.61			1.71			1.40			0.93			0.54			0.12			0.00			6.31
173–4	181,2.9			0.01			0.04			0.04			0.03			0.02			0.01			0.00			0.00			0.14
175	183			0.29			0.83			0.85	1		0.67	1		0.44			0.25			0.06			0.00	2		3.10
176	184			0.06	1		0.18			0.19	1		0.18			0.13			0.10			0.03			0.00	1		0.81
180	189.0–.1			0.11			0.32			0.35			0.31			0.23			0.15			0.04			0.00			1.40
181	188			0.11			0.31			0.34			0.31			0.23			0.17			0.04			0.00			1.40
190	172			0.10			0.27			0.26			0.20			0.13			0.08			0.02			0.00			0.96
191	173	7		1.69	4		4.57	2		4.86	6		4.29	1		3.12	2		2.22			0.63			0.00	15		19.69
192	190			0.02			0.05			0.05			0.04			0.03			0.02			0.00			0.00			0.19
193	191–2			0.08			0.23			0.22			0.17	1		0.10			0.06			0.01			0.00	2		0.79
194	193			0.11			0.30			0.29			0.22			0.13	1		0.08			0.02			0.00			1.04
195	194			0.00			0.01			0.01			0.01			0.01			0.00			0.00			0.00			0.04
196	170			0.01			0.02			0.02			0.02			0.01			0.01			0.00			0.00			0.08
197	171			0.03			0.10			0.10			0.08			0.06			0.04			0.01			0.00			0.39
200,202	200,202			0.14	2		0.41			0.42	2		0.36	1		0.26			0.16	1		0.04			0.00	5		1.65
201	201			0.03			0.08			0.08			0.06			0.05			0.03	1		0.01			0.00	1		0.31
203	203			0.07			0.18			0.19			0.18			0.14			0.10			0.02			0.00			0.81
204.0	204.1,.9			0.05			0.14			0.15			0.14			0.11			0.08			0.02			0.00			0.64
204.1–4	204.0,5–7			0.08			0.21			0.20	1		0.17			0.12			0.08			0.02			0.00	1		0.80
204	204–207			0.13			0.34			0.35	1		0.31			0.23			0.16			0.04			0.00	1		1.43
TOTAL		7		7.00	17		19.67	8		20.57	18		17.45	8		12.28	6		8.11	2		2.08	0		0.00	59		80.16

O : All tumours
O': Histologically confirmed
E : Expected

B. Cases of invasive cervical cancer not treated by radiotherapy

TIME SINCE DIAGNOSIS OF PRIMARY CERVICAL CANCER (IN YEARS)

		<1			1–4			5–9			10–14			15–19			20–24			25–29			30+			Total (excl. <1)		
ICD7	ICD8	O	O'	E	O	O'	E	O	O'	E	O	O'	E	O	O'	E	O	O'	E	O	O'	E	O	O'	E	O	O'	E
Number of women starting intervals		232			190			139			102			52			31			12			0			12		
140	140			0.00			0.01			0.01			0.01			0.01			0.00			0.00			0.00			0.04
141	141			0.00			0.00			0.01			0.01			0.00			0.00			0.00			0.00			0.02
142	142			0.00			0.01			0.01			0.01			0.01			0.00			0.00			0.00			0.04
143-4	143-5			0.00			0.01			0.01			0.01			0.00			0.00			0.00			0.00			0.03
145,7-8	146,8-9			0.00			0.00			0.00			0.00			0.00			0.00			0.00			0.00			0.03
146	147			0.00			0.00			0.00			0.00			0.01			0.00			0.00			0.00			0.00
150	150			0.03			0.01			0.01			0.01			0.06			0.03			0.01			0.00			0.04
151	151			0.00			0.08			0.11			0.09			0.17			0.09			0.00			0.00			0.04
152	152			0.08			0.01		1	0.01			0.25			0.07			0.00			0.02			0.00		1	0.38
153	153			0.00			0.22			0.30		1	0.12			0.07		1	0.09			0.01			0.00		1	0.04
154	154			0.04			0.11			0.15			0.01			0.01			0.04			0.00			0.00		1	1.05
155.0	155			0.01			0.01			0.01			0.04			0.07			0.00			0.00			0.00			0.50
155.1	156			0.00			0.03			0.05			0.07			0.03			0.02			0.00			0.00			0.04
157	157			0.02			0.06			0.08			0.00			0.05			0.03			0.00			0.00			0.17
160	160			0.00			0.00			0.00			0.00			0.00			0.00			0.00			0.00			0.29
161	161			0.00			0.00			0.01			0.00			0.00			0.00			0.00			0.00			0.00
162-3	162-3			0.04			0.12		1	0.15		1	0.10			0.07			0.03			0.01			0.00		1	0.01
170	174			0.26		1	0.83		1	0.97		1	0.65			0.41			0.20			0.04			0.00		4	0.48
172	182.0			0.08			0.26			0.32		2	0.22			0.13			0.06			0.01			0.00			3.10
173-4	181,2.9			0.00			0.01			0.01			0.00			0.00			0.00			0.00			0.00			1.00
175	183			0.04			0.14			0.16			0.11			0.06			0.03			0.01			0.00			0.02
176	184			0.01			0.03			0.04			0.03			0.02			0.01			0.00			0.00			0.51
180	189.0-.1			0.02			0.05		1	0.07			0.05			0.03		1	0.02			0.00			0.00			0.13
181	188			0.02			0.05		1	0.06			0.05			0.04			0.02			0.00			0.00		1	0.22
190	172			0.02			0.05			0.05			0.03			0.02			0.01		1	0.00			0.00		1	0.22
191	173			0.27			0.77			0.92			0.77			0.53			0.29			0.04			0.00			0.16
192	190			0.00			0.01			0.01			0.01			0.00			0.00			0.00			0.00		2	3.26
193	191-2			0.01			0.04			0.04			0.03			0.01			0.01			0.00			0.00			0.03
194	193			0.02			0.05			0.06			0.03			0.02			0.01			0.00			0.00			0.13
195	194			0.00			0.00			0.00			0.00			0.00			0.00			0.00			0.00			0.17
196	170			0.00			0.00			0.00			0.00			0.00			0.00			0.00			0.00			0.00
197	171			0.02			0.02			0.02			0.01			0.01			0.01			0.00			0.00			0.00
200,202	200,202			0.00			0.06			0.08			0.06			0.04			0.02			0.00			0.00			0.06
201	201			0.00			0.01			0.02			0.01			0.01			0.00			0.00			0.00			0.26
203	203			0.01			0.03			0.04			0.03			0.02			0.01			0.00			0.00			0.05
204.0	204.1,.9			0.01			0.02			0.03			0.02			0.02			0.01			0.00			0.00			0.13
204.1-4	204.0,5-7			0.01			0.03			0.04			0.03			0.02			0.01			0.00			0.00			0.10
204	204-207			0.02			0.05			0.07			0.05			0.04			0.02			0.00			0.00			0.23
TOTAL				1.02	1		3.09	4		3.87	4		2.89			1.89	2		0.95	1		0.15			0.00	12		12.84

O : All tumours
O' : Histologically confirmed
E : Expected

Table 3. Breast cancer in women in Saskatchewan by age at diagnosis of cervical cancer, stage and treatment

TIME SINCE DIAGNOSIS OF PRIMARY CERVICAL CANCER (IN YEARS)

INVASIVE — RADIOTHERAPY

Age	<1 (E)	1-4 O'	1-4 E	5-9 O'	5-9 E	10-14 E	15-19 E	20-24 E	25-29 E	30+ E	Total O	Total O'	Total E
<30	0.00		0.01		0.03	0.04	0.05	0.04	0.02	0.00	0.00		0.21
30-39	0.08		0.36		0.58	0.60	0.43	0.29	0.07	0.00	0.00		2.33
40-49	0.38	2	1.37	1	1.58	1.33	0.95	0.62	0.15	0.00	0.00	3	6.01
50-59	0.49		1.54		1.64	1.34	0.86	0.50	0.11	0.00	0.00		5.98
60-69	0.45		1.14	1	0.95	0.62	0.36	0.18	0.03	0.00	0.00	1	3.29
70+	0.39		0.75	1	0.47	0.22	0.07	0.02	0.01	0.00	0.00	1	1.54

INVASIVE — NO RADIOTHERAPY

Age	<1 (E)	1-4 O'	1-4 E	5-9 O'	5-9 E	10-14 E	15-19 E	20-24 E	25-29 E	30+ E	Total O	Total O'	Total E
<30	0.00		0.01		0.01	0.02	0.02	0.01	0.00	0.00	0.00		0.08
30-39	0.01		0.07	1	0.11	0.08	0.08	0.05	0.01	0.00	0.00	1	0.40
40-49	0.05	1	0.22	1	0.26	0.17	0.09	0.04	0.01	0.00	0.00	2	0.80
50-59	0.08		0.30	1	0.32	0.21	0.11	0.05	0.01	0.00	0.00	1	1.01
60-69	0.06		0.16		0.18	0.12	0.07	0.04	0.00	0.00	0.00		0.57
70+	0.06		0.07		0.07	0.05	0.03	0.00	0.00	0.00	0.00		0.23

IN SITU

Age	<1	1-4	5-9	10-14	15-19	20-24	25-29	30+	Total
<30									
30-39									
40-49									
50-59									
60-69									
70+									

O : All tumours
O': Histologically confirmed
E : Expected

SECOND PRIMARY CANCERS AMONG 40 518 WOMEN TREATED FOR CANCER OR CARCINOMA *IN SITU* OF THE CERVIX UTERI IN DENMARK 1943-1976

H.H. Storm & O.M. Jensen

Danish Cancer Registry
Strandboulevarden 49
2100 Copenhagen
Ø, Denmark

Introduction

The Danish Cancer Registry contains information on all patients notified as having cancer in Denmark since 1943. It now covers a population of some 5 100 000 persons in an area of 43 075 km^2 (Danmarks Statistik, 1980). Since the start of the Registry in 1942, notification of cancer cases from clinical departments in hospitals and from pathology institutes has been voluntary. In addition to data from these sources, information from death certificates is added to the Registry files once a year (Clemmesen, 1965).

The Registry is tumour-based, so that patients with multiple primary cancer appear several times in its file, with a record of each tumour. Registered persons are identified by the Danish Central Person Number System, which minimizes the risk of duplicate registrations. All medical information in the Registry is reviewed by the medical coding staff, and particular care is taken before accepting multiple primaries. A second primary is thus defined as a malignancy reported as a new case, and is accepted after review by the medical coding staff. The tumour file is updated at regular intervals, and the originally notified information is kept in a card filing system.

Cancers at the Registry are classified according to a modified version of the 7th Revision of the ICD (Clemmesen, 1977; Danish Cancer Registry, 1982). This classification has been in use since 1957, and cases first diagnosed between 1943 and 1957 were recoded to comply with this classification.

Material and methods

The basis of the present study consists of some 41 412 cases of cervical cancer and carcinoma *in situ* (including severe dysplasia) of the cervix uteri reported, while still alive, to the Danish Cancer Registry between 1943 and 1976 (Table 1). Women with these diagnoses known to the Registry on the basis only of death certificates or autopsy reports are not included.

Table 1. Danish Cancer Registry: Characteristics of the population under study

	Invasive tumours			*In situ* (no radiotherapy)	Total
	Radiotherapy	No radiotherapy	Total invasive		
Number of women	20 024	5 127	25 151	15 367	40 518
Woman-years at risk by time since diagnosis:					
<1 year	18 518.2	4 339.2	22 857.4	14 348.4	37 215.8
1-4 years	47 917.4	13 300.9	61 218.3	38 322.5	99 540.8
5-9 years	39 880.2	11 957.9	51 838.1	15 841.8	67 680.0
10-14 years	27 701.2	7 212.9	34 914.1	1 156.2	36 070.3
15-19 years	17 686.4	3 949.0	21 635.4	138.5	21 773.9
20-24 years	10 163.8	1 431.2	11 595.0	43.2	11 638.2
25-29 years	4 300.3	395.2	4 695.5	16.0	4 711.5
30+	814.3	73.4	887.7	3.5	891.2
All years	166 991.8	42 659.7	209 651.5	69 870.2	279 511.7
Number of women by age at diagnosis:					
<35	1 931	721	2 652	6 247	8 899
35-44	5 148	1 633	6 781	5 565	12 346
45-54	5 854	1 356	7 210	2 784	9 994
55-64	4 129	724	4 853	577	5 430
65-74	2 185	423	2 608	156	2 764
75+	777	270	1 047	38	1 085
Number of women excluded because of:					
- malignancy prior to diagnosis of cervical cancer	293	126	419	238	657
- second cancer (excluding non-melanoma skin) diagnosed simultaneously with cervical cancer	99	46	145	92	237

The material was divided into four treatment and tumour classes, using the following definitions:

- *invasive tumours*: invasive or microinvasive tumours of the cervix uteri;

- *carcinoma* in situ: includes both carcinoma *in situ* and dysplasia of the cervix;

- *radiotherapy*: all types of radiotherapy given to the patient at any time after onset of the malignant disease: thus, no absolute distinction can be made between therapy for a primary tumour and for metastases;

- *no radiotherapy*: notified either as no radiotherapy or treatment unknown.

Exclusions

Patients with cervical cancer or carcinoma *in situ* diagnosed at autopsy or known to the Cancer Registry from death certificates only were excluded, as mentioned above.

Some 240 cases with a primary tumour other than non-melanoma skin cancer that was diagnosed at the same time as the cervical lesion were also excluded, and so were 657 patients in whom the cervical cancer followed another cancer when this was not a non-melanoma skin cancer (Table 1). Furthermore, a few patients who had received radiotherapy for a carcinoma *in situ* were excluded altogether and do not figure in Table 1.

After these exclusions, some 40 518 women remained to be followed up. These consisted of 25 151 women with invasive cancers, of whom 20 024 had received radiotherapy and 5 127 had not received radiotherapy. A total of 15 367 women with carcinoma *in situ* had not received radiation treatment.

Follow-up

Patients were followed in the Cancer Registry from the date of diagnosis (i.e., time of first hospital admission) of the cervical cancer or carcinoma *in situ*, until they developed a second primary cancer, without regard to type (i.e., including non-melanoma skin cancer), until they died or up to 31 December 1976, whichever occurred first. No account was taken of emigration in the computation of years of observation, but this is unlikely to have influenced the results. As part of this investigation, second primary cancers in female genital organs (ICD7: 172, 173, 174, 176) were revised by scrutinizing hospital records in order to exclude recurrences of the cervical cancer erroneously notified as a new, primary, genital cancer.

Person-years of observation were calculated by the life-table method taking account of the ageing of the population as well as calendar time in five-year intervals. Expected numbers of cases for each site were calculated on the basis of incidence rates for all of Denmark, as preliminary analyses had given no indication that adjustments for place of residence had any influence on the expected values obtained.

Observed numbers of cases were computed so as to correspond to the expected values with regard to diagnostic category. The observed numbers were divided into all cases observed (O_1) and histologically verified cases only (O_2). Histological verification in this study included examination of specimens from the primary site or the metastatic site or cytological verification. In the case of leukaemia, confirmation of diagnosis on peripheral blood samples was regarded as histological verification.

The follow-up period was divided into five-year intervals, as shown in Table 1.

In Table 2, the following exceptions were made to the 7th Revision of the ICD, as a result of use of the modified version of the code used in the Danish Cancer Registry:

- site specific diagnoses exclude sarcomas, which are included only in the category 'all sites';

- ICD 146 (nasopharynx) is included with ICD 160 (nasal cavities) and not with pharynx;

- ICD 161 (larynx) includes ICD 162.0 (trachea);

- ICD 162 (lung) excludes trachea;

- ICD 180 (kidney) excludes ureter;

- ICD 181 (bladder, etc.) includes ureter and papilloma of bladder;

- ICD 153 (colon) includes rectosigmoid junction;

- ICD 154 (rectum) includes skin of anus and excludes rectosigmoid junction;

- ICD 191 (skin) excludes skin of anus.

Table 2. Observed and expected numbers of second primary cancers in women diagnosed with primary cervical cancer in Denmark

A. Cases of invasive cervical cancer treated by radiotherapy

TIME SINCE DIAGNOSIS OF PRIMARY CERVICAL CANCER (IN YEARS)

ICD7	ICD8	<1 (20024) O	O'	E	1-4 (16238) O	O'	E	5-9 (9493) O	O'	E	10-14 (6650) O	O'	E	15-19 (4429) O	O'	E	20-24 (2694) O	O'	E	25-29 (1380) O	O'	E	30+ (437) O	O'	E	Total (excl. <1) O	O'	E
140	140			0.15			0.40			0.40			0.34			0.26			0.17			0.09	1	1	0.02	2	2	1.68
141	141			0.16			0.42			0.41			0.35			0.28			0.19			0.10			0.02	2	2	1.77
142	142			0.35			0.94			0.86			0.64			0.43			0.24			0.10			0.02	4	3	3.23
143-4	143-5	1	1	0.20			0.56			0.58			0.52			0.45			0.34			0.19			0.04	3	3	2.68
145,7-8	146,8-9			0.15			0.38			0.37			0.29			0.21			0.14			0.06			0.02	1	1	1.47
146	147																											
150	150	1	1	0.58	5	5	1.53	3	3	1.55	2	2	1.36	1	1	1.13			0.82			0.42			0.09	11	10	6.90
151	151	3	3	6.09	11	6	15.71	13	10	14.88	11	6	12.06	11	10	9.16	2	2	6.22	2	2	3.13			0.65	52	36	61.81
152	152	3	2	0.21			0.57			0.57			0.49			0.38			0.26			0.13			0.03	7	7	2.43
153	153	3	3	6.86	19	16	19.11	24	20	19.67	15	13	17.33	16	13	14.34	5	5	10.34	8	8	5.47			1.22	88	75	87.38
154	154	2	2	4.67	6	4	12.86	6	6	12.72	17	13	10.80	7	6	8.54	6	5	5.95	6	6	3.01	2	2	0.65	53	42	54.53
155.0	155			0.86			2.23	2	2	2.13			1.78			1.45			1.05			0.54			0.11	8	5	9.29
155.1	156	1	1	1.33	3	3	3.81	3	3	4.08	3	3	3.72	2	2	3.14	2	2	2.33			1.23			0.27	17	16	18.58
157	157			2.04	5	4	5.85	7	7	6.25	4	3	5.69	4	4	4.84	3	3	3.62	1	1	1.92			0.42	32	23	28.59
160	160	1	1	0.19			0.53	2	2	0.51	1	1	0.53	2	2	0.31			0.21			0.03			0.03	5	5	2.10
161	161	1	1	0.20			0.58	2	2	0.60			0.52			0.40			0.27			0.12			0.02	5	5	2.51
162-3	162-3	4	4	3.07	38	38	8.98	43	39	9.52	15	15	8.61	9	9	7.15	3	3	5.33	3	3	2.75	1	1	0.58	113	98	42.92
170	174	16	16	20.99	36	36	58.32	39	39	55.37	35	32	43.69	21	20	31.43	10	9	20.23	5	5	9.50	1	1	1.95	147	136	220.49
172	182.0	4	4	5.07	1	1	14.55	3	3	14.44	5	5	11.95	9	9	8.81	7	7	5.58	1	1	2.50			0.49	26	25	58.32
173-4	181,2.9			0.39			0.97			0.86			0.63			0.43			0.28			0.15			0.03	4		3.35
175	183	5	5	5.95	8	8	16.81	4	3	16.21	3	3	12.97	2	2	9.43	6	6	5.99	3	3	2.67			0.52	27	23	64.60
176	184	4	4	0.92	7	7	2.52	3	3	2.47	3	3	2.03	2	2	1.56	3	3	1.06	1	1	0.53			0.11	17	17	10.28
180	189.0-.1	5	4	1.80	6	6	5.16	5	5	5.34	3	3	4.69	2	2	3.76	2	2	2.60	1	1	1.26			0.26	22	18	23.07
181	188	5	5	1.77	10	8	5.10	7	6	5.44	13	11	4.91	16	14	4.12	9	7	3.08	4	4	1.63			0.36	67	51	24.64
190	172	1	1	1.35	8	7	3.85	6	6	3.71	4	4	2.99	4	4	2.16	1	1	1.38	1	1	0.63			0.12	11	10	14.84
191	173	9	7	5.65	19	15	15.85	24	21	16.21	14	13	14.05	15	15	11.43	9	8	8.26	3	3	4.31			0.96	84	75	71.07
192	190			0.28	1	1	0.76	1	1	0.73	3	3	0.59	1	1	0.44			0.28			0.13			0.02	3	3	2.95
193	191-2	1	1	2.51	5	5	7.03	4	3	6.70	3	3	5.39	2	2	3.91	3	3	2.48	1	1	1.10	1	1	0.21	16	14	26.82
194	193			0.54	3	3	1.52			1.50	2	2	1.25	1	1	0.97			0.65			0.31			0.06	7	7	6.26
195	194			0.11			0.30			0.30			0.25			0.20			0.15			0.08			0.02	4	4	1.30
196	170			0.18			0.50			0.44			0.34			0.25			0.17			0.08			0.01	4	4	1.79
197	171			0.38	1	1	0.99	3	3	0.84	1	1	0.61	1	1	0.42			0.26			0.11			0.03	7	7	3.25
200,202	200,202	1	1	1.15	4	4	3.27	5	5	3.36	3	3	2.99	1	1	2.46	1	1	1.78	1	1	0.93			0.21	15	12	15.00
201	201			0.47	1	1	1.25	1	1	1.12			0.84			0.60			0.39			0.19			0.04	8	5	4.43
203	203			0.68			1.95	1	1	2.06			1.86			1.54			1.09			0.54			0.11	7	4	9.15
204,0	204,1,.9	2	2	0.59	2	1	1.63	1	1	1.67	1	1	1.47	2	2	1.22	1	1	0.88			0.46			0.10	12	10	7.43
204,1-4	204,0.5-7	2	2	1.07	5	5	2.94	3	3	2.87	3	3	2.37	2	2	1.80	1	1	1.24	1	1	0.64			0.13	12	10	11.99
204	204-207	2	2	1.66	6	6	4.57	5	5	4.54	3	2	3.84	2	2	3.02	1	1	2.12	1	1	1.10			0.23	14	14	19.42
TOTAL		65	60	78.96	206	180	219.73	228	183	216.74	176	151	180.78	137	123	139.31	82	67	95.31	49	43	47.11	11	8	9.92	889	755	908.90

O : All tumours
O': Histologically confirmed
E : Expected

B. Cases of invasive cervical cancer not treated by radiotherapy

TIME SINCE DIAGNOSIS OF PRIMARY CERVICAL CANCER (IN YEARS)

ICD7	ICD8	<1 (5127) O	O'	E	1-4 (3932) O	O'	E	5-9 (2865) O	O'	E	10-14 (1893) O	O'	E	15-19 (1058) O	O'	E	20-24 (492) O	O'	E	25-29 (141) O	O'	E	30+ (37) O	O'	E	Total (excl. <1) O	O'	E
140	140			0.03			0.08			0.09			0.06			0.04			0.02			0.01			0.00			0.30
141	141			0.03	1		0.07			0.08			0.06			0.05			0.02			0.01			0.00	1	1	0.29
142	142			0.07			0.21			0.19			0.12			0.07			0.03			0.01			0.00			0.63
143-4	143-5			0.04			0.10			0.12			0.10			0.08			0.04			0.02			0.00			0.46
145,7-8	146,8-9			0.03			0.08			0.09			0.06			0.04			0.02			0.00			0.00			0.29
146	147																											
150	150	1	1	0.10	1	1	0.24	1	1	0.27			0.22			0.17			0.09			0.04			0.01	2	2	1.04
151	151	1	1	1.00	2	2	2.33	6	3	2.38	3	2	1.75	3	2	1.23			0.64			0.26			0.05	14	9	8.64
152	152			0.04	1	1	0.11			0.13			0.10			0.06			0.04			0.01			0.00	1	1	0.45
153	153	2	2	1.21	5	5	3.56	3	3	4.12	5	4	3.22	7	7	2.36			1.21	1	1	0.46			0.09	21	20	15.02
154	154			0.80	5	3	2.35	3	2	2.64	4	4	2.04	2	1	1.44			0.70	1	1	0.26			0.05	14	11	9.48
155.0	155			0.14			0.35			0.39	1	1	0.31			0.23	1	1	0.12			0.05			0.01	2	2	1.46
155.1	156			0.22			0.63	1	1	0.75			0.62			0.47	1	1	0.26			0.10			0.02	2	2	2.85
157	157			0.35	2		1.07	1	1	1.30	2	2	1.06	1	1	0.81			0.42			0.16			0.03	6	3	4.85
160	160			0.03			0.10	1	1	0.11	1	1	0.08			0.06			0.03			0.01			0.00	2	1	0.39
161	161			0.04			0.15			0.18			0.14			0.10			0.04			0.01			0.00			0.62
162-3	162-3	1	1	0.58	13	13	1.99	4	4	2.53	9	8	2.04	2	2	1.52	2	2	0.71	2	2	0.24			0.05	30	28	9.08
170	174	3	2	4.26	12	11	14.03	13	13	15.17	9	9	10.63	6	6	6.62	1	1	2.70			0.85			0.16	43	42	50.16
172	182.0	1	1	0.90			3.03			3.54			2.72			1.83			0.76			0.22			0.04			12.14
173-4	181,2.9			0.07			0.17			0.15			0.10			0.06			0.03			0.02			0.00			0.53
175	183	2	2	1.16	3	3	3.84	2	2	4.18	1	1	3.03	2	2	1.91			0.78	1	1	0.23			0.04	10	9	14.01
176	184			0.17			0.48	1	1	0.52	2	2	0.38			0.26			0.13			0.05			0.01	3	3	1.83
180	189.0-.1	2	2	0.33	3	3	1.06	5	5	1.24	2	2	0.98	3	3	0.69	1	1	0.32			0.11			0.02	13	13	4.42
181	188	2	2	0.32	6	5	1.01	1	1	1.23	2	2	0.99	2	2	0.74			0.37			0.14			0.03	13	10	4.51
190	172	2	1	0.35	1	1	1.20	1	1	1.27	1	1	0.85	2	2	0.52			0.20			0.06			0.01	3	3	4.11
191	173	2	1	1.06	4	4	3.17	8	8	3.64	4	4	2.80	2	2	2.00			0.98	1	1	0.37			0.07	19	19	13.03
192	190			0.05			0.16	1	1	0.17			0.12			0.08			0.03			0.01			0.00	1	1	0.57
193	191-2			0.52	3	3	1.71	3	2	1.82	3	3	1.30			0.83			0.35			0.09			0.01	11	10	6.11
194	193			0.11			0.33			0.34			0.24			0.16			0.07			0.03			0.01			1.18
195	194			0.02			0.07			0.09			0.06			0.04			0.02			0.00			0.00			0.28
196	170			0.03			0.11			0.10			0.07			0.04			0.02			0.01			0.00			0.35
197	171			0.07			0.21	1	1	0.20	1	1	0.13			0.08			0.03			0.01			0.00	1	1	0.66
200,202	200,202	1		0.22	2	2	0.71			0.82	1	1	0.64	1	1	0.46	1	1	0.22			0.08			0.02	3	3	2.95
201	201			0.11	2	2	0.33			0.30	1	1	0.19			0.12			0.05			0.02			0.00	3	3	1.01
203	203			0.12			0.36			0.43			0.34			0.25			0.13			0.05			0.01			1.57
204.0	204.0	1	1	0.10	2	2	0.26	2	2	0.30			0.24			0.18			0.10	1	1	0.04			0.01	3	3	1.13
204.1-4	204.1,9	1	1	0.20	2	2	0.64	2	2	0.68	1	1	0.48	1	1	0.34			0.16	1	1	0.06			0.01	4	4	2.37
204	204.0,5-7	1	1	0.30	2	2	0.90	2	2	0.98			0.72			0.52			0.26			0.10			0.02	5	4	3.50
204	204-207																											
TOTAL		17	15	14.88	68	62	46.30	59	54	51.56	52	47	38.27	35	31	25.94	6	5	11.84	7	6	4.10			0.76	227	205	178.77

0 : All tumours
0': Histologically confirmed
E : Expected

C. Cases of carcinoma in situ not treated by radiotherapy

TIME SINCE DIAGNOSIS OF PRIMARY CERVICAL CANCER (IN YEARS)

		<1			1–4			5–9			10–14			15–19			20–24			25–29			30+			Total (excl. <1)		
ICD7	ICD8	O	O'	E	O	O'	E	O	O'	E	O	O'	E	O	O'	E	O	O'	E	O	O'	E	O	O'	E	O	O'	E
140	140			0.04			0.13	1		0.08			0.01			0.01			0.00			0.00			0.00	1		0.22
141	141			0.03			0.12			0.08			0.01			0.01			0.00			0.00			0.00	1		0.21
142	142			0.12			0.30	1		0.12			0.01			0.01			0.00			0.00			0.00	1	1	0.43
143–4	143–5			0.05			0.17			0.12			0.01			0.01			0.00			0.00			0.00			0.30
145,7–8	146,8–9			0.05			0.17			0.11			0.01			0.01			0.00			0.00			0.00			0.29
	147																											
150	150	1	1	0.08			0.30	1		0.21			0.03			0.01			0.01			0.00			0.00	1	1	0.55
151	151			0.69			2.34	1		1.44			0.18			0.04			0.02			0.01			0.00			4.03
152	152	4	4	0.06	6		0.18	2	2	0.12			0.01			0.08			0.03			0.02			0.00	8	8	0.31
153	153			1.57		3	5.55	2	2	3.49	1		0.37			0.08			0.08			0.02			0.01	9	9	9.54
154	154	1	1	0.94			3.32	1	2	2.08			0.23			0.05			0.01			0.01			0.00	7	7	5.71
155.0	155			0.14			0.48			0.30			0.03			0.01			0.01			0.00			0.00	1	1	0.82
155.1	156			0.22			0.82	2	2	0.56			0.07			0.03			0.01			0.01			0.00	2	2	1.47
157	157			0.44	2	2	1.62	2	2	1.08			0.12			0.07			0.03			0.01			0.00	4	4	2.87
160	160			0.05			0.18			0.09			0.02			0.02			0.01			0.00			0.00			0.28
161	161			0.10	1	1	0.37			0.24			0.02			0.00			0.00			0.00			0.00	1	1	0.63
162–3	162–3	3	3	1.23	5	4	4.73	9	8	3.16	2	2	0.31	1	1	0.05			0.02			0.01			0.01	17	14	8.28
170	174	7	7	9.55	22	22	32.59	22	20	18.10	5	5	1.57			0.22			0.07			0.03			0.01	49	47	52.59
172	182.0	3	3	1.40	2	2	5.25	1	1	3.49			0.35			0.00			0.02			0.01			0.00	3	3	9.19
173–4	181,2.9			0.07			0.22			0.10	1	1	0.01			0.01			0.00			0.00			0.00			0.33
175	183	3	3	2.23	3	3	7.48	3	3	4.20	1	1	0.39			0.07			0.02			0.01			0.01	7	7	12.17
176	184			0.23	3	1	0.76	8	8	0.43	1	1	0.04			0.01			0.00			0.00			0.00	12	11	1.24
180	189.0–.1			0.53	3	3	1.87			1.13	1	1	0.11	1	1	0.02			0.02			0.01			0.00	3	2	3.14
181	188			0.51	2	2	1.86	3		1.21			0.13			0.02	2	2	0.02			0.01			0.00	5	4	3.24
190	172	0	0	1.32	4	5	3.99	3	3	1.92	1	1	0.15			0.06			0.03			0.01			0.00	8	7	6.09
191	173	2	2	1.78	7	7	6.19	7	7	3.70			0.37			0.06			0.06			0.03			0.01	14	14	10.36
192	190			0.09			0.28			0.14			0.01			0.04			0.00			0.00			0.00	1	1	0.43
193	191–2			1.23	2	2	3.93			2.15	1	1	0.19			0.00			0.01			0.00			0.00	2	2	6.32
194	193			0.21			0.60			0.29			0.03			0.01			0.00			0.00			0.00			0.93
195	194			0.06			0.21			0.11			0.01			0.00			0.00			0.00			0.00			0.33
196	170			0.08			0.18			0.08			0.01			0.00			0.00			0.00			0.00			0.27
197	171	1	1	0.15	1	1	0.46	1	1	0.23			0.02			0.02			0.00			0.00			0.00	2	2	0.71
200,202	200,202			0.45			1.51	1	1	0.89	1	1	0.08			0.08			0.01			0.01			0.00	2	2	2.50
201	201	1	1	0.35			0.84			0.31			0.02			0.02			0.00			0.00			0.00	1	1	1.17
203	203			0.13	1	1	0.50			0.33	1	1	0.04			0.04			0.00			0.00			0.00	2	2	0.88
204.0	204.1,.9			0.08			0.30			0.20	1	1	0.03			0.03			0.00			0.00			0.00	1	1	0.54
204.1–4	204.0,5–7			0.43			1.32			0.68			0.07			0.07			0.01			0.00			0.00			2.08
204	204–207			0.51			1.62			0.88	1	1	0.10			0.10			0.02			0.00			0.00	1	1	2.62
TOTAL		26	26	26.69	69	63	91.12	69	64	52.97	13	12	5.06	2	2	0.86	2	2	0.30			0.13			0.01	155	143	150.45

O : All tumours
O': Histologically confirmed
E : Expected

Evaluation of information on treatment

The main purpose of the Danish Cancer Registry is to form a basis for epidemiological research. Although treatment given for primary tumours is recorded by the Registry, this information has not received great emphasis and has been used only sporadically in the past. The validity of the coded information is thus unknown.

As misclassification by treatment (i.e., radiotherapy or not) will tend to mask true differences in risks of second primary cancers associated with radiotherapy, the content of the coded information was evaluated on the basis of random samples from each of the cancer treatment categories under study. This would be of particular importance, as the 'no radiotherapy' group in the Danish study corresponds to statements of both no radiotherapy and no information on radiation.

In addition, the risk of gynaecological cancers should be seen in conjunction with the number of organs at risk rather than the number of women at risk, and, if a large number of operations were performed, the denominators should be corrected accordingly. Varying practices in this regard between regions covered by different registries in the international study may influence the comparability of the results.

Invasive/any radiotherapy

Table 3 shows that in a sample of 100 women with cervical cancer treated with radiotherapy, only one case had had radiation to a second primary cancer rather than to the cervical cancer.

Table 3. Evaluation of information on treatment in random samples of cervical cancer treatment categories

Therapy	Invasive/some radiotherapy	Invasive/no radiotherapy	*In situ*/no radiotherapy
Radiotherapy to cervical cancer	99[a]	9	0
Radiotherapy to second primary	1	0	0
No information on radiotherapy	0	19	49
Surgery, no mention of radiotherapy	0	45	-
No radiotherapy	0	19	51

[a] In 10 cases, followed by hysterectomy and oophorectomy

As radiotherapy to a second primary cancer might be reflected in the treatment classification of the cervical cancer, some 700 second primary cancers were checked, as a link between radiotherapy to a second primary and classifications as 'any radiotherapy' would bias the results of the study. Only in 12 cases was there a possibility that treatment of second primary cancers by radiotherapy could have brought the cervical cancer case into the irradiated group. A further review showed that this had been the case in none of the 12 women and that this source of bias could therefore be considered to be minimal.

Invasive/no radiotherapy

A suspicion that this group of women was not homogeneous with regard to treatment was confirmed (Table 3). Only 19 patients (21%) had a positive statement of no radiotherapy; for 64 cases (70%), no information was available as to whether radiotherapy had been given or not, whereas nine women (10%) had in fact received radiotherapy. The majority of the 70%

for whom information is lacking may thus be assumed truly to belong to the non-irradiated group, as two-thirds of this group had undergone radical surgery.

The original information in the card filing system at the Cancer Registry was reviewed for 106 women with second primary cancers belonging to the group of cervical cancer cases with no mention of radiotherapy. Some 24% of these women had in fact received radiotherapy as the initial treatment.

In-situ carcinoma/no radiotherapy

Table 1 shows that only half of the random sample of 100 women in this group had a statement on the notification form of no radiotherapy, the information as to radiotherapy being absent in the remainder of the group. Furthermore, it is noteworthy that 39% had a history of total hysterectomy and 12% also of oophorectomy (Table 4).

Table 4. Recorded surgical treatment in random sample of patients with carcinoma *in situ*

Surgery	No.
Hysterectomy and bilateral oophorectomy	5
Hysterectomy and unilateral oophorectomy	7
Hysterectomy, total [a]	27
Cone excision	55
Biopsy only	6
Total	100

[a] No statement about ovaries; one had later undergone vaginectomy

Treatment evaluation - conclusion

It may thus be concluded that the patients in the radiotherapy group had truly undergone that treatment and furthermore that the radiotherapy was applied to the initial cancer of the cervix uteri. The group of women with invasive cervical cancer in the 'no radiotherapy' group must be considered an unsatisfactory group for comparison in the present material, as at least 10% had received radiotherapy to the cervix uteri, and there is an indication that an even larger proportion of women with second primary cancers in this group had been irradiated as part of their initial treatment requirement. Comparisons of the two groups will thus tend to underestimate any difference in risk of development of a second primary tumour associated with radiotherapy of the cervix uteri. Examination of the in-situ/no radiotherapy group shows that these patients are more likely to be classified correctly.

Tables 3 and 4 further indicate that the risk of gynaecological tumours in the Danish series cannot be evaluated on the basis of woman-years at risk; correction must be made for the loss of uteri and ovaries, which for the former represent some 10, 50 and 40% of the invasive/some radiotherapy, invasive/no radiotherapy and in-situ/no radiotherapy groups, respectively.

Results

Observed and expected numbers of cases by site and time from the diagnosis of cervical cancer/carcinoma *in situ* are given in Table 2.

Observed and expected numbers of breast cancers, by time and age at diagnosis of cervical cancer/carcinoma *in situ* are given in Table 5.

Table 5. Breast cancer in Danish women by age at diagnosis of cervical cancer, stage and treatment

TIME SINCE DIAGNOSIS OF PRIMARY CERVICAL CANCER (IN YEARS)

INVASIVE — RADIOTHERAPY

Age	<1 O	<1 O'	<1 E	1-4 O	1-4 O'	1-4 E	5-9 O	5-9 O'	5-9 E	10-14 O	10-14 O'	10-14 E	15-19 O	15-19 O'	15-19 E	20-24 O	20-24 O'	20-24 E	25-29 O	25-29 O'	25-29 E	30+ O	30+ O'	30+ E	Total O	Total O'	Total E
<30			0.03			0.14			0.37	1	1	0.69			0.92			0.80			0.42			0.08	1	1	3.42
30-39			1.12	1	1	4.80	3	2	7.81	3	3	8.61	1	1	6.94	1	1	4.96			2.65	1	1	0.64	10	9	36.41
40-49	3	3	5.61	8	8	17.14	13	13	17.31	10	9	13.95	11	11	10.68	5	4	7.73	3	3	3.96			0.89	50	48	71.66
50-59	4	4	6.05	11	11	17.02	10	10	15.82	16	16	12.56	6	6	8.98	3	3	5.33	2	2	2.20			0.26	48	48	62.17
60-69	8	8	4.84	13	13	12.60	9	7	10.07	4	3	6.35	3	2	3.49	1	1	1.24			0.21			0.04	30	26	34.00
70+	1	1	3.35	3	3	6.62	4	2	3.99	1	1	1.54			0.40			0.17			0.08			0.02	8	6	12.82

INVASIVE — NO RADIOTHERAPY

Age	<1 O	<1 O'	<1 E	1-4 O	1-4 O'	1-4 E	5-9 O	5-9 O'	5-9 E	10-14 O	10-14 O'	10-14 E	15-19 O	15-19 O'	15-19 E	20-24 O	20-24 O'	20-24 E	25-29 O	25-29 O'	25-29 E	30+ O	30+ O'	30+ E	Total O	Total O'	Total E
<30			0.01			0.07			0.19	1	1	0.32	1	1	0.38			0.24			0.09			0.03	2	2	1.32
30-39	1	1	0.40	1	1	2.10	2	2	3.63	5	5	3.43	2	2	2.36			0.82			0.21			0.04	10	10	12.59
40-49	1	1	1.54	5	4	5.78	3	3	6.04	1	1	3.92	3	3	2.32	1	1	0.99			0.32			0.07	13	12	19.44
50-59	1	1	1.10	4	4	3.35	4	4	3.43	1	1	2.09	1	1	1.19	1	1	0.49			0.17			0.02	11	11	10.74
60-69			0.64	2	2	1.71	2	2	1.51	1	1	0.71			0.32			0.13			0.05			0.00	5	5	4.43
70+	2	1	0.57			0.82	2	2	0.46			0.15			0.05			0.03			0.00			0.00	2	2	1.51

IN SITU

Age	<1 O	<1 O'	<1 E	1-4 O	1-4 O'	1-4 E	5-9 O	5-9 O'	5-9 E	10-14 O	10-14 O'	10-14 E	15-19 O	15-19 O'	15-19 E	20-24 O	20-24 O'	20-24 E	25-29 O	25-29 O'	25-29 E	30+ O	30+ O'	30+ E	Total O	Total O'	Total E
<30			0.17	1	1	0.77			0.60			0.10			0.01			0.00			0.00			0.00	1	1	1.48
30-39	1	1	1.92	4	4	7.54	8	7	5.27	2	2	0.55			0.07			0.02			0.01			0.00	14	13	13.46
40-49	3	3	5.06	13	13	17.27	9	9	8.93	1	1	0.64			0.09			0.05			0.02			0.00	23	23	27.00
50-59	1	1	1.73	3	3	5.10	3	3	2.49	1	1	0.20			0.04			0.00			0.00			0.00	7	7	7.83
60-69	1	1	0.49	1	1	1.43	1	1	0.62	1	1	0.03			0.00			0.00			0.00			0.00	3	3	2.08
70+			0.18	1	1	0.49			0.19			0.05			0.01			0.00			0.00			0.00	1	1	0.74

O : All tumours
O': Histologically confirmed
E : Expected

Total cancer morbidity

The total risk of incurring a second primary cancer after treatment for invasive cervical cancers and carcinoma *in situ* shows no excess.

In the different time periods following the diagnosis of cervical cancer or in-situ carcinoma, the observed and expected numbers are similar, with no excesses or deficits found.

Site-specific morbidity

Tumour sites at which there was an overall excess represent increased risks for all time periods since diagnosis of the cervical cancer. Even tumours for which there was a deficit in the observed numbers, like breast cancer, show a consistent deficit throughout the different time periods.

The same pattern of excesses and deficits emerges for tumour sites in the two groups of patients with invasive tumours, whereas the pattern seen for the in-situ group is slightly different. Statistically significant excess risks are summarized in Table 6. Significant deficits in the observed numbers are found for the sites given in Table 7.

Table 6. Sites at which excess risks of second primary cancers were seen following cancer of the cervix uteri or carcinoma *in situ*

Site	Invasive		*In-situ*
	Some radiotherapy	No radiotherapy	
Oesophagus	1.6	2.0	-
Pancreas	1.3	1.5	1.4
Nose and sinus	2.4	5.1	-
Larynx	2.0	1.6	1.6
Lung	2.7	3.3	2.2
Other genital	1.7	1.6	9.7
Bladder	2.9	2.9	1.5
Other skin	1.2	1.5	1.5
Bone	2.8	-	-
Small intestine	2.9	2.2	3.2

Table 7. Sites at which decreased risks of second primary cancers were seen following cancer of the cervix uteri or carcinoma *in situ*

Site	Invasive		*In-situ*
	Some radiotherapy	No radiotherapy	
Breast	0.67	0.86	0.93
Corpus uteri	0.45	-	0.33
Ovary, etc	0.42	0.71	0.58

In the case of breast cancer, a deficit is found in the patients with invasive cancers. The observed/expected ratio (O/E) for the irradiated invasive cervical cancer group is 0.67 and that for the non-irradiated group 0.86. In the in-situ group, the O/E ratio is 0.93. When the results are broken down by age at irradiation (Table 5), a deficit of breast cancers in patients irradiated at under age 40 is seen (O/E = 0.30), whereas no deficit is found in either of the non-irradiated groups in relation to age at first treatment for cervical cancer.

The deficits of corpus uterine and ovarian cancers may be explained in part by surgical treatment (Table 3).

Summary and conclusions

The procedure by which the Registry dealt with multiple notification of cancers would appear to underestimate rather than overestimate the number of second primary cancers. The problem is not regarded as a major one and would not bias the analysis, since errors would not be correlated with the division of the material into two treatment groups.

There is no overall excess of second primary cancers in either of the treatment groups, and only slight increases are found in relative risks for cancers of specific organs in the irradiated group. It is important to emphasize, however, that the division of the Danish material into an irradiated and a non-irradiated group is subject to misclassification, since at least 10% of the non-irradiated group and possibly a larger proportion of the patients with second primary cancers had in fact been radiated. The non-irradiated group should thus be disregarded as a potential reference group.

The cancer sites for which deficits are found must be seen in conjunction with both ovarian status (e.g., breast cancer) and organs at risk (uterus, ovary), since pelvic surgery in combination with radiation treatment has been extensive.

It is noteworthy that most of the excess risks observed at particular sites - respiratory organs, oesophagus and bladder - may indicate the presence of confounding or a degree of common etiology between these cancers and the cervical cancer. This may tend to hide the presence of a possible radiation effect, which is indicated by increased risks of cancers of the bone and small intestine. Only more detailed studies with regard to radiotherapy will determine the possible, small fraction associated with radiation.

Acknowledgements

Mr P. Troelsen assisted with the programming and Miss P. Toft and Mrs A. Falck with the tabulations.

References

Clemmesen, J. (1965) Statistical studies in malignant neoplasms, Vol. I. *Acta pathol. microbiol. Scand.*, *Suppl. 174*

Clemmesen, J. (1977) Statistical studies in malignant neoplasms, Vol. V. *Acta pathol. microbiol. Scand.*, *Suppl. 261*

Danish Cancer Registry (1982) *Incidence of Cancer in Denmark 1973-1977*, Copenhagen

Danmarks Statistik (1980) *Statistical Yearbook, 1980*, Copenhagen

RADIATION AND MULTIPLE PRIMARY CANCERS AMONG CERVICAL CANCER PATIENTS DIAGNOSED IN FINLAND BETWEEN 1953 AND 1977

M. Hakama, T. Hakulinen & K. Mäkelä

Finnish Cancer Registry
00170 Helsinki 17, Finland

Introduction

The Finnish Cancer Registry covers the whole of Finland and is population-based (Teppo *et al.*, 1975). New cases of cancer have been reported since 1953 by hospitals, pathology laboratories and private practitioners. In addition, all deaths occurring in Finland are matched annually against the Cancer Registry files: if the report is in any way incomplete, inquiries are sent to the sender of the pathology specimen or to the writer of the death certificate. Reporting is practically complete for all cancer cases diagnosed in Finland.

Follow-up of the patients is based on cross checking of the Registry files against all death certificates issued in Finland. Until the beginning of the 1970s, this was done manually, by comparing annual alphabetical lists of deaths with a similar list of cancer patients assumed to be alive. Since 1967, every person resident in Finland has been issued with a personal identification number, and in recent years the follow-up has been computerized on the basis of this 11-digit number.

The follow-up described here was completed in 1974 by identifying manually from the national population registry all those patients assumed still to be alive. At the same time, the personal identification number was recorded for those cases diagnosed before 1967. Of more than 200 000 cancer patients, 22 were lost for follow-up (Hakulinen *et al.*, 1981). Follow-up for 1975 to 1977 was also virtually complete, because it was based on personal identification number and on linkage of the cancer registry computer tapes with those giving annual deaths in Finland. Whenever the personal identification numbers was erroneous on the cancer registry tapes, it was corrected manually using information from the national population registry.

The Finnish population numbered four million in 1950 and remained very stable, at about 4.7 million, throughout the 1970s. The annual number of new cases of cancer of the cervix uteri was around 400 (15 per 10^5 person-years, adjusted to the world standard population) up to the mid 1960s. Since then, there has been a continuous decrease in the incidence of this disease, the most recent figure being 233 cases in 1977. This reduction is probably due to an organized mass screening programme which covers the entire country (Hakama, 1982). In consequence, the detection rate of carcinoma *in situ* increased from almost zero to more than 10 per 10^5 person-years in 1953-1968, and has since decreased.

The cancers found most commonly among females in Finland, other than that of the cervix uteri, are, in order of descending incidence, breast, stomach, corpus uteri, ovary, colon and rectum. The total number of female cancer cases diagnosed in Finland was 4200 in 1953 and

6700 in 1977 (carcinoma *in situ* of the cervix included and basal-cell carcinomas of the skin excluded). The proportion of cases confirmed microscopically (by autopsy histology or cytology) has increased continuously among females, being 60% in 1954 and 93% in 1977 (Saxen *et al.*, 1969; Finnish Cancer Registry, 1981).

Material and methods

The basic material consists of all cases of invasive or in-situ cervical cancer diagnosed between 1953 and 1977 in Finland. New primary cancers in these patients were recorded if diagnosed during the same perod of time. Only cases with at least one year between the diagnoses of the two primary cancers (and the person-years) were included in the analysis. A patient was excluded from the series if the cervical cancer or carcinoma *in situ* had been preceded by a prior malignancy: there were 178 such females, 171 of whom had two primary cancers and seven who had three or more primaries. Furthermore, if two primary cancers (cervix, other than cervix) were diagnosed within one month, they were regarded as simultaneous cancers and were not included in the material. After exclusions, the series comprised 12 296 women, of whom 8491 had invasive cancer; 515 who had carcinoma *in situ* and were treated with radiotherapy were included only in the Finnish analysis and were excluded from the combined cancer registry material reported in the Appendix. The total number of woman-years at risk was 88 837 (Table 1).

Table 1. Finnish Cancer Registry: Characteristics of the population under study

	Invasive tumours			*In-situ* tumours			Total
	Radiotherapy	No radiotherapy	Total invasive	Radiotherapy	No radiotherapy	Total *in-situ*	
Number of women by age at diagnosis:	7 285	1 206	8 491	515	3 290	3 805	12 296
Woman-years at risk by time since diagnosis:							
<1 year	6 716	886	7 602	511	3 195	3 706	11 308
1-4 years	17 079	2 543	19 622	1 898	11 004	12 902	32 524
5-9 years	13 507	1 991	15 498	2 085	8 537	10 622	26 120
10-14 years	7 990	825	8 815	1 162	2 669	3 831	12 646
15-19 years	3 802	321	4 123	347	614	961	5 084
20-24 years	972	66	1 038	57	60	117	1 155
25-29 years							
30+ years							
All years	50 090	6 629	56 718	6 059	26 078	32 137	88 837
Number of women by age at diagnosis:							
<35	307	100	407	25	700	725	1 132
35-44	1 398	262	1 660	180	1 254	1 434	3 094
45-54	2 217	291	2 508	193	1 038	1 231	3 739
55-64	1 912	209	2 121	89	223	312	2 433
65-74	1 130	196	1 326	25	69	94	1 420
75+	321	148	469	3	6	9	478

	Invasive tumours			In-situ tumours			Total
	Radiotherapy	No radiotherapy	Total invasive	Radiotherapy	No radiotherapy	Total in-situ	
Number of women excluded because of:							
- malignancy prior to diagnosis of cervical cancer	3	2	5	-	2	2	7
- second cancer (excluding non-melanoma skin) diagnosed simultaneously with cervical cancer	3	2	5	-	8	8	13
- two primary cancers with cervical cancer as second primary (total, 171)							
Number of women with three or more primary cancers	3	1	4	1	1	2	6

Follow-up to estimate the number of subsequent primary cancers and the number of woman-years at risk was started at the time of diagnosis of cervical cancer or carcinoma in situ and was terminated either at the death of the patient or at the end of 1977. Altogether, 351 multiple primary cancers were diagnosed in 345 patients.

The expected numbers of cases were estimated by multiplying age-calendar time-specific incidence rates for each anatomical site by the number of age-calendar time-specific person-years. Three calendar time periods, 1953-1959, 1960-1969 and 1970-1977, and a five-year age classification were used. The incidence rates were derived from figures for the whole of Finland.

The results were reported by five-year follow-up intervals, excluding the new primary cancers diagnosed and person-years accumulated less than one year after diagnosis of a cervical lesion.

The material was divided into invasive cancers and carcinomas in situ. Cases with unknown extent of disease were regarded as invasive. Severe dysplasias are not reported to the Finnish Cancer Registry.

Histological verification of cases included microscopical examination of biopsy or autopsy samples of either the primary tumour or a metastasis. For leukaemias, a study of bone marrow or peripheral blood was regarded as histological confirmation.

Crude data on the first course of treatment are recorded in the Cancer Registry material. First course of treatment was defined as interventions made during the first four months after diagnosis. The following classification was used in this study:

(i) Surgery (possibly combined with treatment other than radiation);

(ii) Radiation (alone or combined with any other treatment);

(iii) Treatment other than surgery or radiation or no known treatment.

The third group comprised less than 2% of all person-years and was combined with the first group. The radiation group was divided into radiation with or without surgery for a closer analysis of selected primary sites.

The 7th Revision of the ICD was used for definition of primary sites. Basal-cell carcinomas of the skin and papillomas of the urinary bladder were not included in the material.

HAKAMA *et al.*

Table 2. Observed and expected numbers of second primary cancers in women diagnosed with primary cervical cancer in Finland

A. Cases of invasive cervical cancer treated by radiotherapy

TIME SINCE DIAGNOSIS OF PRIMARY CERVICAL CANCER (IN YEARS)

ICD7	ICD8	<1 O	<1 O'	<1 E	1-4 O	1-4 O'	1-4 E	5-9 O	5-9 O'	5-9 E	10-14 O	10-14 O'	10-14 E	15-19 O	15-19 O'	15-19 E	20-24 O	20-24 O'	20-24 E	25-29 O	25-29 O'	25-29 E	30+ O	30+ O'	30+ E	Total O	Total O'	Total E
		7285			5986			3360			2153			1133			447									5986		
140	140			0.08			0.21			0.18			0.13			0.08			0.02									0.62
141	141			0.10			0.27			0.24			0.17			0.09			0.03							2	2	0.80
142	142	1	1	0.15	1	1	0.38	1	1	0.29			0.17			0.07			0.02							1	1	0.93
143-4	143-5			0.09			0.23			0.20			0.14	1	1	0.08			0.02									0.67
145,7-8	146,8-9			0.12			0.30			0.26			0.18			0.10			0.03							1	1	0.87
146	147			0.03			0.09			0.08			0.05			0.03			0.01									0.26
150	150	1	1	0.79			2.00			1.67	1	1	1.16			0.62	3	3	0.19							5	5	5.64
151	151			4.05	9	4	10.13	6	6	8.12	7	5	5.48	5	3	2.82			0.86							31	21	27.41
152	152			0.10			0.27			0.24			0.16			0.09			0.03							1	1	0.79
153	153			1.38	5	1	3.77	4	4	3.57	5	5	2.61			1.55			0.48							15	14	11.98
154	154			1.15	1		3.13	2	2	2.96	6	5	2.13	5	3	1.21			0.37							16	13	9.80
155.0	155			0.22			0.61			0.58	1	1	0.44			0.28			0.09							1	1	2.00
155.1	156			0.46	1	2	1.29	1	1	1.29	3	3	1.00			0.64			0.20							5	5	4.42
157	157			0.99	3		2.72	4	4	2.62	3	3	1.95	2	1	1.16			0.36							13	10	8.81
160	160			0.11			0.28			0.23			0.14			0.06			0.02									0.73
161	161			0.06			0.16			0.14			0.09			0.04			0.01									0.44
162-3	162-3	1		0.91	12	11	2.50	7	7	2.38	6	3	1.71	4	3	0.99	1	2	0.29							32	24	7.87
170	174	2	2	5.75	12	12	15.68	17	17	14.13	10	8	9.36	3	3	5.04	1	2	1.38							44	42	45.59
172	182.0			1.90	2	2	5.14	1	1	4.66	2	2	3.14	1	1	1.69			0.45							6	6	15.08
173-4	181,2.9			0.20			0.52			0.42	1	1	0.24			0.10			0.02							1	1	1.30
175	183	5	5	1.77	2	2	4.77	3	3	4.23	4	4	2.78	3	4	1.46			0.39							10	9	13.63
176	184			0.39	1	1	1.02	1	1	0.90	1	1	0.63	3	4	0.35			0.11							9	9	3.01
180	189.0-.1	3	3	0.60	2	2	1.66	2	2	1.66	1	1	1.14			0.65	1		0.19							4	4	5.23
181	188			0.36	1	1	0.99			0.99			0.74			0.46			0.14							2	2	3.31
190	172			0.39	1	1	1.09	2	2	1.09	1	1	0.68			0.37			0.10							2	2	3.25
191	173	3	3	0.58	2	2	1.52	2	2	1.52			0.91			0.49			0.15							4	4	4.40
192	190			0.11			0.29			0.29			0.17			0.09			0.02									0.83
193	191-2			0.67	1	1	1.83	4	4	1.83	1	1	1.05			0.55	1	1	0.14							6	6	5.21
194	193			0.42			1.15	1	1	1.15	3	3	0.71			0.39	1	1	0.11							6	6	3.40
195	194			0.03			0.08			0.07			0.04			0.02			0.01									0.22
196	170			0.12			0.28			0.28			0.13			0.06			0.02							1		0.70
197	171	1	1	0.19	1		0.52	1	1	0.47	2	2	0.31			0.17	1	1	0.05							6	6	1.52
200,202	200,202			0.32			0.89			0.86			0.62	2	2	0.37	1	1	0.11							2	2	2.85
201	201			0.16			0.42	2	2	0.42			0.24			0.14			0.04									1.21
203	203			0.31			0.85	1	1	0.84			0.62	1	1	0.37	1		0.11							4	4	2.79
204.0	204.1,.9			0.20	5	5	0.53	1	1	0.50			0.36			0.14			0.07							1		1.67
204.1-4	204.0,5-7	5	5	0.51	5	5	1.35	2	2	1.18	1	1	0.78			0.41	1	1	0.12							8	7	3.84
204	204-207	5	5	0.71	5	5	1.88	2	2	1.68	1	1	1.15	1	1	0.62	1	1	0.18							9	8	5.51
TOTAL		17	17	25.77	67	59	68.92	66	62	61.74	60	51	42.37	33	26	23.30	14	12	6.75							240	210	203.08

O : All tumours
O': Histologically confirmed
E : Expected

B. Cases of invasive cervical cancer not treated by radiotherapy

TIME SINCE DIAGNOSIS OF PRIMARY CERVICAL CANCER (IN YEARS)

ICD7	ICD8	<1 (1206) O	O'	E	1-4 (785) O	O'	E	5-9 (529) O	O'	E	10-14 (273) O	O'	E	15-19 (90) O	O'	E	20-24 (39) O	O'	E	25-29 O	O'	E	30+ O	O'	E	Total (excl. <1) (785) O	O'	E
140	140			0.01			0.02			0.02			0.01	1	1	0.01			0.00									0.06
141	141			0.01			0.03			0.03			0.01			0.01			0.00							1	1	0.08
142	142			0.02			0.04			0.03			0.01			0.01			0.00									0.09
143-4	143-5			0.01			0.02			0.02			0.01			0.01			0.00									0.06
145,7-8	146,8-9			0.00			0.03			0.03			0.02			0.00			0.00									0.09
146	147			0.10			0.01			0.01			0.00			0.04			0.01									0.02
150	150			0.50	1	1	0.17	1		0.13			0.08			0.19			0.06							1	1	0.43
151	151			0.01	1		0.92	1	1	0.69			0.38			0.01			0.00							2	2	2.24
152	152			0.17			0.03			0.03			0.01			0.11			0.03									0.08
153	153			0.14	1	1	0.39			0.36			0.20	1	1	0.09			0.03							1	1	1.09
154	154			0.03			0.32	2	2	0.30			0.17			0.02			0.01							4	4	0.91
155.0	155	1	1	0.05			0.06			0.06	1	1	0.04			0.04			0.01									0.19
155.1	156			0.12			0.13			0.13			0.08			0.08			0.01									0.39
157	157			0.01			0.26			0.25			0.15	1	1	0.00			0.02							1	1	0.76
160	160			0.01			0.03			0.02			0.01			0.00			0.00									0.06
161	161			0.11			0.02			0.02			0.01			0.00			0.00									0.05
162-3	162-3			0.70	2	2	0.28			0.27	1	1	0.15			0.08			0.02							2	2	0.80
170	174			0.20	5	5	2.10			1.94			0.92	1	1	0.41			0.09							7	7	5.46
172	182.0			0.03			0.62			0.62			0.31	1	1	0.14			0.03							1	1	1.72
173-4	181,2.9			0.20			0.06			0.05			0.02			0.01			0.00									0.14
175	183			0.05			0.59			0.55			0.27			0.12			0.03									1.56
176	184			0.07			0.10			0.09			0.05			0.03			0.01									0.28
180	189.0-.1			0.04			0.19	1	1	0.18			0.10			0.05			0.01							1	1	0.53
181	188			0.05			0.10	1	1	0.10			0.06			0.03			0.01							1	1	0.30
190	172			0.07			0.16			0.15			0.07			0.03			0.01									0.42
191	173			0.01			0.15			0.12			0.07			0.01			0.01									0.38
192	190			0.08			0.03			0.03			0.02			0.02			0.01									0.09
193	191-2			0.05	1	1	0.26			0.24			0.11			0.05			0.01							1	1	0.67
194	193			0.00			0.16			0.14			0.07			0.03			0.00									0.41
195	194			0.01			0.01			0.01			0.00			0.00			0.01									0.02
196	170			0.02			0.03			0.02			0.01			0.01			0.00									0.06
197	171			0.04			0.06			0.06			0.03			0.03			0.00									0.16
200,202	200,202			0.02			0.10			0.10			0.05			0.01			0.01									0.29
201	201			0.04			0.05			0.05			0.02			0.01			0.00									0.13
203	203			0.02			0.09			0.09			0.05			0.01			0.01									0.27
204.0	204.1..9			0.03			0.05			0.05			0.03			0.00			0.00									0.14
204.1-4	204.0.5-7			0.06	1		0.15			0.13			0.07			0.03			0.01							1	1	0.39
204	204-207			0.08	1		0.20			0.18			0.09			0.05			0.01							1	1	0.53
TOTAL		1	1	3.06	12	9	7.82	6	5	7.12	2	2	3.66	5	5	1.78			0.44							25	21	20.82

O : All tumours
O': Histologically confirmed
E : Expected

HAKAMA *et al.*

C. Cases of carcinoma <u>in situ</u> not treated by radiotherapy

TIME SINCE DIAGNOSIS OF PRIMARY CERVICAL CANCER (IN YEARS)

		<1			1-4			5-9			10-14			15-19			20-24			25-29			30+			Total (excl. <1)		
Number of women starting intervals		3290			3128			2347			1033			215			38									3128		
ICD7	ICD8	O	O'	E	O	O'	E	O	O'	E	O	O'	E	O	O'	E	O	O'	E	O	O'	E	O	O'	E	O	O'	E
140	140			0.01			0.04			0.04			0.02			0.01			0.00											0.11
141	141			0.02	1	1	0.08			0.09			0.04			0.01			0.00								1		0.22
142	142			0.04			0.14			0.11			0.04			0.01			0.00										0.30
143-4	143-5			0.02			0.06			0.06			0.03			0.01			0.00										0.16
145,7-8	146,8-9			0.01			0.09			0.09			0.04			0.00			0.00										0.23
146	147			0.01			0.02			0.02			0.01			0.05			0.00										0.05
150	150			0.08	2	2	0.30	2		0.33			0.17			0.26			0.01							1	1	0.86
151	151	1	1	0.49			1.88			1.92	1	1	0.86			0.04			0.04							4	3	4.96
152	152			0.02			0.08			0.09			0.04			0.01			0.00									0.22
153	153			0.25	1	1	1.05	3	1	1.14	1	1	0.50	1	1	0.02			0.02							6	6	2.87
154	154			0.20			0.85	1		0.97			0.42			0.13			0.02							1	1	2.39
155.0	155			0.03	1	1	0.15			0.19			0.09			0.03			0.00							2	2	0.46
155.1	156			0.07	1	1	0.30	1		0.37			0.18			0.06			0.01							2	2	0.92
157	157			0.14	1	1	0.60			0.73	1	1	0.35			0.12			0.02							2	2	1.82
160	160			0.02			0.08			0.07			0.03			0.01			0.00							1	1	0.19
161	161			0.02			0.06			0.07			0.02			0.00			0.00									0.16
162-3	162-3	1	1	0.18			0.79	2	2	0.94	3	3	0.40	1	1	0.12			0.02							3	3	2.27
170	174			1.94	9	9	7.90	4	4	7.80	3	3	2.81	1	1	0.72			0.08							17	17	19.31
172	182.0			0.49	1	1	2.09			2.36			0.91			0.25			0.03							1	1	5.64
173-4	181,2.9			0.06			0.23			0.21			0.07			0.02			0.00									0.53
175	183	5	5	0.53	2	2	2.08	3	1	2.09			0.78			0.21	1	1	0.02							5	4	5.18
176	184			0.06	1		0.26	2	1	0.26	1	1	0.12			0.04			0.01							3	3	0.69
180	189.0-.1			0.13			0.56	1		0.64			0.27			0.08			0.01							1	1	1.56
181	188			0.06			0.25			0.32			0.15			0.05			0.05									0.78
190	172			0.17	2		0.68			0.68			0.22			0.06			0.06									1.61
191	173			0.09	1	1	0.33	1	1	0.32			0.15			0.05			0.05							2	2	0.86
192	190			0.03			0.12			0.12			0.04			0.01			0.01							1	1	0.29
193	191-2			0.28	2	2	1.05	1		1.00			0.35			0.09			0.01							3	3	2.50
194	193			0.15	2	2	0.60			0.55			0.20			0.05			0.01							2	2	1.41
195	194			0.01			0.05			0.04			0.01			0.00			0.00									0.10
196	170			0.03			0.10			0.09			0.03			0.01			0.00									0.23
197	171			0.06			0.22			0.21			0.08			0.02			0.01									0.53
200,202	200,202			0.08	1		0.31	1		0.34			0.14			0.04			0.02							1	1	0.84
201	201			0.06			0.21			0.17			0.06			0.02			0.02							1	1	0.46
203	203			0.06			0.24			0.28			0.13			0.04			0.04									0.70
204.0	204.1,.9			0.02			0.10			0.12			0.06			0.02			0.00									0.30
204.1-4	204.0,5-7			0.13	1	1	0.48			0.45			0.17			0.05			0.05							1	1	1.16
204	204-207			0.16	1	1	0.58			0.57			0.23			0.07			0.07							1	1	1.46
TOTAL		7	7	6.07	29	29	24.43	19	17	25.24	7	7	9.99	3	3	2.84	1	1	0.37							59	57	62.87

O : All tumours
O' : Histologically confirmed
E : Expected

Table 3. Breast cancer in women in Finland by age at diagnosis of cervical cancer, stage and treatment

TIME SINCE DIAGNOSIS OF PRIMARY CERVICAL CANCER (IN YEARS)

INVASIVE — RADIOTHERAPY

Age	<1 O'	<1 :O	<1 E	1-4 :O	1-4 E	5-9 :O	5-9 E	10-14 :O	10-14 E	15-19 :O	15-19 E	20-24 :O	20-24 E	25-29 E	30+ E	Total :O	Total E
<30			0.00		0.00		0.00		0.1		0.10		0.00	0.00	0.00		0.00
30-39	1		0.20		0.80		1.40	1	1.40		0.90		0.30	0.00	0.00	2	4.80
40-49		4	1.20	7	3.90	2	4.30	1	3.10	1	2.00	1	0.70	0.00	0.00	17	14.00
50-59		1	1.80	7	5.10	2	4.90	1	3.40	1	1.60	1	0.40	0.00	0.00	12	15.40
60-69	1	5	1.60	2	4.00	1	2.80	1	1.40	1	0.50	1	0.10	0.00	0.00	10	8.80
70+		2	1.00	1	1.90		0.80		0.20		0.00		0.00	0.00	0.00	3	2.90

INVASIVE — NO THERAPY

Age	<1 :O	<1 E	1-4 :O	1-4 E	5-9 :O	5-9 E	10-14 :O	10-14 E	15-19 :O	15-19 E	20-24 :O	20-24 E	25-29 E	30+ E	Total :O	Total E
<30		0.00		0.00		0.00		0.00		0.00		0.00	0.00	0.00		0.00
30-39		0.00		0.20		0.30		0.20		0.10		0.00	0.00	0.00	1	0.80
40-49	2	0.20		0.80		0.80	1	0.40		0.20		0.10	0.00	0.00	3	2.30
50-59	2	0.20		0.60		0.50		0.30		0.10		0.00	0.00	0.00	2	1.50
60-69	1	0.10		0.30		0.20		0.10		0.00		0.00	0.00	0.00	1	0.60
70+	1	0.10		0.20		0.00		0.00		0.00		0.00	0.00	0.00		0.20

IN-SITU

Age	<1 :O	<1 E	1-4 :O	1-4 E	5-9 :O	5-9 E	10-14 :O	10-14 E	15-19 :O	15-19 E	20-24 E	25-29 E	30+ E	Total :O	Total E
<30		0.00		0.10		0.10		0.10		0.00	0.00	0.00	0.00		0.30
30-39		0.30		1.30		1.70		0.80		0.30	0.00	0.00	0.00	1	4.10
40-49	7	1.00	1	4.10	1	4.10	1	1.30		0.30	0.00	0.00	0.00	9	9.80
50-59	1	0.50	3	1.90	1	1.80	1	0.60	1	0.10	0.00	0.00	0.00	6	4.40
60-69		0.20		0.50		0.30	1	0.10		0.00	0.00	0.00	0.00	1	0.90
70+		0.00		0.10		0.00		0.00		0.00	0.00	0.00	0.00		0.10

O : All tumours
O': Histologically confirmed
E : Expected

The relative risks of developing a second primary cancer were estimated for irradiated patients and for non-irradiated patients as the ratio of observed to expected numbers of second primary cancers. The ratio of the relative risk for irradiated to the relative risk for non-irradiated patients was used as an indicator of the effect of radiation.

Results

Altogether, 351 multiple primary cancers were diagnosed in 345 patients among the 12 296 with cervical cancer or carcinoma *in situ*. The observed and expected numbers of cases are given in Table 2, according to year of follow-up and primary site for in-situ and invasive tumours and irradiated and non-irradiated cases. An additional breakdown by age was made for breast cancer cases only (Table 3). Six patients had a third primary cancer.

The relative risks (observed to expected ratios) of total cancer were close to unity and varied from 0.9 (in-situ, non-irradiated group) to 1.1 (invasive, irradiated and non-irradiated groups), indicating no major overall radiation hazard. There was also very little difference in relative risk between invasive and in-situ cases (Table 4) with regard to primary site. The only exception was genital cancer, which showed a higher effect of radiation in invasive than in in-situ cases. The invasive and in-situ groups were therefore pooled.

Table 4. Observed numbers (O) and relative risks (RR, observed/expected) of cancers at selected anatomical sites by extent of disease and treatment

| Anatomical | ICD7 code | Invasive | | | | | In-situ | | | | |
| | | Radiotherapy | | No radiotherapy | | Ratio of RRs | Radiotherapy | | No radiotherapy | | Ratio of RRs |
		O	RR	O	RR		O	RR	O	RR	
Stomach	151	31	1.1	2	0.9	1.3	3	1.3	4	0.8	1.7
Lung	162	32	4.1	2	2.5	1.6	2	2.5	3	1.3	1.9
Breast	170	44	1.0	7	1.3	0.8	6	1.1	17	0.9	1.2
Other genital	172-4,176	26	0.8	1	0.3	2.9	3	0.8	09	0.7	1.1
Other		111	1.1	13	1.4	0.8	09	0.9	26	1.0	0.9
All		244	1.1	25	1.1	1.0	23	1.0	59	0.9	1.1

The relative risks of total cancer showed a consistent increase with time since diagnosis of cervical cancer among the irradiated group, whereas the trend was more irregular in the non-irradiated group (Table 5).

Table 5. Observed numbers (O) and relative risks (RR, observed/expected) of total cancer by time between diagnosis of cervical cancer and the second primary, by treatment

| Treatment | Time since diagnosis of cervical cancer (years) | | | | | | | | | | | |
| | <1 | | 1-4 | | 5-9 | | 10-14 | | 15-19 | | 20+ | |
	O	RR	O	RR	O	RR	O	RR	O	RR	O	RR
Radiotherapy	21	0.7	75	1.0	77	1.0	64	1.3	36	1.4	15	2.0
No radiotherapy	9	0.9	41	1.2	25	0.7	9	0.6	8	1.6	1	1.1
All	30	0.8	116	1.0	102	1.0	73	1.1	44	1.4	1	1.1

The ratio of the relative risk of cancer in the irradiated group to the relative risk of cancer in the non-irradiated group was used as an indicator of the radiation effect (Table 6). Only selected primary sites with observed or expected numbers higher than 10 were considered. The highest ratios were found for cancers of the lung, thyroid gland and leukaemia. There was very little indication of any radiation effect on gastrointestinal and genital cancers.

Table 6. Observed numbers (O) and relative risks (RR, observed/expected) of cancer at selected anatomical sites, by treatment

Anatomical site	ICD7 code	Radiotherapy		No radiotherapy		Ratio of RRs
		O	RR	O	RR	
Stomach	151	34	1.1	6	0.8	1.4
Colon	153	16	1.2	7	1.8	0.7
Rectum	154	16	1.5	5	1.5	1.0
Pancreas	157	13	1.4	3	1.2	1.2
Lung	162	34	3.9	5	1.6	2.4
Breast	170	50	1.0	24	1.0	1.0
Corpus uteri	172	6	0.4	2	0.3	1.3
Ovary	175	12	0.8	5	0.7	1.1
Other genital	173-4, 176	11	2.3	3	1.9	1.3
Thyroid	194	7	1.8	2	1.1	1.7
Leukaemia	204	09	1.5	2	1.0	1.6
All sites		267	1.1	84	1.0	1.2

Discussion

An overall discussion of the limitations of the material and the implications of these results is given elsewhere in this monograph. Only aspects pertinent to the Finnish material are given here.

Distinguishing between a second primary cancer and a metastasis is an especially difficult problem at any cancer registry, where only limited cancer registry reports are available and when detailed medical records are not available. In Finland, coding, which requires medical expertise, is done by a pathologist, and hence such errors are minimized. Furthermore, it is unlikely that metastases would be classified as second primary cancers more often in irradiated patients than in non-irradiated patients.

Because patients with two or more primary cancers tend to be the most complicated cases in any cancer registry material, direct errors in coding, punching and other routine manoeuvres are more likely to occur in those cases than in cases with one primary tumour only. The material was corrected for obvious errors resulting from routine handling of the material.

The potential effect of radiation was very similar for cases of invasive cancer and cases of carcinoma *in situ*. The exception was cases of genital organ cancer, in which the risk from radiation seemed to be greater for invasive cases than for in-situ cases. This may be due to more frequent surgical removal of genital organs other than the cervix among invasive cases at the primary operation. In fact, all cases of corpus and ovarian cancer among the invasive cases with irradiation were in the subgroup that received radiation only.

The increase in the ratio of relative risk for the radiation group to relative risk for the non-irradiated females with follow-up time is consistent with the hypothesis that radiation is an etiological factor for second primary tumours. This indicator was greater than one and almost consistently less than two for a few anatomical sites only. Therefore, the number of tumours due to radiation appears to be relatively small.

Summary

All new cases of cervical cancer or carcinoma *in situ* diagnosed in Finland between 1953 and 1977 were followed up to 1977, and multiple primary cancers were recorded to evaluate the effect of radiation on the risk of subsequent cancer. Among the 12 296 patients, 345 second cancers and six third cancers were diagnosed. The numbers of observed cases were compared with those expected on the basis of incidence rates for the whole Finnish population. The relative risks were close to unity for invasive and in-situ cancers and for those subjected to radiation and other treatment. Among those irradiated, the relative risk increased from one to two by time since diagnosis of cervical cancer; nevertheless, the effect of radiation on the risk of subsequent cancers seemed to be relatively small, and only a small fraction of the multiple primary cancers can be ascribed to radiation.

References

Finnish Cancer Registry (1981) *Cancer Incidence in Finland 1977* (*Cancer Society of Finland Publication No. 28*), Helsinki

Hakama, M. (1982) *Trends in the incidence of cervical cancer in the Nordic countries.* In: Magnus, K., ed., *Trends in Cancer Incidence: Causes and Practical Implications*, New York, Hemisphere Publishing Corp., pp. 279-292

Hakulinen, T., Pukkala, E., Hakama, M., Lehtonen, M., Saxen, E. & Teppo, L. (1981) Survival of cancer patients in Finland in 1953-1974. *Ann. clin. Res., 13*, Supplement 31

Saxen, E., Hakama, M. & Lehtonen, M. (1969) Cancer in Finland 1964-1963. *Ann. clin. Res., 1*, 291-300

Teppo, L., Hakama, M., Hakulinen, T., Lehtonen, M. & Saxen, E. (1975) Cancer in Finland 1953-1970. Incidence, mortality, prevalence. *Acta pathol. microbiol. Scand., Section A*, Supplement 252

SECOND PRIMARY CANCERS AMONG CASES WITH INVASIVE CANCER OR CARCINOMA *IN SITU* OF THE CERVIX DIAGNOSED IN NORWAY BETWEEN 1953 AND 1969

K. Magnus, A. Andersen & J.E. Skjerven

The Cancer Registry of Norway
The Norwegian Radium Hospital
Oslo 3, Norway

The cancer registry

All new cases of cancer in Norway are subject to compulsory reporting, by hospital departments and institutes of pathology. In addition, general practitioners may be asked for information when cancer is mentioned on a death certificate. Reports are submitted whenever a new cancer patient is seen in hospital in-patient or out-patient departments and whenever a cancer patient is readmitted to hospital and there is a change in status.

The Cancer Registry data file is matched at regular intervals against all deaths registered in the files of the Central Bureau of Statistics to obtain an updated mortality follow-up. All reports on cancer patients are checked for completeness and classified by personal identification numbers.

Material

A total of 6069 new cases of invasive cervical cancer were diagnosed in Norway during the period 1953-1969, of which 81% had been treated in the Norwegian Radium Hospital. Second cancers were diagnosed in 49 of these patients before and in 14 patients within one month after diagnosis of the cervical cancer; these were excluded, leaving 6006 cases for follow-up. In the period 1953-1969, 2143 cases of carcinoma *in situ* were diagnosed. In this group, second cancers were diagnosed in six patients before and in seven patients within one month after the diagnosis; when these 13 were excluded, 2130 cases were left for follow-up.

Classification of cases

Invasive cancer: Invasive or microinvasive tumour

Cancer *in situ*: Intraepithelial atypia corresponding to the 4th digit 2 in the SNOP code.

Radiotherapy

Whenever radiological treatment was noted on a report, the patient was allocated to the radiotherapy group, irrespective of the dose and source of radiation.

The 'No radiotherapy' group includes all other patients.

Follow-up

Each patient was followed until 31 December 1978 or until death, whichever was earlier. If not reported dead, it was verified that the patient was alive at 31 December 1978.

Estimation of expected numbers

Estimation of expected numbers of second primary cancers was based on the continuous incidence rates for the whole country throughout the follow-up period. There are large regional as well as urban-rural differences in the incidence of cervical cancer in Norway, implying that for other types of cancer with obvious geographical variations in incidence, the estimated numbers are biased. This must be taken into consideration in interpreting the data.

Table 1. Norwegian Cancer Registry: Characteristics of the population under study

	Invasive tumours			*In situ* (no radiotherapy)	Total
	Radiotherapy	No radiotherapy	Total invasive		
Number of women	5 282	724	6 006	2 130	8 136
Woman-years at risk by time since diagnosis:					
<1 year	5 152.0	648.0	5 800.0	2 127.0	7 927.0
1-4 years	15 227.0	1 766.5	16 993.5	8 549.5	25 543.0
5-9 years	14 828.5	1 714.5	16 543.0	10 334.5	26 877.5
10-14 years	10 314.0	960.5	11 274.5	6 500.5	17 775.0
15-19 years	5 454.5	362.5	5 817.0	2 289.0	8 106.0
20-24 years	1 862.5	80.0	1 942.5	505.5	2 448.0
25-29 years	76.5	3.0	79.5	15.0	94.5
30+ years	-	-	-	-	-
All years	52 915.0	5 535.0	58 450.0	30 321.0	88 771.0
Number of women by age at diagnosis:					
<35	377	83	460	465	925
35-44	1 369	214	1 583	920	2 503
45-54	1 488	177	1 665	568	2 233
55-64	1 164	79	1 243	126	1 369
65-74	653	84	737	43	780
75+	231	87	318	8	326
Number of women excluded because of:					
- malignancy prior to diagnosis of cervical cancer	48	1	49	6	55
- second cancer (excluding non-melanoma skin) diagnosed simultaneously with cervical cancer	11	3	14	7	21

Table 2. Observed and expected numbers of second primary cancers in women diagnosed with primary cervical cancer in Norway

A. Cases of invasive cervical cancer treated by radiotherapy

TIME SINCE DIAGNOSIS OF PRIMARY CERVICAL CANCER (IN YEARS)

		<1 (5282)			1-4 (5094)			5-9 (3168)			10-14 (2531)			15-19 (1415)			20-24 (621)			25-29 (79)			30+			Total (excl. <1)		
ICD7	ICD8	O	O'	E	O	O'	E	O	O'	E	O	O'	E	O	O'	E	O	O'	E	O	O'	E	O	O'	E	O	O'	E
140	140			0.01			0.06			0.08			0.07			0.05			0.02			0.00						0.28
141	141			0.03			0.17	1		0.19	1	1	0.16	1	1	0.10			0.04			0.00				1	1	0.66
142	142			0.02			0.16			0.17	1	1	0.13			0.07			0.03			0.00				1	1	0.56
143-4	143-5	1	1	0.03	1	1	0.18	1	1	0.26	1	1	0.21	1	1	0.13			0.05			0.00				4	4	0.88
145,7-8	146,8-9			0.02	4	4	0.18	1	1	0.19	1	1	0.14	1	1	0.07			0.03			0.00				4	4	0.61
146	147			0.01			0.07			0.07			0.06			0.03			0.01			0.00						0.24
150	150			0.05	1	1	0.32	2	2	0.38	1	1	0.32			0.20			0.09			0.00				4	4	1.31
151	151			1.05	8	8	6.46	12	11	6.24	8	6	4.54	3	2	2.63	1	1	0.99			0.05				32	24	20.91
152	152			0.02			0.16	1	1	0.21	1	1	0.21			0.11			0.04			0.00				1	1	0.70
153	153	1	1	0.68	5	3	4.70	11	10	6.10	7	6	5.46	5	5	3.60	2	2	1.55			0.08				30	26	21.49
154	154	1	1	0.29	2	2	2.06	2	2	2.72	5	5	2.53	4	4	1.69	1	1	0.73			0.04				14	14	9.77
155.0	155																											
155.1	156			0.13	1	1	0.87	1	1	1.00	2	2	0.84	3	1	0.54			0.22			0.01				8	3	3.48
157	157			0.24	1	1	1.66			2.13	2	2	1.86		1	1.24			0.51			0.02	3	3	7.42
160	160			0.03			0.17	1	1	0.18	2	2	0.14			0.09	1	1	0.03			0.00	2	2	0.61
161	161			0.01			0.06			0.08			0.08			0.05			0.02			0.00	1	1	0.29
162-3	162-3			0.20	5	4	1.43	8	6	2.00	3	2	1.85	4	3	1.20			0.48			0.02	20	15	6.98
170	174	3	3	2.46	12	12	16.37	14	14	18.95	10	9	15.03	6	6	8.76	1	1	3.28			0.15	43	42	62.54
172	182.0			0.51			3.56	3	3	4.50	6	6	3.81	1	1	2.27	1	1	3.83			0.04	11	11	15.01
173-4	181,2.9			0.03			0.23			0.19			0.11			0.05			0.02			0.00				0.60
175	183	2	2	0.70	4	4	4.71	2	2	5.47	1	1	4.37	2	2	2.49	2	2	0.89			0.04	11	11	17.97
176	184			0.13	3	2	0.82	3	3	0.93	6	6	0.77	1	1	0.51	1	1	0.21			0.01	14	13	3.25
180	189.0-1	1	1	0.22	2	2	1.45	1	1	1.74			1.48	1	1	0.94	2	2	0.38			0.02	4	18	6.01
181	188	1	1	0.14	2	2	1.00	2	2	1.42	1	1	1.34	6	6	0.96	5	5	0.41			0.02	20	2	5.15
190	172			0.16			1.21	1	1	1.70	1	1	1.49			0.89			0.36			0.02	2	2	5.67
191	173																								
192	190			0.03	1	1	0.21	3	3	0.23			0.18	1	1	0.10	1	1	0.04			0.00	1	1	0.76
193	191-2			0.16	1	1	0.99	3	2	1.04			0.79	1	1	0.45			0.17	1	1	0.01	5	5	3.45
194	193	1		0.13	3	3	0.88	2		1.06			0.86			0.51			0.18			0.01	5	5	3.50
195	194			0.01			0.06			0.09			0.05			0.03			0.01			0.00				0.21
196	170	1	1	0.01			0.08			0.38	1		0.07			0.04			0.02			0.00	1	1	0.30
197	171			0.04			0.29	2	2	1.32			0.32			0.21			0.08			0.00	2	2	1.28
200,202	200,202	2	2	0.15	2	2	1.01			0.45	2	2	1.16	1	1	0.74			0.31			0.02	5	5	4.56
201	201	2	1	0.07	2	1	0.42	2	2	1.07	2	2	0.34	1	1	0.18			0.07				5	2	1.46
203	203			0.11	1	1	0.80	2	2	0.44	2	2	0.92	2	2	0.59			0.22	1		0.01	4	4	3.61
204.0	204.1,.9	1	1	0.06			0.36	2	2	1.25	1	1	0.36			0.24			0.10				3	3	1.50
204.1-4	204.0,5-7	1	1	0.18			1.16	2	2	1.69	2	2	1.00			0.61			0.24			0.01	3	3	4.27
204	204-207	1	1	0.24			1.52				3	3	1.36	2	2	0.85			0.34			0.01	7	7	5.77
TOTAL		8	8	8.12	57	47	54.37	78	71	64.29	68	62	53.02	44	40	32.37	15	15	12.66	1	1	0.58				263	236	217.29

O : All tumours
O': Histologically confirmed
E : Expected

B. Cases of invasive cervical cancer not treated by radiotherapy

TIME SINCE DIAGNOSIS OF PRIMARY CERVICAL CANCER (IN YEARS)

		<1 (724)			1–4 (572)			5–9 (368)			10–14 (271)			15–19 (105)			20–24 (27)			25–29 (3)			30+			Total (excl. <1)		
ICD7	ICD8	O	O'	E	O	O'	E	O	O'	E	O	O'	E	O	O'	E	O	O'	E	O	O'	E	O	O'	E	O	O'	E
140	140			0.00			0.01			0.01			0.01						0.00			0.00						0.03
141	141			0.00			0.01			0.01			0.01						0.00			0.00						0.03
142	142			0.00			0.01			0.02			0.01						0.00			0.00						0.04
143-4	143-5			0.00			0.02			0.02			0.01						0.00			0.00						0.05
145,7-8	146,8-9			0.00			0.01			0.01			0.00						0.00			0.00						0.04
146	147			0.00			0.01			0.01			0.00						0.00			0.00						0.02
150	150			0.09		1	0.02		1	0.03			0.02			0.01			0.01			0.00				1	1	0.08
151	151			0.09			0.47			0.43	1	1	0.27			0.00			0.03			0.00				1	1	1.32
152	152			0.00			0.02			0.02			0.01			0.00			0.00								1	0.06
153	153			0.06			0.39			0.52			0.41			0.18			0.05			0.00					1	1.55
154	154			0.02			0.17			0.24	1	1	0.20			0.09			0.03							1	1	0.73
155.0	155			0.01			0.06			0.07			0.05			0.02			0.01			0.00						0.21
155.1	156			0.02			0.12			0.17			0.13			0.06			0.02			0.00				2	2	0.50
157	157			0.00		1	0.01		1	0.02			0.01			0.00			0.00			0.00						0.04
160	160			0.00			0.01			0.01			0.01			0.00			0.00			0.00						0.03
161	161			0.02																								0.03
162-3	162-3			0.24	2	1	0.13	2		0.20			0.16	1	1	0.07			0.02			0.01				3	3	0.58
170	174			0.04	2	1	1.64		2	2.00	1	1	1.32	1	1	0.55			0.13			0.04				3	5	5.65
172	182.0			0.00			0.34			0.48			0.35			0.15			0.04			0.00				1	1	1.36
173-4	181,2.9			0.06		1	0.01			0.01			0.00	1	1	0.00			0.00			0.00				2	1	0.02
175	183	1	1	0.01			0.46	2	1	0.58			0.38			0.16			0.16			0.00				2	1	1.62
176	184			0.02			0.07			0.08			0.06			0.00			0.00			0.01				1	1	0.25
180	189.0-.1	1	1	0.01		1	0.12		1	0.15			0.11			0.03			0.01			0.01				1		0.44
181	188			0.02			0.08			0.12			0.10			0.05			0.01			0.01				1		0.36
190	172			0.00			0.16	1	1	0.23			0.16			0.07			0.02			0.02				1	1	0.64
191	173																											
192	190			0.01		1	0.02			0.02			0.02			0.01			0.00			0.00					1	0.07
193	191-2			0.00			0.10			0.11			0.07	1		0.03			0.01			0.01					1	0.32
194	193			0.00			0.09			0.12			0.08			0.03			0.03			0.00						0.33
195	194			0.00			0.01			0.01			0.00			0.00			0.00			0.00						0.02
196	170			0.01			0.01			0.01			0.01			0.00			0.00			0.00						0.03
197	171			0.01			0.03	1		0.04			0.03			0.01			0.01			0.00				1		0.11
200,202	200,202			0.00			0.09			0.12			0.09			0.04			0.04			0.01						0.35
201	201			0.01			0.04			0.04			0.03			0.01			0.01									0.12
203	203			0.00			0.06			0.09			0.06			0.03			0.03									0.25
204.0	204.1.,9			0.02			0.03			0.03			0.02			0.01			0.01			0.01						0.09
204.1-4	204.0,5-7			0.02	1	1	0.10			0.11			0.07			0.03			0.01			0.01				1	1	0.32
204	204-207				1	1	0.13			0.14			0.09			0.04			0.01			0.01				1	1	0.41
TOTAL		2	2	0.70	7	7	4.93	8	7	6.15	4	3	4.28	4	4	1.82			0.47			0.01				23	21	17.66

O : All tumours
O': Histologically confirmed
E : Expected

C. Cases of carcinoma in situ not treated by radiotherapy

TIME SINCE DIAGNOSIS OF PRIMARY CERVICAL CANCER (IN YEARS)

ICD7	ICD8	<1 O	<1 O'	<1 E	1-4 O	1-4 O'	1-4 E	5-9 O	5-9 O'	5-9 E	10-14 O	10-14 O'	10-14 E	15-19 O	15-19 O'	15-19 E	20-24 O	20-24 O'	20-24 E	25-29 O	25-29 O'	25-29 E	30+ O	30+ O'	30+ E	Total O	Total O'	Total E
	Number of women starting intervals		2130			2128			2079			1747			722			175			15							
140	140			0.00			0.02			0.03			0.03			0.01			0.00			0.00						0.09
141	141			0.00			0.04			0.06			0.05			0.03			0.01			0.00						0.19
142	142			0.01			0.06			0.08			0.05			0.02			0.01			0.01						0.22
143-4	143-5			0.00			0.05			0.09			0.08			0.03			0.01			0.01						0.26
145,7-8	146,8-9			0.00			0.04			0.07	1	1	0.07	1	1	0.02			0.00			0.00				2	2	0.20
146	147			0.00			0.02			0.03	3	3	0.03			0.01			0.02			0.00				1	1	0.09
150	150			0.01			0.05	1		0.09	3	3	0.10			0.05	1	1	0.02			0.01				4	3	0.31
151	151			0.14			1.19			1.78			1.44			0.68			0.20			0.01						5.30
152	152			0.00			0.05			0.09			0.08			0.04			0.01									0.27
153	153			0.12	1	1	1.21	2	2	2.34	2	2	2.24	1	1	1.13			0.35			0.01				6	6	7.28
154	154			0.05			0.53	1		1.09			1.12			0.58	1	1	0.18			0.01				2	1	3.51
155.0	155																											
155.1	156			0.02			0.17			0.30	2		0.28	1	1	0.14			0.05			0.00				1	1	0.94
157	157			0.03			0.35			0.69	1	1	0.67	1	1	0.35			0.11			0.00				5	1	2.17
160	160			0.00			0.04			0.07			0.06	1		0.03			0.01			0.00				1		0.21
161	161			0.00			0.03			0.04			0.03			0.02			0.00			0.00						0.12
162-3	162-3	1	1	0.04	4	4	0.46	2	2	0.98	3	2	0.97	5	5	0.46	1	1	0.13			0.00				10	9	3.00
170	174	1	1	0.74	8	8	6.85	10	10	10.87	15	15	8.47	5	5	3.45	1	1	0.85			0.03				38	38	30.52
172	182.0			0.13	1	1	1.34			2.56	2	1	2.30			0.97			0.23			0.01				3	2	7.41
173-4	181,2,9			0.00			0.05			0.05			0.04			0.01			0.00									0.15
175	183			0.20	3	3	1.89	4	4	3.14	2	2	2.50	2	2	1.02	1	1	0.25			0.01				12	12	8.81
176	184			0.02			0.20	1	1	0.34	2	2	0.32			0.16			0.05			0.00				3	3	1.07
180	189.0-1			0.04			0.37	1	1	0.71	1	1	0.67			0.32			0.09			0.00				3	3	2.16
181	188			0.02			0.20	1	1	0.48	1		0.51			0.28			0.09			0.00				1	1	1.56
190	172			0.08			0.78	1	1	1.42	1	1	1.11			0.42			0.10			0.00				3	3	3.83
191	173																											
192	190			0.01	1	1	0.07	1	1	0.12	1	1	0.10			0.04			0.01			0.00				1	1	0.34
193	191-2			0.05	2	2	0.43	1	1	0.63	1	1	0.49	1	1	0.20			0.05			0.00				2	2	1.80
194	193			0.04	2	2	0.42	1	1	0.70	1	1	0.52			0.20			0.05			0.00				5	5	1.89
195	194			0.00			0.02			0.04			0.02			0.01			0.00			0.00						0.09
196	170			0.00			0.03			0.05			0.03			0.01			0.00			0.00						0.12
197	171			0.01	1	1	0.12	1		0.20	1		0.16			0.07	1	1	0.08			0.00				1	1	0.57
200,202	200,202			0.04	1	1	0.34			0.61			0.55			0.26	1	1	0.08			0.00				2	2	1.84
201	201			0.03			0.19			0.25			0.17			0.07			0.02									0.70
203	203			0.02			0.18			0.36			0.34			0.17			0.05			0.00						1.10
204.0	204.1,.9			0.01			0.07			0.13			0.12			0.06			0.02		0.00						0.40
204.1-4	204.0,5-7			0.04	1	1	0.36	1	1	0.51	1	1	0.39			0.18			0.05							3	3	1.49
204	204-207			0.05	1	1	0.43	1	1	0.64	1	1	0.51			0.24			0.07		0.00				3	3	1.89
TOTAL		2	2	1.90	25	23	18.22	25	23	31.00	38	35	26.11	13	12	11.50	6	6	3.10			0.08				107	99	90.01

O : All tumours
O': Histologically confirmed
E : Expected

Table 3. Breast cancer in women in Norway by age at diagnosis of cervical cancer, stage and treatment

TIME SINCE DIAGNOSIS OF PRIMARY CERVICAL CANCER (IN YEARS)

INVASIVE — RADIOTHERAPY

Age	<1 O	<1 O'	<1 E	1-4 O	1-4 O'	1-4 E	5-9 O	5-9 O'	5-9 E	10-14 O	10-14 O'	10-14 E	15-19 O	15-19 O'	15-19 E	20-24 O	20-24 O'	20-24 E	25-29 O	25-29 O'	25-29 E	30+ O	30+ O'	30+ E	Total O	Total O'	Total E
<30						0.02			0.07			0.11			0.13			0.10			0.00			0.00			0.43
30-39			0.11			1.25	1	1	2.42	1	1	2.86			2.15			0.93			0.04			0.00	2	2	9.65
40-49	1	1	0.68	1	1	4.81	4	4	6.09	2	2	5.18	1	1	3.10			1.23			0.07			0.00	8	8	20.48
50-59			0.65	4	4	4.57	7	7	5.35	3	3	4.10	2	2	2.29	1	1	0.80			0.03			0.00	17	17	17.14
60-69	2	2	0.63	3	3	3.67	3	3	3.70	2	2	2.31	2	2	0.97			0.21			0.01			0.00	10	10	10.87
70+			0.37	4	4	2.04	1		1.32	1	1	0.48			0.11			0.01			0.00			0.00	6	5	3.96

INVASIVE — NO RADIOTHERAPY

Age	<1 O	<1 O'	<1 E	1-4 O	1-4 O'	1-4 E	5-9 O	5-9 O'	5-9 E	10-14 O	10-14 O'	10-14 E	15-19 O	15-19 O'	15-19 E	20-24 O	20-24 O'	20-24 E	25-29 O	25-29 O'	25-29 E	30+ O	30+ O'	30+ E	Total O	Total O'	Total E
<30			0.00			0.00			0.01			0.02			0.01			0.00			0.00			0.00			0.04
30-39			0.02			0.22			0.40			0.37			0.24			0.06			0.00			0.00			1.29
40-49			0.10			0.67	1	1	0.82			0.53			0.17			0.05			0.00			0.00	1	1	2.24
50-59	1	1	0.06	1	1	0.42	1	1	0.48	1	1	0.26			0.10			0.02			0.00			0.00	3	3	1.28
60-69			0.03			0.19			0.22	1	1	0.12			0.04			0.00			0.00			0.00	1	1	0.57
70+			0.04			0.13			0.06			0.01			0.00			0.00			0.00			0.00			0.20

IN-SITU

Age	<1 O	<1 O'	<1 E	1-4 O	1-4 O'	1-4 E	5-9 O	5-9 O'	5-9 E	10-14 O	10-14 O'	10-14 E	15-19 O	15-19 O'	15-19 E	20-24 O	20-24 O'	20-24 E	25-29 O	25-29 O'	25-29 E	30+ O	30+ O'	30+ E	Total O	Total O'	Total E
<30						0.05	1	1	0.19				1	1	0.21			0.07			0.00			0.00	2	2	0.66
30-39			0.10	1	1	1.38	2	2	2.99	7	7	2.71	1	1	1.15			0.25			0.00			0.00	12	12	8.48
40-49	1	1	0.41	5	5	3.62	5	5	5.22	5	5	3.89	2	2	1.60			0.39			0.02			0.00	16	16	14.74
50-59			0.16	2	2	1.25	2	2	1.77	3	3	1.28	1	1	0.44			0.13			0.00			0.00	8	8	4.87
60-69			0.04			0.38			0.51			0.28			0.10			0.01			0.00			0.00			1.28
70+			0.02			0.16			0.17			0.09			0.02			0.00			0.00			0.00			0.44

O : All tumours
O': Histologically confirmed
E : Expected

SECOND PRIMARY CANCERS AFTER TREATMENT FOR CERVICAL CANCER A STUDY OF 58 731 SWEDISH WOMEN WITH INVASIVE OR IN-SITU CANCER

B. Malker & F. Pettersson

The Cancer Registry
National Board of Health and Welfare
106 30 Stockholm, Sweden

Introduction

This study is based on data obtained from the Swedish Cancer Registry, which was initiated in 1958. The Swedish Medical Statute 1968:1 stipulates that doctors working in hospitals or in any other publicly controlled establishment for the care of the sick in Sweden must report all cases of diagnosed cancer to the Cancer Registry. In addition, pathologists and cytologists must report separately to the Registry all diagnoses of cancer made on the basis of examinations of surgically removed organs, biopsies, cytological specimens or at autopsy.

Information on dates and causes of death is obtained from death certificates at the National Central Bureau of Statistics. Cancer diagnoses notified only from death certificates, however, are not accepted by the Cancer Registry.

For this study of the incidence of second primary cancer following cancer of the cervix uteri, death certificates up to 1 January 1977 were checked against the files at the Cancer Registry. Cancer patients not certified as dead were assumed to be alive at the end of the study period. Emigration from Sweden and incorrectly noted personal identification numbers may have led to some overestimation of the calculated person-years at risk. The extent of this uncertainty in follow-up is assessed as about 5%.

Patient series

In the period 1958 through 1976, 14 760 new cases of invasive cervical cancer were reported to the Swedish Cancer Registry; in the same period 43 971 cases of carcinoma *in situ* were registered.

The annual notifications of carcinoma *in situ* to the Registry increased during the study period from some 200 to about 4000 in 1976. The incidence of invasive cervical carcinoma rose slightly up to 1965, but thereafter decreased by about 5% annually. In 1960, approximately 20 cases of invasive cervical carcinoma per 100 000 mean female population were reported to the Registry, i.e., about 850 cases.

The cohort of women with cervical carcinoma diagnosed in the period 1958 through 1976 was followed up from the date of diagnosis until January 1977. The maximum period of observation was thus 19 years.

The age distribution of patients with invasive and in-situ cancer is displayed in Table 1. As expected, women with in-situ cancer are younger than the patients with invasive tumour.

A total of 1074 cases were excluded from the series studied, due to previous other malignancy (604 women), incomplete personal identification number (367 women), or simultaneously diagnosed other cancer (103 women).

Table 1. Swedish Cancer Registry: Characteristics of the population under study

	Invasive tumours			*In situe* (no radiotherapy)	Total
	Radiotherapy	No radiotherapy	Total invasive		
Number of women			14 760	43 971	58 371
Woman-years at risk by time since diagnosis:					
<1 year			13 299.9	41 820.6	55 120.5
1-4 years			35 860.8	131 558.6	167 419.4
5-9 years			27 562.3	75 866.8	103 429.1
10-14 years			13 173.4	12 991.9	26 165.3
15+ years			2 934.4	1 432.2	4 366.6
All years			92 830.9	263 670.1	356 500.9
Number of women by age at diagnosis:					
<35			1 364	23 036	24 400
35-44			3 649	12 800	16 449
45-54			4 046	6 210	10 256
55-64			3 050	1 397	4 447
65-74			1 798	434	2 232
75+			853	94	947
Number of women excluded because of:					
- malignancy prior to diagnosis of cervical cancer			237	367	604
- second cancer (excluding non-melanoma skin) diagnosed simultaneously with cervical cancer			59	44	103
- other causes, incomplete identification			121	246	367

Treatment and follow-up of cervical cancer in Sweden

Treatment and follow-up of invasive carcinoma of the cervix uteri in Sweden are centralized in seven regional hospitals. The approximate populations they serve range from 700 000 to 1 600 000. (The total population of Sweden is about eight million.) In the early years of the study, however, there were only five centres for the treatment of cervical cancer.

Follow-up of patients treated for carcinoma of the cervix uteri, by examinations at regular intervals by specialists in gynaecological oncology, is usually continued for ten years, but longer observation times are not uncommon. When this active phase of follow-up is discontinued, information on the patient's health is obtained from correspondence with her, with her local doctor, or *via* civic registers. When a patient dies, records (including autopsy reports) are requested from the hospital she last attended. Cancer Registry follow-up comprises only records of deaths and notifications of new primary tumours.

Treatment techniques used in Swedish regional hospitals

The original 'Stockholm method' for treating cancer of the uterine cervix has been adopted throughout Sweden, with a few modifications. In our study period (1958 through 1976), primary treatment consisted of a combination of intracavitary radium and external X-ray or telecobalt therapy to the parametrium. Towards the end of the period, betatron X-ray and linear accelerators were introduced. In most cases of Stage I or Stage II cancer the radium treatment was divided into two applications with an interval of three weeks. Each dose consisted of 53-88 mg radium distributed homogeneously in an intrauterine applicator with an active length of 44-60 mm, filter 3 mm Pb. Vaginal applications of radium were placed as near the tumour as possible but were spread over a larger surface, 60-90 mg of radium being introduced into the vagina. The application time varied from case to case (20-30 hours), taking into consideration many factors. The dose in the bladder and in the rectum served as a basis for estimating application time.

Since 1963, radical hysterectomy using a modified Wertheim technique was performed in many cases of Stage Ib and IIa, about four weeks after the last radium treatment. External irradiation was given only when histological examination revealed a malignant tumour in the parametrium or in the lymph nodes. In relatively advanced cases, irradiation was begun with cobalt[60] or with a linear accelerator. A therapy plan for each individual patient was evolved in collaboration with the centre's physicists.

The great majority of Stage III and Stage IV tumours were treated by external irradiation through one anterior and two lateral portals. In the latter part of the study period, radiation was given with two opposite beams by means of accelerators, to give a dose of 4500-5000 rads over a period of five to six weeks. Following external irradiation, radium or caesium was introduced into the uterine cavity and the vagina. As a rule, these patients also received one intracavitary irradiation. Finally, additional irradiation was given to residual tumour tissue on the pelvic wall. Electrofulguration was performed on radioresistant and recurrent tumours.

These programmes are by and large standard practice at all Swedish treatment centres.

Management of carcinoma in situ

Treatment of non-invasive cervical cancer in Sweden is less centralized and is conducted at departments of gynaecology throughout the country. Conization is the usual procedure. Hysterectomy is carried out in relatively few cases, and intracavitary radium is seldom given. Follow-up is supervised by the patient's gynaecologist, and the intensity of surveillance may therefore vary widely.

Changes in stage distribution of invasive cervical carcinoma

The rapid extension of gynaecological services in Sweden and the advent of screening programmes for cervical cancer led to an appreciable shift in the distribution of cancer stages during the study period. The numbers of Stage I tumours thus rose from about 20% to 40%, while Stages II and III showed a decreasing trend. Stage IV cases showed little numerical change (Fig. 1). This altered stage distribution obviously influenced treatment, since the increase in the number of localized tumours reduced the need for massive doses of radiation.

Figure 1. Distribution by stage for cases of carcinoma of the cervix
treated at Radiumhemmet, Stockholm, 1914-1973

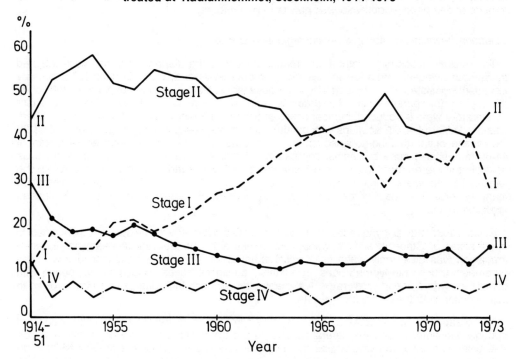

Second primary cancers

Only tumours appearing one month or more after the cervical cancer was diagnosed were classified as second primary cancers. 'Synchronous' malignancies - 59 in patients with invasive cervical cancer and 44 with cancer *in situ* were therefore excluded from this classification.

Since the study was based solely on information available to the Cancer Registry, no estimate can at present be given of the extent of errors in case reporting or coding. A modified version of ICD7 is used for coding at the Cancer Registry. Thus, myelofibrosis, but not polycythaemia rubra vera, is included in the leukaemia group; mycosis fungoides is classed with lymphosarcoma. Since 1975, the leukaemias (204) have been coded in accordance with ICD8.

Expected numbers

The expected numbers of new primary cancers among the cohort were calculated on the basis of five-year age and five-year calendar-year incidence rates for each site of notification to the Cancer Registry. Whether such notifications concerned a first, second or subsequent tumour was not taken into account.

Results

The number of women observed for at least one year after treatment for invasive carcinoma of the cervix uteri was 12 075, and the woman-years at risk contributed by these patients totalled 79 531. A second primary tumour had been notified to the Cancer Registry in 464 cases, with histological confirmation in 413. The expected number of tumours was 397.8. Carcinomas of the rectum, bladder, bronchus and trachea were found in numbers exceeding that expected, even when only histologically confirmed cases were taken into account. When tumours without histological confirmation were included in the calculations, pancreatic cancers also exceeded the expected number. For cancers of the breast, corpus uteri and ovaries, however, there was a deficit. The number of leukaemias, all of which are considered to be histologically confirmed, was higher than could have been expected. Excess numbers of kidney and of bladder tumours were observed within the first four years after treatment.

Among the 40 640 women with in-situ cervical carcinoma who were observed for at least one year, and who contributed 221 850 woman-years at risk, 530 second primary tumours were registered and histologically confirmed. The expected number was 512.7. Excess numbers were found of cancers of the pharynx, rectum, pancreas, trachea and bronchus and urinary bladder, and also of leukaemia. There was a deficit of breast cancer among women treated for in-situ cervical cancer.

The numbers of breast cancers occurring in the population of women treated for invasive cervical cancer are analysed in Table 3 with respect to age at treatment for cervical cancer and interval between this treatment and detection of breast cancer. Altogether, 92 breast cancers were observed, whereas 116 were expected. In women up to the age of 49, there were 37 cases observed (33 histologically confirmed) but 54.2 expected; in women aged 50 or more, the corresponding figures were 55 (48) and 61.9.

Table 2. Observed and expected numbers of second primary cancers in women diagnosed with primary cervical cancer in Sweden

A. Cases of invasive cervical cancer treated by radiotherapy

TIME SINCE DIAGNOSIS OF PRIMARY CERVICAL CANCER (IN YEARS)

		<1 (14760)			1-4 (12075)			5-9 (7066)			10-14 (4033)			15-19 (1491)			20-24			25-29			30+			Total (exel. <1)		
ICD7	ICD8	O	O'	E	O	O'	E	O	O'	E	O	O'	E	O	O'	E	O	O'	E	O	O'	E	O	O'	E	O	O'	E
140	140		1	0.07			0.19			0.16			0.10			0.03												1	0.48
141	141		1	0.13			0.34			0.30			0.18			0.05												1	0.87
142	142			0.19			0.52			0.45			0.24			0.06										2	2	1.27
143-4	143-5	1	1	0.19	1	1	0.50	1	1	0.45			0.27			0.07										3	3	1.29
145,7-8	146,8-9			0.17	1	1	0.46	2	2	0.38			0.22			0.06										3	3	1.12
146	147			0.09			0.24			0.20			0.11			0.03										1	1	0.58
150	150			0.33			0.86	10	9	0.74	1	1	0.44			0.12										2	2	2.16
151	151	2	2	3.52			8.98	9	9	7.41			4.19	3	3	1.09										22	19	21.67
152	152	1	1	0.24			0.68			0.63			0.38	1	1	0.10										2	2	1.79
153	153	5	4	4.45	12	11	12.00	14	12	10.81	7	7	6.58	1	1	1.80										34	31	31.19
154	154	3	3	2.18	9	9	5.96	9	9	5.37	9	9	3.23	1	1	0.88										28	28	15.44
155.0	155			0.42			1.17	4	4	1.13	3	2	0.75			0.23										4	3	3.28
155.1	156	1	1	1.07	3	3	2.85	5	1	2.55			1.53			0.42										8	8	7.35
157	157	1	1	1.71	9	6	4.65	5	1	4.34	5	4	2.74	1		0.79										19	12	12.52
160	160			0.12			0.32	1	1	0.26			0.15			0.04										1	1	0.77
161	161			0.07			0.21	1	1	0.20			0.13			0.03										1	1	0.57
162-3	162-3	14	12	16.43	29	26	4.65	25	23	4.47	5	3	2.81	3	3	0.78										62	55	12.71
170	174	8	8	4.04	33	31	46.61	35	30	41.22	21	19	22.69	3	2	5.59										92	82	116.11
172	182,0			0.67	3	3	11.67	7	7	10.66	5	5	6.07	1	1	1.52										16	16	29.92
173-4	181,2,9	9	8	4.63	3	3	1.82	7	1	1.48	1	1	0.73			0.16										9	8	4.19
175	183	5	5	0.62	6	6	13.14	7	7	11.61	10	9	6.43	3	2	1.57										26	24	32.75
176	184	9	9	1.77	9	7	1.64	3	3	1.39	1	1	0.78			0.20										13	11	4.01
180	189,0-1	2	1	1.24	9	9	4.95	5	5	4.57	1	1	2.72	2	2	0.73										17	17	12.97
181	188			1.16	11	10	3.43	3	3	3.22	8	6	2.04	2	1	0.57										23	20	9.26
190	172			0.92	4	4	3.46	3	3	3.16	1	1	1.76	1	1	0.43										9	9	8.81
191	173			0.21	7	7	2.42	2	2	2.23			1.43			0.41										9	9	6.49
192	190			2.19			0.57			0.48			0.25			0.06												1.36
193	191-2	1	1	0.88	9	9	6.15	3	3	5.33	1	1	2.91			0.71										13	13	15.10
194	193			0.91	2	2	2.46	4	4	2.12	1		1.15			0.29										7	6	6.02
195	194	1	1	0.12	2	2	2.81	5	5	2.90	2	2	1.86			0.49										9	8	8.06
196	170			0.40			0.32			0.26	1	1	0.14			0.03										2	1	0.75
197	171	1	1	1.05	1	1	1.07	2	2	0.92	1	1	0.52			0.13										4	3	2.64
200,202	200,202			0.41	2	1	2.93	2	2	2.71	5	4	1.65			0.45										9	7	7.74
201	201			0.71	1	1	1.08	1	1	0.89			0.49			0.12										2	2	2.58
203	203			0.42	1	1	1.96			1.83			1.16			0.32										5	7	5.27
204,0	204,1,9	2	2	0.88	4	4	1.10	3	3	0.97	1		0.58			0.16										1	1	2.81
204,1-4	204,0,5-7	2	1	1.29	9	4	2.40	3	3	2.06			1.17			0.30										13	7	5.93
204	204-207				10	5	3.50	3	3	3.04	1		1.75			0.45										14	8	8.74
TOTAL		67	61	56.24	185	164	156.57	160	145	139.87	98	85	80.58	21	19	20.81										464	413	397.83

0 : All tumours
0': Histologically confirmed
E : Expected

B. Cases of invasive cervical cancer not treated by radiotherapy

TIME SINCE DIAGNOSIS OF PRIMARY CERVICAL CANCER (IN YEARS)

Number of women starting intervals		<1 43971			1-4 40640			5-9 25243			10-14 6448			15-19 843			20-24			25-29			30+			Total (excl. <1)		
ICD7	ICD8	O	O'	E	O	O'	E	O	O'	E	O	O'	E	O	O'	E	O	O'	E	O	O'	E	O	O'	E	O	O'	E
140	140	1	1	0.06			0.22			0.18			0.05			0.01											0.46
141	141	1	1	0.09			0.34	1		0.28			0.08			0.01									1	1	0.71
142	142			0.28			1.00	1		0.71			0.16			0.02											1.89
143-4	143-5			0.16	2		0.62			0.53	1	1	0.15			0.02									2	1	1.32
145,7-8	146,8-9	1		0.12	1	1	0.48	4	4	0.44			0.13			0.02									5	5	1.07
146	147			0.08			0.29	1	1	0.23			0.06			0.01									2	2	0.59
150	150			0.16			0.63			0.55			0.17			0.03											1.38
151	151	4	1	2.05	6	5	7.87	5	5	6.50	4	4	1.85	1		0.30									16	15	16.52
152	152	1		0.22			0.89	1	1	0.74			0.20			0.03									1	1	1.86
153	153	2	2	3.44	20	20	13.54	9	9	11.65	4	4	3.40	2	2	0.55									31	31	29.14
154	154	1		1.63	8	8	6.65	11	11	6.02			1.78	1	1	0.28									24	24	14.73
155.0	155			0.30			1.25	2	2	1.14			0.34			0.06									2	2	2.79
155.1	156			0.53			2.19	1	1	2.08			0.65			0.11									2	2	5.03
157	157	1		0.97	8	7	4.16	5	5	3.99	1	1	1.28	2	2	0.23									16	15	9.66
160	160			0.10	1		0.36			0.28			0.09			0.01									1	1	0.74
161	161			0.10	1	1	0.42			0.37			0.10			0.01									1	1	0.91
162-3	162-3	2	2	1.42	11	11	6.16	11	11	5.91	6	6	1.75	1	1	0.27									31	29	14.09
170	174	10	9	20.96	83	80	84.90	62	57	71.56	14	14	17.45	3	3	2.28									162	154	176.19
172	182.0	5	5	4.02	12	12	17.50	17	17	16.56	5	5	4.71			0.64									34	34	39.41
173-4	181,2.9	1		0.93	2	2	3.50	3	3	2.67	1	1	0.60			0.07									6	6	6.84
175	183	8	7	6.05	20	20	23.67	24	22	19.55	2	2	4.96			0.66									48	46	48.84
176	184	4	4	0.49	13	13	1.85	12	12	1.47	2	2	0.39			0.06									27	27	3.77
180	189,0--.1	3	3	1.43	6	6	5.88	7	7	5.26	5	5	1.57			0.24									10	10	12.95
181	188	1		0.87	6	6	3.59	5	5	3.35	2	2	1.06			0.18									18	17	8.18
190	172	1	1	3.01	11	11	10.94	5	5	7.77	2	2	1.60			0.20									18	18	20.51
191	173	1	1	0.62	2	2	2.44	1	1	2.10			0.62			0.10									9	9	5.26
192	190			0.27	1	1	0.98	2	2	0.73			0.18			0.02									2	2	1.91
193	191-2			3.47	14	12	12.52	12	12	9.23	2	2	2.19			0.29									27	25	24.23
194	193	1		1.90	3	3	6.70	3	3	4.55			0.93	1	1	0.12									7	7	12.30
195	194	2	2	1.69	6	6	6.74	3	3	5.78	3	3	1.52			0.21									12	12	14.25
196	170			0.27			0.91	1	1	0.55			0.21			0.01									1	1	1.58
197	171	3	3	0.59	1	1	2.09			1.56			0.11			0.05									1	1	4.07
200,202	200,202			1.14	6	5	4.47	2	2	3.73	2	2	0.37			0.15									10	9	9.33
201	201			0.85	4	4	2.69			1.61			0.98			0.04									4	4	4.67
203	203			0.44	1	1	1.93			1.93			0.33			0.10									4	1	4.57
204.0	204.1,.9	1		0.23	2	2	0.96	1	1	0.91			0.61			0.05									3	1	2.20
204.1-4	204.0,5-7	1		1.30	10	9	4.60	9	9	3.25	1	1	0.28			0.10									20	16	8.68
204	204-207			1.53	12	10	5.56	10	10	4.16	1	1	0.73			0.15									23	17	10.89
TOTAL		58	56	62.24	262	251	245.93	224	210	205.72	58	58	53.44	11	11	7.55									555	530	512.64

O : All tumours
O': Histologically confirmed
E : Expected

Table 3. Breast cancer in women in Sweden by age at diagnosis of cervical cancer, stage and treatment

TIME SINCE DIAGNOSIS OF PRIMARY CERVICAL CANCER (IN YEARS)

INVASIVE — RADIOTHERAPY

Age	<1 O	<1 O'	<1 E	1-4 O	1-4 O'	1-4 E	5-9 O	5-9 O'	5-9 E	10-14 O	10-14 O'	10-14 E	15-19 O	15-19 O'	15-19 E	20-24 O	20-24 O'	20-24 E	25-29 O	25-29 O'	25-29 E	30+ O	30+ O'	30+ E	Total O	Total O'	Total E
<30			0.02			0.11			0.18			0.19			0.09												0.57
30-39			0.74	2	2	3.55	3	2	5.74	2	2	4.54	1	1	1.29										8	7	15.12
40-49	3	2	4.15	10	10	14.21	12	11	14.34	5	5	7.88	2	1	2.06										29	27	38.50
50-59	5	4	4.55	11	9	13.23	5	4	11.21	12	11	6.04			1.41										28	24	31.88
60-69	3	3	3.82	8	8	9.79	10	8	6.93	1	1	3.15			0.65										19	17	20.53
70+	3	3	3.14	2	2	5.72	5	5	2.83	1	1	0.88			0.10										8	7	9.52

INVASIVE — (no data)

Age	<1	1-4	5-9	10-14	15-19	20-24	25-29	30+	Total
<30									
30-39									
40-49									
50-59									
60-69									
70+									

IN SITU — SURGERY

Age	<1 O	<1 O'	<1 E	1-4 O	1-4 O'	1-4 E	5-9 O	5-9 O'	5-9 E	10-14 O	10-14 O'	10-14 E	15-19 O	15-19 O'	15-19 E	20-24	25-29	30+	Total O	Total O'	Total E
<30	1		0.54	4	3	3.26	4	4	3.60			0.87			0.16				8	7	7.89
30-39	3	3	4.32	18	18	21.32	21	19	23.52	6	6	6.16	1	1	0.83				46	44	51.83
40-49	4	4	10.31	33	33	40.65	27	26	31.88	5	5	7.66			0.91				65	64	81.10
50-59	2	2	3.80	20	18	13.45	8	7	9.21	2	2	2.22	1	1	0.30				31	28	25.18
60-69			1.40	7	7	4.54	1	1	2.77	1	1	0.49	1	1	0.07				10	10	7.86
70+			0.59	1	1	1.67	1	1	0.59			0.06			0.01				2	1	2.33

O : All tumours
O': Histologically confirmed
E : Expected

Among the population of women treated for carcinoma *in situ*, 162 cases of breast cancer were subsequently registered (154 histologically confirmed), and 176.2 were expected. Among women under 30 years of age, there were 8 notifications (7.9 expected); at ages 30-39 there were 46 cases (51.8 expected); and at ages 40-49 the figures were 65 (81). In women aged 50 or more, the observed numbers slightly exceeded those expected.

Discussion

In the statistical analysis, the total number of histologically confirmed new cancers found in the cohort of women treated for invasive cancer of the cervix uteri slightly exceeded the expected number. This was also true in the cohort treated for cancer *in situ*.

The overall distribution of second primary cancers observed in the cohort with invasive cancer and that in the cohort with cancer *in situ* were similar. Thus, in both cohorts there was a deficit of breast cancer but excesses of rectal and urinary bladder cancer and of leukaemia.

The excess of bronchogenic cancer, especially among the women with invasive carcinoma of the cervix, was probably to some extent attributable to pulmonary metastases mistaken for primary tumours. The corresponding excess among women treated for in-situ carcinoma is less easily explained. Possibly these women, and also the women with invasive cervical cancer, belonged to a high-risk category as regards bronchogenic carcinoma, with smoking habits as the most likely common factor. The occupational patterns of the women with invasive and those with in-situ cervical cancer were similar (Table 4).

The excess numbers of kidney tumours, and also to some extent of bladder tumours, found after the short follow-up period can probably be ascribed to the fact that urographic and cystoscopic examinations are carried out routinely on all patients with invasive cervical carcinoma.

Table 4. Invasive and in-situ carcinoma of the cervix uteri in women in certain occupational groups in Sweden[a]

Occupational group	Invasive cancer		In-situ cancer	
	Observed cases	% observed/ expected	Observed cases	% observed/ expected
Farming, forestry	82	57	209	67
Technique, natural science	208	73	992	104
Transport, communications	114	82	631	121
Medicine	265	85	1264	98
Administration	1236	108	5497	124
Manufacturing	783	131	2315	142
Graphic work	31	141	131	168
Service	1249	142	2984	139

[a] Data from the period 1960-1973 (Swedish Cancer-Environment Register)

The deficit as regards endometrial and ovarian carcinomas may be explained by the treatment - combination of irradiation and surgery - for the original tumours. There is also a possibility that these women belonged to a low-risk group for those cancers.

The total numbers of registrations of breast cancer in the women with invasive cervical carcinoma and in those with cervical carcinoma *in situ* were lower than the expected rates. The deficit was more pronounced among women treated in the premenopausal period than among those treated after the menopause. In the women who received irradiation for invasive cancer, this difference indicates a preventive effect of the withdrawal of ovarian hormones. Among the cohort treated for cancer *in situ*, with the deficit obvious only in the age group 30-49 years, the explanation is obscure. Most of these cervical lesions were treated only with conization, and only a few by hysterectomy or irradiation.

SECOND PRIMARY CANCERS FOLLOWING INVASIVE AND IN-SITU CARCINOMA OF THE CERVIX UTERI: BIRMINGHAM CANCER REGISTRY

P. Prior & R. Brown

Birmingham and West Midlands Regional Cancer Registry
Cancer Epidemiology Research Unit
University of Birmingham
Birmingham B15 2TH, UK

The Registry

Cancer registration in Birmingham dates back to 1936. Based originally on a single hospital in the city, its scope was gradually extended, until by 1957 it included the whole of the region, which now has a population of just over five million.

Cases are registered, mainly by clerical staff, who are instructed to copy certain items from records of hospital in-patient and out-patients and of radiotherapy and pathology departments. Registrations are also obtained from doctors who attend cases at home (domiciliary visits) and from coroners. Information derived from death certificates leads to registration only if it is possible to obtain further information by inquiries to hospitals or general practitioners. Multiple-source registration and a variety of systems of cross-checking help to ensure the high degree of registration efficiency now achieved, and the available evidence suggests that fewer than 2% escape record.

The information recorded includes, in addition to items of identification (name, age, sex, residence, occupation, etc.) and of the clinicians and hospitals involved in the patient's treatment, a full description of the clinical findings and of the details of the treatment given. Except for basal-cell carcinoma and squamous-cell cancers of the skin, all cases are followed up until death; the successive reports provided after each follow-up visit thus furnish a useful chronicle of the subsequent course of the disease.

Analyses of the records of the Registry are used in both undergraduate and postgraduate medical teaching to illustrate the natural history of the disease, with special reference to the local situation, and to show its prognosis by site and treatment. The records of the Registry have also been used for an exhaustive on-going study of the incidence of multiple primary carcinoma, for various studies of childhood cancer, and for a number of studies of specific tumour sites. More recently, the Registry has been engaged in several epidemiological investigations of environmental health, particularly those involving carcinogenic hazards in certain industries. Other areas of interest include joint epidemiological and clinical studies of cancers at various sites; studies of the malignant sequelae of certain chronic diseases; and the organization of and participation in clinical therapeutic trials.

The Registry covers the whole of the five West Midland counties: Warwickshire, Worcestershire, Staffordshire, Shropshire and Herefordshire, in the central part of England. Since 1974, the counties of Worcester and Hereford have been amalgamated to form 'Hereford Worcester', and much of the urbanized central area has been put together as the 'West Midland Metropolitan County'; fortunately, however, the outer boundaries have not been changed. The region includes not only some of the most highly industrialized sections of the country, but also large areas of farmland. It lies between latitudes 52° 08′ and 53° 00′ north, and longitudes 1° 10′ and 3° 03′ west. The total registration area is 13 014 km².

The main occupational groups in which the total population is employed are: industry (63.0%), commerce (28.8%), agriculture (1.5%) and personal service (6.7%). Over 40% of the population live in conurbations of more than 100 000.

Multiple primary cancers

Multiple primary tumours have been considered of special interest since the inception of the Registry and have been the subject of surveys since 1960. The Registry operates an active follow-up system. Annual reports are requested from the hospitals concerned during the time when the patient continues under observation; and, when hospital follow-up is terminated, the patient's general practitioner is contacted annually.

Notifications for registration are checked initially against the main alphabetical index file primarily to guard against duplicate registration. This procedure also allows identification of possible candidates for a subsequent primary registration. In general, second primary cancers are reported by the hospital involved in treatment; but, in addition, the annual reports, subsequent pathology reports, post-mortem results and death certificates are scrutinized, and additional information is requested to ascertain the nature - whether primary or recurrent - of any subsequent sign of malignancy.

Seminars, informal talks and demonstrations on multiple primary cancers are organized for the Registry staff and for groups of visiting personnel who are involved in data collection and abstraction to stimulate their interest in the topic and to bring to their attention the problems involved in identifying and reporting possible cases.

The majority of second primary cancers are confirmed histologically; that is, a copy of the signed pathology report is received at the Registry. For cases with less precise information, a registration may be made after the clinical, X-ray and cytological evidence has been referred to the consultant for the Registry.

Information for registration is abstracted centrally. This procedure makes it possible for all the available information to be reviewed before a registration for a second primary is effected and also provides a second check of possible duplicate registrations. A separate record is made for each primary tumour, and each record carries a code to indicate that another registration has been made. The pro-forma records are cross-referenced manually, and the new registration number is added to the existing alphabetical index card.

When a specific analysis is to be undertaken, the 'flagged' records are listed, and linkage is effected by means of the pro-forma records and/or index cards. The records are again reviewed, and a new pro-forma record is prepared for each patient, bringing together summary information on all primary tumours diagnosed in that patient. This procedure enables similar cases to be viewed as a group. The consistency in registration can be assessed, and any necessary exclusions can be made at this time: for example, those patients who developed a first primary while resident outside the region or in whom the first lesion was non-malignant. This procedure acts as an additional safeguard against duplicate registration. With this intensive method of follow-up and review, it is considered that a high level of identification and confirmation of subsequent primary cancers is achieved.

Material and methods

The composition of the series in relation to stage, treatment and age is given in Table 1. The stage of the cancer was confirmed in all cases from biopsy and/or resected tissue. 'Treatment' refers to first planned treatment; no allowance has been made for later treatment of a recurrence or of metastases.

Table 1. Birmingham and West Midlands Regional Cancer Registry: Characteristics of the population under study

	Invasive tumours			*In situ* (no radiotherapy)	Total
	Radiotherapy	No radiotherapy	Total invasive		
Number of women	3 808	819	4 627	2 034	6 661
Woman-years at risk by time since diagnosis:					
<1 year	3 333.5	590.0	3 923.5	2 030.0	5 953.5
1-4 years	8 357.0	1 129.5	9 486.5	8 058.0	17 544.5
5-9 years	7 351.0	1 045.5	8 396.5	3 883.5	12 280.0
10-14 years	5 792.0	856.5	6 648.5	708.5	7 357.0
15-19 years	2 679.5	293.5	2 973.0	-	2 973.0
20-24 years	492.5	49.5	542.0	-	542.0
All years	28 005.5	3 964.5	31 970.0	14 680.0	46 650.0
Number of women by age at diagnosis:					
<35	204	44	248	496	744
35-44	853	124	977	852	1 829
45-54	1 035	167	1 202	531	1 733
55-64	919	169	1 088	111	1 199
65-74	588	181	769	37	806
75+	209	134	343	7	350
Number of women excluded because of:					
- malignancy prior to diagnosis of cervical cancer	29	8	37	11	48
- second cancer (excluding non-melanoma skin) diagnosed simultaneously with cervical cancer	15	10	25	11	36

For the current survey of cervical cancers, registrations of a malignant tumour of the cervix were selected for the years 1950-1964. The records were updated to the 25th anniversary of registration in the years 1950-1953, the 20th anniversary for 1954-1959 and the 15th anniversary for 1960-1964 - anniversary date being the date of first treatment. For the cervix *in situ* series, records were available from 1957 to 1970, and these cases were updated to the appropriate 5th, 10th or 15th anniversary. Termination date varied, therefore, from 1974-1979, depending on the year of registration. Follow-up reports are recorded on the punch-card/computer record for years one to seven inclusive. From the 10th year, only quinquennial reports are recorded. The analysis has been confined to those points, as opposed to a specific calendar date, to ensure that maximum follow-up and therefore optimal reporting of second primaries, has been obtained. This approach facilitates data processing, and it is considered to give a more accurate result than when patients are dropped from the analysis at 'date of last contact'.

Expected numbers

The number of years of survival was computed for each patient from the date of first treatment to the selected anniversary date, or to death if it occurred before the end of the survey period. 'Person-years' at risk were tabulated by stage, treatment, age at first primary and year from first treatment. The incidence rates used for computing expected numbers were based on registrations for 1960-1962 and on population figures for the region from the Population Census (1961) and were classified according to the 7th Revision of the ICD. The classification was adhered to as closely as possible, but some local rulings on registrations may affect inter-registry comparisons:

ICD 140	includes cases specified as 'lip',
ICD 142	includes all salivary-gland tumours,
ICD 163	includes implied primary tumours,
ICD 180.1	excludes benign papillomas,
ICD 191	includes 'rodent ulcers' (basal-cell carcinomas) and squamous-cell carcinomas,
ICD 193	includes ICD 223 and 237,
ICD 204	comprises all leukaemias - no separation by specific cell type was made.

Patients were not excluded from the 'person-years' at risk after developing a second primary cancer, but all other exclusions laid down in the guidelines for the survey were implemented.

It should be noted, however, that the longer established registries exclude a greater proportion of cases with primary cancers that occurred previous to the cervical cancer and, because of the long period of observation, those cases with third and subsequent primary cancers occurring after the cervical primary.

Results

All sites

The small excess of 16 second primary cancers which was observed when all three groups of patients were combined (Table 2) was not of statistical significance (relative risk, RR=1.09; t=1.18). Radiotherapy was not associated with a significant excess (RR=1.04), nor was the excess of tumours in the groups that received no radiotherapy significant (62 observed, 51.14 expected; RR=1.21; t=1.52). In terms of stage (invasive *versus* non-invasive), the relative risks were 1.00 (153 observed, 153.21 expected; t=0.02) and 1.47 (t=2.75; $p<0.01$), respectively.

Table 2. Observed and expected numbers of second primary cancers in women diagnosed with primary cervical cancer in Birmingham and West Midlands

A. Cases of invasive cervical cancer treated by radiotherapy

TIME SINCE DIAGNOSIS OF PRIMARY CERVICAL CANCER (IN YEARS)

Number of women starting intervals

ICD7	ICD8	<1 (3808) O	O'	E	1-4 (2859) O	O'	E	5-9 (1654) O	O'	E	10-14 (1301) O	O'	E	15-19 (613) O	O'	E	20-24 (269) O	O'	E	25-29 O	O'	E	30+ O	O'	E	Total (excl. <1) O	O'	E
140	140			0.03			0.09			0.09			0.09			0.05			0.01									0.33
141	141			0.04			0.12			0.12			0.11			0.06			0.01							1	1	0.42
142	142			0.09			0.23			0.21			0.18			0.09			0.01									0.72
143-4	143-5			0.05			0.14			0.15			0.13	1		0.07			0.02							1	1	0.51
145,7-8	146,8-9			0.08			0.23			0.22			0.20			0.10			0.02									0.77
146	147			0.01			0.04			0.03			0.03			0.01												0.11
150	150			0.21	1		0.58	1		0.60	1		0.57	1		0.32			0.08							2	2	2.15
151	151	1	1	1.32			3.61	3	2	3.79			3.67			2.10			0.50							5	4	13.67
152	152			0.04			0.11			0.11			0.10			0.05												0.38
153	153	1	1	1.34	3	3	3.65	6	5	3.80	6	3	3.64	1	1	2.06			0.48							16	12	13.63
154	154	1	1	0.77	3	1	2.11	3	1	2.18	3	3	2.06	2	1	1.16			0.26							9	7	7.77
155.0	155			0.02			0.06			0.07	1		0.06			0.03			0.01							1	1	0.23
155.1	156			0.19			0.52			0.55			0.53			0.31			0.07							1		1.98
157	157			0.38	2		1.04	1		1.09	1		1.05	2	1	0.61			0.14							6	3	3.93
160	160			0.04			0.11			0.11			0.10			0.06			0.01									0.39
161	161			0.03			0.07			0.07			0.06			0.03			0.01							1		0.24
162-3	162-3	1		0.68	7	6	1.81	8	7	1.79	7	5	1.61	7	7	0.84			0.18							29	21	6.23
170-	174			3.99	10	8	10.46	13	12	10.05	9	7	8.66	7	3	4.31	1		0.87							34	27	34.35
172	182.0	1		0.74			1.96			1.91	1	1	1.68	1		0.83	1	1	0.16							2	2	6.54
173-4	181,2.9			0.10			0.26			0.26	1		0.24			0.12			0.02									0.90
175	183	1	1	0.86	1		2.26	1	1	2.17			1.84			0.90			0.17							1	1	7.34
176	184			0.19			0.52			0.53			0.51			0.28			0.06							1	1	1.90
180	189.0--1	1	1	0.14	1	1	0.37	1	1	0.38	2	2	0.34			0.19			0.04							1	1	1.32
181	188	1	1	0.22	1	1	0.60			0.63	1	1	0.61	2	2	0.35			0.08							5	5	2.27
190	172			0.10			0.25			0.22			0.17			0.09			0.02							1	1	0.75
191	173	4	4	1.28	5	4	3.44	3	1	3.51	3	3	3.28	1	1	1.81			0.40							12	9	12.44
192	190			0.03			0.08			0.08			0.06			0.03			0.01									0.26
193	191-2			0.24	1	1	0.61	2	2	0.56			0.46			0.21			0.03							2	2	1.87
194	193			0.10			0.26			0.25			0.22	1	1	0.12			0.03							1	1	0.88
195	194			0.03			0.08			0.07			0.06			0.03			0.00									0.24
196	170			0.03	1		0.08			0.08	1		0.07			0.04			0.01							1		0.28
197	171			0.08			0.20	1		0.20			0.17			0.09			0.02							1		0.68
200,202	200,202			0.15	1	1	0.40			0.39	1		0.35			0.19			0.04							1	1	1.37
201	201			0.06			0.15			0.14	2	2	0.13			0.07			0.01							2	2	0.50
203	203			0.08	1	1	0.21	2	2	0.20	2		0.18			0.09	1	1	0.02							3	3	0.70
204.0	204.1,.9																											
204.1-4	204.0,5-7																											
204	204-207										1	1														1	1	2.26
TOTAL		8	8	13.99	34	28	37.37	43	35	37.25	38	29	33.80	21	14	18.01	3	2	3.88			0.07				139	108	130.31

O : All tumours
O': Histologically confirmed
E : Expected

B. Cases of invasive cervical cancer not treated by radiotherapy

TIME SINCE DIAGNOSIS OF PRIMARY CERVICAL CANCER (IN YEARS)

ICD7	ICD8	<1 O	<1 O'	<1 E	1-4 O	1-4 O'	1-4 E	5-9 O	5-9 O'	5-9 E	10-14 O	10-14 O'	10-14 E	15-19 O	15-19 O'	15-19 E	20-24 O	20-24 O'	20-24 E	25-29 O	25-29 O'	25-29 E	30+ O	30+ O'	30+ E	Total (excl. <1) O	Total (excl. <1) O'	Total (excl. <1) E
Number of women starting intervals				819			362			242			189			66			12									
140	140			0.01			0.01			0.01			0.01			0.00			0.00									0.03
141	141			0.01			0.01			0.01			0.01			0.01			0.00									0.04
142	142			0.02			0.03			0.03			0.02			0.01			0.01									0.09
143-4	143-5			0.01			0.02			0.02			0.02			0.01			0.01									0.07
145,7-8	146,8-9			0.02			0.03			0.03			0.03			0.01			0.01									0.10
146	147			0.00			0.00			0.00			0.00			0.00			0.00									0.00
150	150			0.05			0.07			0.07			0.07			0.03			0.01									0.25
151	151			0.34			0.45			0.44	1	1	0.42			0.20			0.04							1	1	1.55
152	152			0.01			0.01			0.01			0.01			0.01			0.01									0.04
153	153			0.34			0.46	1	1	0.46			0.43	1	1	0.20			0.04							2	2	1.59
154	154			0.19			0.27			0.26			0.25			0.11			0.02									0.91
155.0	155			0.05			0.01			0.01			0.01			0.00			0.00									0.03
155.1	156			0.06			0.06			0.06			0.06			0.03			0.01									0.22
157	157			0.10			0.13			0.13			0.12			0.06			0.01									0.45
160	160			0.01			0.01			0.01			0.01			0.01			0.01									0.04
161	161			0.01			0.01			0.01			0.01			0.00			0.00									0.03
162-3	162-3			0.14	1	1	0.22	1	1	0.21			0.20			0.08			0.01							2	2	0.72
170	174			0.79			1.33	1	1	1.32			1.18	1	1	0.45			0.08							2	2	4.36
172	182.0			0.13			0.24			0.23			0.23			0.09			0.02									0.81
173-4	181,2.9			0.16			0.03			0.03			0.03			0.01			0.01									0.10
175	183			0.05			0.28			0.28			0.26			0.09			0.02									0.93
176	184			0.07			0.07	1	1	0.06	1	1	0.06			0.03			0.01							2	2	0.23
180	189.0-.1			0.03			0.05			0.05			0.04			0.02			0.00									0.16
181	188			0.06			0.07			0.08			0.07			0.03			0.01									0.26
190	172			0.02			0.03			0.03			0.03			0.01			0.00									0.10
191	173			0.32			0.44	1	1	0.43			0.40			0.18			0.04							1	1	1.49
192	190			0.01			0.01			0.01			0.01			0.00			0.00									0.03
193	191-2	1	1	0.04			0.08			0.08			0.07			0.02			0.02									0.25
194	193			0.02			0.03			0.03			0.03			0.01			0.01									0.10
195	194			0.01			0.01			0.01			0.01			0.00			0.00									0.03
196	170			0.01			0.01			0.01			0.01			0.00			0.00									0.03
197	171			0.02			0.03			0.02			0.02			0.01			0.01									0.08
200,202	200,202			0.03			0.05			0.05			0.04			0.02			0.02									0.16
201	201			0.01			0.02			0.02			0.02			0.01			0.01									0.07
203	203			0.01			0.02			0.02			0.02			0.01			0.00									0.07
204.0	204.1,.9																											
204.1-4	204.0,5-7																											
204	204-207										1	1														1	1	0.27
TOTAL		1	1	3.11	1	1	4.68	5	5	4.61	3	3	4.28	2	2	1.79			0.33							11	11	15.69

O : All tumours
O' : Histologically confirmed
E : Expected

C. Cases of carcinoma in situ not treated by radiotherapy

TIME SINCE DIAGNOSIS OF PRIMARY CERVICAL CANCER (IN YEARS)

ICD7	ICD8	<1 O	<1 O'	<1 E	1-4 O	1-4 O'	1-4 E	5-9 O	5-9 O'	5-9 E	10-14 O	10-14 O'	10-14 E	15-19 O	15-19 O'	15-19 E	20-24 O	20-24 O'	20-24 E	25-29 O	25-29 O'	25-29 E	30+ O	30+ O'	30+ E	Total O	Total O'	Total E
		(2034)			(2026)			(786)			(143)																	
140	140			0.01			0.03			0.03			0.01															0.07
141	141			0.01			0.05			0.03			0.01															0.09
142	142			0.04			0.18	1	1	0.10			0.02													1	1	0.30
143-4	143-5			0.01			0.06			0.04			0.01														1	0.11
145,7-8	146,8-9			0.02			0.10			0.07			0.02															0.19
146	147			0.00			0.02			0.01			0.00															0.03
150	150			0.04			0.21			0.16			0.04															0.41
151	151			0.20			1.04			0.88			0.21															2.13
152	152			0.01			0.04			0.03			0.01															0.08
153	153			0.25	4	3	1.27	1	1	1.00	1	1	0.24													6	5	2.51
154	154			0.15			0.78			0.59			0.14															1.51
155.0	155			0.00			0.02			0.01			0.00															0.03
155.1	156			0.02			0.13			0.12			0.03															0.28
157	157			0.05	1		0.28			0.25			0.06													1		0.59
160	160			0.01			0.05			0.03			0.01															0.09
161	161			0.01			0.04			0.03			0.01															0.08
162-3	162-3			0.17	2		0.83			0.58			0.13													2		1.54
170	174			1.46	9	8	6.69	8	7	4.13	1	1	0.85													17	15	11.67
172	182.0			0.19			0.98			0.71			0.16														1	1.85
173-4	181,2.9			0.03			0.15			0.10			0.02															0.27
175	183			0.30	1	1	1.40	2	2	0.89			0.19													3	3	2.48
176	184			0.04	2	2	0.19	4	4	0.14			0.03													6	6	0.36
180	189.0-.1	1	1	0.03			0.16			0.16			0.03													1	1	0.37
181	188			0.03			0.18			0.15			0.04													1	1	0.30
190	172			0.06			0.23			0.11			0.02															0.36
191	173	1	1	0.31	1	1	1.50	1		1.05			0.23													2	2	2.78
192	190			0.11			0.06			0.03			0.01															0.10
193	191-2			0.04			0.48			0.28			0.06															0.82
194	193			0.02			0.15			0.09			0.02															0.26
195	194			0.01			0.06			0.03			0.01															0.10
196	170			0.03			0.04			0.02			0.01															0.07
197	171			0.05			0.12	1	1	0.07			0.02															0.21
200,202	200,202			0.02	1	1	0.21			0.13			0.03													1	1	0.37
201	201			0.02	1	1	0.09			0.05			0.01													1	1	0.15
203	203																											
204.0	204.1,.9																											
204.1-4	204.0,5-7																											
204	204-207	1	1	0.07	1	1	0.34	1	1	0.22			0.05													1	1	0.61
TOTAL		3	3	3.83	22	19	18.26	21	18	12.34	2	2	2.76													45	39	33.36

O   : All tumours
O' : Histologically confirmed
E   : Expected

Leukaemia (ICD 204)

No excess of leukaemia was observed (3 observed, 3.13 expected). Two of the observed cases had been treated by surgery only.

Colon, rectum, kidney and bladder (ICD 153, 154, 180, 181.0)

For these heavily irradiated areas, the relative risk was higher in the later years of the survey, but the effect appeared to be related to age at first primary rather than to radiotherapy (R+). The invasive group not treated by radiotherapy was combined with in-situ cases in assessing the effect of no radiotherapy (R-).

1-9 years	:	RR=1.12	—
10+ years	:	RR=1.55	p<0.05
R+	:	RR=1.27	—
R-	:	RR=1.45	—
Age <50 years	:	RR=1.71	p<0.05
Age +50 years	:	RR=1.11	—

Breast (ICD 170)

For all three groups of patients in Table 3, the observed number was close to that expected (53 observed, 50.38 expected; RR=1.05). A small negative trend over time was observed, and no effect of radiation could be demonstrated. A negative trend with age at first primary was again found.

1-9 years	:	RR=1.21	—
10+ years	:	RR=0.73	—
R+	:	RR=1.18	—
R-	:	RR=1.18	—
Age <50 years	:	RR=1.35	—
Age 50+ years	:	RR=0.77	—

Bronchus (ICD 162, 163)

Although there was a highly significant excess of tumours in the bronchus overall (33 observed, 8.5 expected; RR=3.88; p<0.001) and an apparent effect of radiation, the increase in risk over time was small and was not significant. The risk was also related to age at first primary.

1-9 years	:	RR=3.49	p<0.001
10+ years	:	RR=4.59	p<0.001
R+	:	RR=4.65	p<0.001
R-	:	RR=1.77	—
Age <50 years	:	RR=6.19	p<0.001
Age 50+ years	:	RR=2.58	p<0.01

Table 3. Breast cancer in women in Birmingham and the West Midlands by age at diagnosis of cervical cancer, stage and treatment

TIME SINCE DIAGNOSIS OF PRIMARY CERVICAL CANCER (IN YEARS)

	<1			1-4			5-9			10-14			15-19			20-24			25-29			30+			Total (excl. <1)		
	O	O'	E	O	O'	E	O	O'	E	O	O'	E	O	O'	E	O	O'	E	O	O'	E	O	O'	E	O	O'	E
INVASIVE — RADIOTHERAPY																											
<30			0.00			0.01			0.03			0.05			0.05			0.02										0.16
30-39			0.16	1	1	0.67			1.13	3	3	1.34			0.83			0.14							4	4	4.11
40-49			1.92	4	3	2.63	9	9	2.82			2.64	1	1	1.27			0.30							14	13	9.66
50-59			1.12	3	2	2.84	1	1	2.78	3	1	2.46	2	1	1.41			0.35							9	5	9.84
60-69	1	1	1.01	2	2	2.70	3	2	2.29			1.63			0.60			0.06							5	4	7.28
70+			0.78	2	1	1.61			1.00			0.54			0.15			0.00							2	1	3.30
INVASIVE — NOT RADIOTHERAPY																											
<30			0.00			0.00			0.00			0.01			0.01			0.00									0.02
30-39			0.03			0.14			0.26			0.33			0.16			0.04									0.93
40-49			0.11			0.30			0.35			0.34			0.09			0.01									1.09
50-59			0.18			0.40	2	2	0.32			0.28			0.12			0.02							2	2	1.14
60-69			0.16			0.26			0.24			0.19			0.07			0.02									0.78
70+			0.31			0.24			0.14			0.04			0.01			0.00									0.43
IN-SITU																											
<30			0.01			0.09			0.09			0.03															0.21
30-39			0.21	1	1	1.27	1	1	1.05			0.30													2	2	2.62
40-49			0.81	8	7	3.59	5	5	1.84			0.34													13	12	5.77
50-59			0.31			1.27			0.76			0.12															2.15
60-69			0.08	1	1	0.33			0.28			0.06													1	1	0.67
70+			0.04	1	1	0.15			0.11			0.00													1	1	0.26

O : All tumours
O': Histologically confirmed
E : Expected

Lymphomas and multiple myeloma (ICD 200,203)

The risk of developing these tumours was not so markedly dependent on age, but the increased risk over time was confined to the group treated by radiotherapy.

1-9 years   : RR=0.54 —
10+ years   : RR=4.89 $p<0.01$
R+   : RR=2.43 —
R-   : RR=1.22 —
Age <50 years : RR=1.77 —
Age 50+ years : RR=2.29 —

Other genital sites (ICD 176)

A significant excess was found only in the in-situ group, and the effect was due to primary tumours in the vagina. Such tumours would be more difficult to diagnose in the group with invasive cancer.

Corpus uteri, ovary (ICD 172, 175)

Deficits of cancers in these organs seen in the groups with invasive cancer are probably due in part to the difficulty of recognizing new primary cancers in heavily irradiated tissue and in part to surgical removal of the organs as treatment for the cervical cancer.

Stomach (ICD 151)

A significant deficit of stomach cancers was observed overall (5 observed, 17.36 expected; $p<0.001$). The effect was common to each of the three groups.

Discussion

The results from the Birmingham Cancer Registry are broadly in line with those found for other areas. No excess of leukaemias could be demonstrated, but the results are suggestive of an increased risk of lymphomas and multiple myeloma in the later years of observation in patients treated by radiotherapy. The results for bronchus are more difficult to interpret, but they do not exclude a possible effect of radiation. In general, a deficit of breast tumours has been observed in other series; this effect was not apparent in the Birmingham data.

SECOND PRIMARY CANCERS FOLLOWING CERVICAL CANCER: SOUTH THAMES CANCER REGISTRY, 1961-1976

L.A. Brinton

Imperial Cancer Research Fund
Cancer Epidemiology and Clinical Trials Unit
Oxford, UK[1]

P.G. Smith, C.C. Patterson & M.P. Coleman

Department of Medical Statistics and Epidemiology
London School of Hygiene and Tropical Medicine
London, UK

R.G. Skeet & G.W.O. Tomkins

South Thames Cancer Registry
Sutton, Surrey, UK

Study population and methods

The study population comprised those patients who were registered in the South Thames Cancer Registry with invasive or in-situ cervical cancer during the period 1961-1976 and whose usual place of residence was in the area covered by the Registry. This area includes the part of Greater London south of the River Thames, and the counties of Kent, Surrey and Sussex. Over six million people live in the area served by the Registry, and over 30 000 tumours are registered each year. The staff of the Registry regularly follow up all patients who are registered with them, even if a patient leaves the area. Information about any subsequent primary cancers or death is sought at follow-up. The analyses we present are based upon the follow-up of patients to 1 January 1977.

Since a cancer registration may be initiated from several possible sources, all registrations are checked against the alphabetical index to exclude double registration of one tumour; this check also serves to link two primary cancers registered for the same person. A second cancer will not be accepted as a separate primary cancer unless both the site and the histology are

---

[1]Present address: Environmental Epidemiology Branch, National Cancer Institute, Bethesda, MD 20205, USA

different from that of the first cancer; if the site is different but the histology is the same as that of the first cancer, the new cancer will be registered as a second cancer only if the hospital record states explicitly that the new tumour is a primary, distinct from the previous cancer.

During the period 1961 to 1976, 12 259 women with cervical cancer were registered. Women were excluded from the analysis if they had had a primary cancer diagnosed before (173 women) or at the same time (48 women) as the diagnosis of cervical cancer, or if they were aged 85 or older at diagnosis of cervical cancer (238 women), or if the histology of the primary cervical cancer had not been recorded (578 women, 4.7%). Of those women who had in-situ cervical cancer, 99 (2.6%) received radiotherapy as their first treatment; these women were also excluded. Registration records for 22 women either contained defective data or contributed no follow-up (registered at death); these women were also excluded. A total of 1158 women (9.4%) were excluded in these ways (see Table 1), leaving 11 101 women eligible for analysis. Of these, 7327 (66%) had invasive cancer, 6110 of whom (83%) were treated with radiotherapy; 3774 women had in-situ cancer of the cervix.

Table 1. South Thames Cancer Registry: Characteristics of the population under study

	Invasive tumours			*In situ* (no radiotherapy)	Total
	Radiotherapy	No radiotherapy	Total invasive		
Number of women	6 110	1 217	7 327	3 774	11 101
Woman-years at risk by time since diagnosis:					
<1 year	5 324	1 040	6 364	3 470	9 834
1-4 years	11 670	2 781	14 451	10 446	24 897
5-9 years	7 278	2 167	9 445	6 819	16 264
10-14 years	2 514	663	3 177	996	4 172
15-16 years	66	18	84	18	102
All years	26 852	6 669	33 521	21 749	55 269
Number of women by age at diagnosis:					
<45	1 169	446	1 615	2 721	4 336
45-54	1 680	295	1 975	763	2 738
55-64	1 655	200	1 855	213	2 068
65-74	1 085	136	1 221	61	1 282
75-84	521	140	661	16	677
Number of women excluded because of:					
- malignancy prior to diagnosis of cervical cancer					173
- second cancer (excluding non-melanoma skin) diagnosed simultaneously with cervical cancer					48
- cervical cancer diagnosed at death					2
- missing or incorrect information:					
- histology of cervix					578
- other					12
- survival for less than one day					8
- aged 85 or over at diagnosis of cervical cancer					238
- in-situ cervical cancer irradiated immediately					99

Each woman was included in the analysis from the date she was first treated for cervical cancer until the earliest date of her date of death, her 85th birthday, or the date she developed a second primary tumour, if any of these dates preceded the end of the study period (1 January 1977). Only the *year* of birth and the *year* of developing a second tumour were coded on the computer record, and in the analysis these events were assumed to have occurred on 2 July in the relevant year.

Some women (363, 3.3%) were not followed up to the end of the study period, but we have included them in the analysis until the end of the study period on the assumption that they did not develop a second tumour. If such patients had developed a second tumour, it is very likely that this tumour would have been linked to the patient's original record at the time the second tumour was registered, through the alphabetical index of all registrations that is maintained by the Registry. This link is less likely to have been made if the patient was not resident in the area covered by the Registry at the time the second tumour was diagnosed, but this has probably biased our results only slightly.

Of the 6110 patients with invasive cervical tumours who were treated with radiotherapy, 1035 (17%) did not receive radiotherapy as their first treatment. On average, these patients received radiotherapy about three months after first diagnosis (most were treated within a few weeks, but a small number received radiotherapy some years after first presentation). In the analysis, these patients were included in the 'no radiotherapy' group until they received radiotherapy and, subsequently, were included in the 'radiotherapy' group. Similarly, 135 (3.6%) of the women with in-situ cancer received delayed radiotherapy; these women were included in the 'in situ, no radiotherapy' group until they received radiotherapy and were then censored from the study.

The total number of woman-years of follow-up was 55 269 - an average of five years per woman. Of these, 37% were five or more years after first treatment and 8% were 10 or more years after first treatment. Most of the women with in-situ cancer (72%) were diagnosed before the age of 45 years, whereas only 22% of women with invasive cancer were diagnosed before this age (Table 1).

Expected numbers of second primary tumours following the diagnosis of cervical cancer were calculated on the assumption that such tumours would occur with the same frequency among cervical cancer patients as do first primary cancers among women of similar age in the population of the area covered by the Registry. Female age-specific cancer incidence rates for each site among residents of the South Thames Cancer Registry area were taken from published tables (Payne, 1976) for the period 1967-1971; these rates were similar to those for the entire study period, 1961-1976. Woman-years at risk were accumulated within five-year age groups for all women in the study. Expected numbers of second tumours at each site were then calculated by multiplying the total woman-years at risk in each age group by the female age-specific incidence rate for that tumour. The statistical significance of the difference between the observed and the expected numbers of second tumours at a particular site was calculated by assuming the observed number to be drawn from a Poisson distribution with mean equal to the expected number. Statistical tests were one-sided, in the direction of the observed difference.

Results

The results of our analyses are shown in Tables 2A, B, C, in a format similar to that of other contributions to this publication.

Table 2. Observed and expected numbers of second primary cancers in women diagnosed with primary cervical cancer in the South Thames area

A. Cases of invasive cervical cancer treated by radiotherapy

TIME SINCE DIAGNOSIS OF PRIMARY CERVICAL CANCER (IN YEARS)

Number of women starting intervals		<1			1-4			5-9			10-14			15-16									Total (excl. <1)		
		6110			4510			2030			959			127									4510		
ICD7	ICD8	O	O'	E	O	O'	E	O	O'	E	O	O'	E	O	O'	E							O	O'	E
140	140			0.02			0.04			0.03			0.01			0.00										0.08
141	141			0.07	1		0.16			0.11			0.05			0.00							1		0.32
142	142			0.08			0.19	1		0.12			0.04			0.00							1		0.35
143-4	143-5			0.09			0.21			0.15			0.06			0.00									0.42
145,7-8	146,8-9			0.12			0.27			0.19			0.08			0.00									0.54
146	147			0.03			0.08			0.05			0.02			0.01									0.15
150	150			0.39	1		0.90			0.66			0.28			0.04							3		1.85
151	151	1		1.38	2		3.12	2		2.32	1		1.00			0.01							6		6.48
152	152			0.07			0.16			0.11			0.04			0.01									0.32
153	153			2.30	1		5.23	1		3.79	2		1.57			0.05							8		10.64
154	154	1		1.19	5		2.72	5		1.97	2		0.81			0.03							10		5.53
155,0	155			0.08			0.18			0.13			0.05			0.00									0.36
155,1	156			0.23			0.52			0.38			0.16			0.01									1.07
157	157			0.80	2		1.83	1		1.34	1		0.56			0.02							3		3.75
160	160			0.06			0.14			0.13			0.04			0.00									0.31
161	161			0.09			0.22			0.15			0.06			0.00									0.43
162-3	162-3	1		2.43	20		5.61	13		3.91	1		1.54			0.05							34		11.11
170	174	13		7.04	12		15.91	10		10.56	2		3.85			0.11							24		30.43
172	182,0	3		1.34			3.07	1		2.09			0.80			0.02							1		5.98
173-4	181,2.9			0.00			0.00			0.00			0.00			0.00									0.00
175	183	2		1.67	1		3.82	2		2.57			0.96			0.03							3		7.38
176	184			0.26	1		0.59			0.43			0.18			0.01							2		1.21
180	189,0-,1	1		0.29	2		0.65	1		0.46			0.19			0.01							2		1.31
181	188			0.72	4		1.65			1.20	2		0.50			0.02							7		3.37
190	172	3		0.30			0.66			0.41			0.14			0.00									1.21
191	173	5		2.37	3		5.38	4		3.80	3		1.52			0.05							10		10.75
192	190			0.05			0.13	1		0.63			0.03			0.00							1		0.25
193	191-2			0.43			0.97			0.24			0.22			0.01									1.83
194	193			0.16			0.35			0.09			0.09			0.00									0.68
195	194			0.04			0.09			0.09			0.02			0.00									0.16
196	170			0.06			0.13			0.13			0.04			0.00									0.26
197	171			0.08	1		0.18	1		0.47			0.05			0.00							1		0.36
200,202	200,202			0.30			0.68			0.19			0.19			0.01									1.35
201	201			0.13			0.28			0.07			0.07			0.00									0.54
203	203			0.25			0.57			0.41			0.17			0.01									1.16
204,0	204,1,9	1		0.16			0.36			0.27			0.11			0.00							1		0.74
204,1-4	204,0.5-7			0.28	2		0.64	1		0.44			0.17			0.01							3		1.26
204	204-207	1		0.44	3		1.00	1		0.71			0.28			0.01							4		2.00
TOTAL		31		25.36	59		57.69	48		40.07	15		15.67			0.51							122		113.94

O : All tumours
O': Histologically confirmed
E : Expected

B. Cases of invasive cervical cancer not treated by radiotherapy

TIME SINCE DIAGNOSIS OF PRIMARY CERVICAL CANCER (IN YEARS)

ICD7	ICD8	<1 (2252) O	O'	E	1-4 (874) O	O'	E	5-9 (559) O	O'	E	10-14 (272) O	O'	E	15-16 (37) O	O'	E	Total (excl. <1) (874) O	O'	E
140	140			0.00			0.01			0.01			0.00			0.00			0.02
141	141			0.01			0.02			0.02			0.01			0.00			0.05
142	142			0.01			0.04	1		0.03			0.01			0.00	1		0.08
143-4	143-5			0.01			0.03			0.03			0.01			0.00			0.07
145,7-8	146,8-9			0.02			0.04			0.04			0.01			0.00			0.09
146	147			0.00			0.01			0.01			0.01			0.00			0.03
150	150			0.05			0.12			0.10			0.04			0.00			0.26
151	151			0.19			0.40			0.35			0.14			0.01			0.90
152	152			0.01			0.02			0.02			0.01			0.00			0.05
153	153			0.31	1		0.72	1		0.64			0.26			0.01	2		1.63
154	154			0.16			0.37			0.34			0.14			0.01			0.86
155.0	155			0.01			0.03			0.03			0.01			0.00			0.07
155.1	156			0.03			0.07			0.06			0.02			0.00			0.15
157	157			0.11			0.24			0.22			0.09			0.00			0.55
160	160			0.01			0.02			0.02			0.01			0.00			0.05
161	161			0.01			0.03			0.03			0.01			0.00			0.07
162-3	162-3	2		0.32	1		0.80	4		0.76			0.30			0.01	5		1.87
170	174	1		1.11	3		3.01	4		2.65			0.91			0.03	7		6.60
172	182.0			0.18			0.48			0.46			0.18			0.01			1.13
173-4	181,2.9			0.00			0.00			0.00			0.00			0.00			0.00
175	183	1		0.24	1		0.66			0.61			0.22			0.01	1		1.50
176	184			0.04			0.08			0.07			0.03			0.00			0.18
180	189.0-.1	1		0.10			0.10			0.09			0.03			0.00			0.22
181	188	1		0.06			0.22			0.20			0.08			0.00			0.50
190	172			0.33			0.16			0.13			0.04			0.00			0.33
191	173			0.01	1		0.82	2		0.73			0.28			0.01	3		1.84
192	190			0.07			0.02			0.02			0.01			0.00			0.05
193	191-2			0.03			0.18			0.16			0.06			0.00			0.40
194	193			0.01			0.06			0.05			0.02			0.00			0.13
195	194			0.01			0.02			0.02			0.01			0.00			0.05
196	170			0.01			0.03			0.02			0.01			0.00			0.06
197	171			0.04	1		0.03	1		0.03			0.01			0.00	2		0.07
200,202	200,202			0.02			0.11			0.09			0.04			0.00			0.24
201	201			0.03			0.06			0.05			0.02			0.00			0.13
203	203			0.02			0.07			0.07			0.03			0.00			0.17
204.0	204.1..9			0.04	1		0.05			0.05			0.02			0.00	1		0.12
204.1-4	204.0.5-7			0.06			0.11			0.09			0.03			0.00			0.23
204	204-207				1		0.16			0.14			0.05			0.00	1		0.35
TOTAL		5		3.65	10		9.24	13		8.30			3.11			0.10	23		20.75

O : All tumours
O': Histologically confirmed
E : Expected

C. Cases of carcinoma in situ not treated by radiotherapy

TIME SINCE DIAGNOSIS OF PRIMARY CERVICAL CANCER (IN YEARS)

Number of women starting intervals		<1 (3774)			1–4 (3231)			5–9 (2079)			10–14 (571)			15–16 (36)			Total (excl. <1) (3231)		
ICD7	ICD8	O	O'	E	O	O'	E	O	O'	E	O	O'	E	O	O'	E	O	O'	E
140	140			0.00			0.01			0.01			0.00			0.00			0.02
141	141			0.01	1		0.05			0.05			0.01			0.01	1		0.11
142	142			0.03			0.12			0.09			0.02			0.02			0.23
143–4	143–5			0.02			0.07			0.08			0.01			0.01			0.14
145,7–8	146,8–9			0.02			0.09			0.03			0.02			0.02			0.19
146	147			0.01			0.04			0.03			0.01			0.00			0.08
150	150			0.05	1		0.19	3		0.20			0.04			0.00	4		0.43
151	151			0.17			0.66			0.64			0.14			0.00			1.44
152	152			0.01	2		0.05			0.05			0.01			0.00	2		0.11
153	153	1		0.35	2		1.37			1.32			0.27			0.01	2		2.97
154	154			0.18			0.71			0.69			0.15			0.00			1.55
155.0	155			0.02	1		0.06			0.06			0.01			0.00	1		0.13
155.1	156			0.03			0.12			0.12			0.02			0.00			0.26
157	157			0.10			0.41			0.42			0.09			0.00			0.92
160	160			0.01			0.04	1		0.04	1		0.01			0.00	1		0.09
161	161			0.02			0.08			0.07			0.02			0.00			0.17
162–3	162–3			0.41			1.66	6		1.64			0.35			0.01	7		3.66
170	174			2.24	9		8.29	9		7.05			1.24			0.02	18		16.60
172	182.0			0.27			1.09			1.07			0.23			0.00			2.39
173–4	181,2.9			0.00			0.01			0.00			0.00			0.00			0.01
175	183			0.45	1		1.70	3		1.52			0.29			0.01	4		3.52
176	184			0.04	3		0.16	1		0.15			0.03			0.00	4		0.34
180	189.0–1	3		0.06			0.22			0.20			0.04			0.00			0.46
181	188			0.10	2		0.38			0.38			0.09			0.00			0.85
188	172			0.17	1		0.55	1		0.39			0.06			0.00	2		1.00
190	173			0.47			1.80			1.66	1		0.33			0.00	2		3.80
191	190			0.02			0.06			0.05			0.01			0.00			0.12
192	191–2			0.16			0.54	1		0.43			0.08			0.00			1.05
193	193			0.06			0.19			0.14			0.02			0.00			0.35
194	194			0.02			0.07			0.05			0.01			0.00			0.13
195	170			0.02			0.07			0.06			0.01			0.00			0.14
196	171			0.03			0.09			0.07			0.01			0.00			0.17
197				0.07			0.26			0.22			0.04			0.00			0.52
200,202	200,202			0.07	1		0.22			0.14			0.02			0.00	1		0.38
201	201			0.03	1		0.13			0.13			0.03			0.00	1		0.29
203	203			0.03			0.10			0.09			0.02			0.00			0.21
204.0	204.1,.9	1		0.09	2		0.29	2		0.23			0.04			0.00	3		0.56
204.1–4	204.0,5–7	1		0.12	1		0.39	2		0.32			0.06			0.00	3		0.77
204	204–207																		
TOTAL		5		5.84	27		21.95	27		19.60	2		3.78			0.06	56		45.39

O : All tumours
O': Histologically confirmed
E : Expected

Among patients with invasive cancer treated with radiotherapy, there were 122 second tumours at all sites, a 7% excess over the expected number (113.9), although the difference is not statistically significant (Table 2A). The only sites at which there were significant excesses of second primary cancers were lung (34 observed, 11.1 expected; $p < 0.001$) and bladder (7 observed, 3.4 expected; $p = 0.06$); for both of these sites there was evidence of a substantial excess within five years of radiotherapy, suggesting that the effect may not have been due to radiation. Four women developed leukaemia, whereas only 2.0 would have been expected.

Among women with invasive cancer not treated with radiotherapy (Table 2B), there were 23 second primary cancers at all sites, compared with 20.8 expected. No patient developed cancer of the bladder, but five (1.9 expected; $p = 0.04$) developed cancer of the lung.

Among women with in-situ cancer who were not treated with radiotherapy (Table 2C), there were 56 second cancers at all sites (45.4 expected). There were slight excesses of lung cancer (7 observed, 3.7 expected) and stomach cancer (4 observed, 1.4 expected; $p = 0.06$) and marked excesses of leukaemia (3 observed, 0.8 expected; $p = 0.04$) and 'other female genital' tumours (4 observed, 0.3 expected; $p < 0.001$). Three of the four tumours in this last group occurred within five years of diagnosis of in-situ carcinoma.

In none of the three groups of patients was there a notable excess of breast cancer. Among women with invasive cancer not treated with radiotherapy, there was evidence of a differential incidence of second breast cancers according to their age at treatment of the cervical cancer (Table 3). Among women first treated at age 50 or more, there were five breast cancers (2.6 expected), while among women first treated at less than 50 years of age, there were fewer breast cancers than expected (2 observed, 3.96 expected). These differences are not statistically significant, and no similar difference was apparent among women treated with radiotherapy for invasive cancer, or among those with in-situ cancer.

The computations of woman-years at risk were performed using a computer programme kindly supplied by Julian Peto.

Reference

Payne, P. (1976) *UK, England, South Metropolitan Region*. In: Waterhouse, J., Muir, C., Correa, P. & Powell, J., eds, *Cancer Incidence in Five Continents*, Volume III (*IARC Scientific Publications No. 15*), Lyon, International Agency for Research on Cancer, pp. 388-395

Table 3. Breast cancer in women in the South Thames area by age at diagnosis of cervical cancer, stage and treatment

TIME SINCE DIAGNOSIS OF PRIMARY CERVICAL CANCER (IN YEARS)

INVASIVE — RADIOTHERAPY

Age	<1 O	<1 E	1–4 O	1–4 E	5–9 O	5–9 E	10–14 O	10–14 E	15–19 E	20–24 E	Total O	Total E
<30		0.00		0.02		0.02		0.01	0.00	0.00		0.05
30–39		0.17		0.60	1	0.73		0.40	0.01		1	1.74
40–49	2	1.39	5	3.68	1	2.90	1	1.09	0.02		7	7.69
50–59	5	2.11	4	4.96	3	3.32		1.28	0.04		7	9.59
60–69	4	1.93	2	4.24	3	2.53	1	0.90	0.04		6	7.70
70+	2	1.43	1	2.42	2	1.05		0.18	0.00		3	3.65

INVASIVE — OTHER THERAPY

Age	<1 O	<1 E	1–4 O	1–4 E	5–9 O	5–9 E	10–14 O	10–14 E	15–19 E	Total O	Total E
<30		0.00		0.02		0.03		0.02	0.00		0.07
30–39		0.07	1	0.30		0.43		0.19	0.00	1	0.92
40–49	1	0.37		1.28	1	1.26		0.41	0.02	1	2.97
50–59	1	0.27		0.76	3	0.56		0.20	0.00	3	1.51
60–69	1	0.21		0.40	1	0.27		0.09	0.00	1	0.76
70+	1	0.19		0.26		0.10		0.00	0.00		0.36

IN SITU — OTHER THERAPY

Age	<1 O	<1 E	1–4 O	1–4 E	5–9 O	5–9 E	10–14 E	15–19 E	Total O	Total E
<30		0.03	1	0.18		0.21	0.05	0.00	1	0.44
30–39	2	0.40	2	1.71	2	1.90	0.41	0.01	4	4.03
40–49	3	1.13	3	4.22	5	3.52	0.60	0.01	8	8.35
50–59	3	0.48	2	1.58	3	1.04	0.14	0.00	5	2.76
60–69		0.15		0.44		0.25	0.04	0.00		0.73
70+		0.06		0.16		0.12	0.00	0.00		0.28

O: All tumours
O': Histologically confirmed
E: Expected

THE CONNECTICUT TUMOR REGISTRY

J.T. Flannery

Connecticut Tumor Registry
Hartford, CT, USA

J.D. Boice, Jr & R.A. Kleinerman

Radiation Studies Section
Environmental Epidemiology Branch
National Cancer Institute
Bethesda, MD, USA

R.E. Curtis

Biometry Branch
National Cancer Institute
Bethesda, MD, USA

The Connecticut Tumor Registry was established in 1941 within the Connecticut State Department of Health Services. It includes records on all malignant neoplasms diagnosed in residents of Connecticut since 1935. The population of Connecticut is approximately 3.1 million, with 93% white and 7% non-white people. All hospitals in Connecticut routinely report to the Registry information on all newly diagnosed cancers as well as annual follow-up information on previously reported cases. In addition, Registry staff visit selected out-of-state hospitals and abstract cancer data on Connecticut residents admitted to those institutions for diagnosis and/or treatment. Death certificates that list cancer as a cause of death are also reviewed and used to find cases. There are currently 371 000 cases in the Registry. All patients are followed annually from diagnosis to death, and of the 87 000 individuals under active follow-up, less than 5% are lost.

The Registry maintains stringent quality control internally to avoid duplication of case reporting and data errors. Quality control measures range from recording of samples of records to sophisticated data processing-editing procedures. Quality control efforts at the hospital level include cancer case-finding audits and reabstracting projects. Currently, the guidelines of the SEER (Surveillance, Epidemiology and End Results) Program of the National Cancer Institute (USA) are being followed to judge whether a new lesion should be considered a second primary cancer. Multiple lesions of different histological types occurring in different sites are considered to be separate primary cancers, whether they occur simultaneously or at different times.

Multiple lesions of the same histological type occurring at different sites are considered to be separate primary cancers unless stated to be metastatic by the reporting physician.

Of 8247 women with a primary diagnosis of invasive cancer of the cervix uteri diagnosed between 1935 and 1978, 1120 were excluded from this analysis because of identification by death certificate or autopsy only (349), unknown treatment category (442), the occurrence of a second primary cancer within three months of the diagnosis of cervical cancer (48), survival or follow-up less than three months (236) and incomplete follow-up (45). Incidence of second primary cancer was evaluated in 7127 women. Histological confirmation was available for 96% of the cervical cancers and for 85% of all second primary cancers. At the closing date of the study, 31 December 1978, 65% of the cervical cancer patients had died. Overall, 84% of the women received some radiation treatment. Radiation treatment was by external beam (22%), radium implant (20%) or a combination of both (58%). The non-irradiated group included women who had had surgery alone (52%), surgery and chemotherapy or hormones (46%), or chemotherapy or hormones or both (1%). The mean age of the group that received radiotherapy was 53 years at the time of treatment, in contrast to 45 years for the non-irradiated group. Maximum follow-up was 38 years for both groups. The women who received radiotherapy contributed 45 400 woman-years of observation, and the women who did not receive radiotherapy accumulated 11 000 woman-years.

A sample of medical records of 622 women with invasive cervical cancer treated in Connecticut indicated that 4% of the women never married, 11% were nulliparous, 10% had six or more children, and 43% of those who had children gave birth before age 20. The average weight at diagnosis was 140 lbs (63.5 kg), and the average height was 62 inches (1.57 m); 33% received surgical treatment, 34% were known to have had a hysterectomy, and 7% were known to have taken oestrogens.

Among 5997 women with invasive tumours treated by radiation, 398 had developed second primary cancers by one year after treatment, compared with 286 expected (relative risk, 1.4). The excess incidence was attributable to cancers of the lung (59 versus 11.7), bladder (23 versus 7.1), kidney (13 versus 4.8), uterine corpus (32 versus 20.4) and rectum (29 versus 16.7). The excess of cancers of the bladder (9 versus 2.8), kidney (9 versus 1.7) and rectum (16 versus 5.5) observed 15 or more years after radiotherapy is consistent with the expected long latent period for radiation-induced solid tumours. Despite the large radiation dose received by the pelvic bone marrow, only a slight excess of leukaemia was observed (9 versus 6.7). An excess of cancer of the uterine corpus (13 versus 6.5) and ovary (10 versus 4.1) which occurred 15 years after treatment is consistent with a radiation etiology; however, metastases to these sites may account for a portion of the excess. Among 1130 women with invasive tumours not treated by radiation, a slight excess of cancer was also observed (69 versus 57); the excess was due primarily to breast cancer (26 versus 17). In contrast, a deficit of breast cancer occurred in the irradiated group (54 versus 78), due possibly to radiation-induced menopause or to reproductive factors (e.g., early first pregnancy) that may be protective.

The incidence of second primary cancers was also evaluated in 7260 women diagnosed with in-situ cervical cancer during the same time period. The mean age at diagnosis of in-situ cervical cancer was 37 years, and 54 000 woman-years of observation were accrued. Overall, 223 second primary cancers were diagnosed at least one year after treatment, whereas 166 cancers were expected (relative risk, 1.3). The excess was attributable mainly to cancers of the lung (26 versus 9.7), other genital tumours (28 versus 3.4), kidney tumours (8 versus 2.3), and non-Hodgkin's lymphoma (7 versus 1.6). No excess of leukaemia was observed (4 versus 3.3); the number of breast cancers was as expected (61 versus 63); and no striking deficit of cancer at any site occurred.

Table 1. Connecticut Tumor Registry: Characteristics of the population under study

	Invasive tumours			*In situ* (no radiotherapy)	Total
	Radiotherapy	No radiotherapy	Total invasive		
Number of women	5 997	1 130	7 127	7 260	14 387
Woman-years at risk by time since diagnosis:					
<1 year	5 257	1 064	6 321	6 908	13 229
1-4 years	12 896	3 152	16 048	21 057	37 105
5-9 years	10 548	2 658	13 206	14 894	28 100
10-14 years	7 205	1 849	9 054	7 128	16 182
15-19 years	4 698	1 282	5 980	2 901	8 881
20-24 years	2 714	686	3 400	927	4 327
25-29 years	1 344	262	1 606	204	1 810
30+ years	730	88	818	21	839
Total	45 392	11 041	56 433	54 040	110 473
Number of women by age at diagnosis:					
<45	438	233	671	3 461	4 132
45-54	1 273	371	1 644	2 258	3 902
55-64	1 640	283	1 923	1 001	2 924
65-74	1 486	156	1 642	357	1 999
75-84	1 160	87	1 247	183	1 430
Number of women excluded because of:					
- second cancer (excluding non-melanoma skin) diagnosed simultaneously with cervical cancer	36	9	45	37	82
- cervical cancer diagnosed by autopsy or death certificate			349	5	354
- missing information on treatment			442	0	442
- survival for less than three months	190	46	236	221	457
- insufficient follow-up			45	224	269

Table 2. Observed and expected numbers of second primary cancers in women diagnosed with primary cervical cancer in Connecticut

A. Cases of invasive cervical cancer treated by radiotherapy

TIME SINCE DIAGNOSIS OF PRIMARY CERVICAL CANCER (IN YEARS)

ICD7	ICD8	<1 (5997) O	O'	E	1-4 (4518) O	O'	E	5-9 (2580) O	O'	E	10-14 (1736) O	O'	E	15-19 (1176) O	O'	E	20-24 (727) O	O'	E	25-29 (386) O	O'	E	30+ (180) O	O'	E	Total (excl. <1) O	O'	E
140	140			0.03			0.08			0.07			0.06			0.04			0.03			0.01			0.01	1	1	0.30
141	141			0.09	1	1	0.26	1	1	0.25			0.22			0.17			0.11			0.07			0.04	1	1	1.12
142	142			0.08	1	1	0.21	1	1	0.18			0.14			0.10			0.07			0.04			0.03	4	4	0.77
143-4	143-5			0.14	1	1	0.38	1	1	0.38	2	2	0.32	2	2	0.25			0.17			0.10			0.06	5	5	1.66
145,7-8	146,8-9			0.09			0.26			0.25			0.20	1	1	0.16			0.10			0.04			0.02	5	5	1.03
146	147			0.02			0.06			0.05			0.04			0.03			0.02			0.01			0.01	1	1	0.22
150	150	1		0.20	2	2	0.40	1	1	0.40	1	1	0.40	1	1	0.30			0.20			0.10			0.10	5	5	1.90
151	151	3	3	1.40	2	2	3.40	2	2	3.10	6	4	2.40	2	2	1.80	3		1.20	1	1	0.70			0.40	16	10	13.00
152	152			0.08			0.21	1	1	0.20	1	1	0.17			0.12			0.08			0.05			0.03	2	2	0.86
153	153	3		3.40	5	3	9.40	7	7	9.10	12	11	8.40	8	8	6.30	4	3	4.50	3	3	2.70	2	1	1.80	44	34	42.20
154	154	1		1.50	3	3	4.10	5	5	3.90	4	3	3.20	9	9	2.40			1.60	1	1	0.90	2	1	0.60	29	22	16.70
155,0	155			0.16			0.16			0.33	1	1	0.25			0.19			0.13			0.07			0.05	3	3	1.42
155,1	156			0.43			1.15	2	2	1.12			0.95	2	2	0.74	1	1	0.52			0.30			0.20	6	6	4.98
157	157			0.70	2	2	2.00	2	1	1.90			1.60			1.30			1.00			0.60			0.40	10	10	8.80
160	160			0.06	2	2	0.14			0.13			0.10			0.80			0.05			0.03			0.02	3	3	1.27
161	161			0.08	2	2	0.22	1	1	0.21	1	1	0.17	2	2	0.13			0.09			0.04			0.02	3	3	0.88
162-3	162-3	5	3	0.90	18	15	2.60	17	11	2.60	16	14	2.30	6	4	1.80	1	1	1.30	1	1	0.70	1	1	0.40	59	46	11.70
170	174	4	4	7.80	17	16	20.80	11	10	19.10	12	12	14.80	5	5	10.70	6	4	6.90	1	1	3.80	1	1	2.30	55	51	78.40
172	182.0,	1	1	1.80	3	3	5.00	10	9	4.85	6	6	4.02	5	5	3.01	4	4	1.91	2	1	1.01	3	2	0.56	32	31	20.36
173-4	181,2,9	1	1	0.71	1	1	1.71	1	1	1.42	1	1	0.90			0.49	1	1	0.29			0.09			0.04	5	5	4.94
175	183	2	2	1.50	4	4	4.10	6	6	3.60	3	3	2.70	3	3	1.90	2	2	1.20	2	2	0.60	3	3	0.40	23	23	14.50
176	184	1		1.10	5	5	2.70	3	3	2.20	4	3	1.60	1	1	1.10	5	5	1.20	1	1	0.60			0.30	18	17	9.70
180	189.0-.1	1	1	0.39	3	3	1.08			1.05	1	1	0.87	1	1	0.68	1	1	0.47			0.27			0.16	13	12	4.58
181	188	3	3	0.60	3	2	1.50	2	2	1.50	7	7	1.30	3	2	1.10	2	2	0.80	2	2	0.50	2	2	0.40	23	19	7.10
190	172	1	1	0.30	2	2	0.70	4		0.70			0.50			0.40	1		0.30			0.10			0.10	2	2	2.80
191	173																											
192	190			0.06	1	1	0.16			0.14	1		0.11			0.08			0.06			0.03			0.01	1	1	0.59
193	191-2			0.30	2	2	0.90			0.80	3	3	0.60	1	1	0.40			0.30			0.10	3	3	0.10	3	3	3.20
194	193			0.24			0.63			0.58			0.43			0.30			0.18			0.10	2	2	0.05			2.27
195	194			0.02			0.05			0.04			0.03			0.02			0.01			0.00			0.00			0.15
196	170			0.07	1	1	0.18	1	1	0.15	1	1	0.11	1	1	0.08	1	1	0.05			0.02			0.01	1	1	0.60
197	171			0.14	1	1	0.37	1	1	0.33	1	1	0.25	1	1	0.18			0.12			0.06			0.04	2	2	1.35
200,202	200,202	1	1	0.40	5	4	1.10	2	2	0.80	3	3	0.90	1	1	0.80	1	1	0.60	2	2	0.50			0.30	12	11	5.00
201	201			0.20	1	1	0.50	1	1	0.50			0.40			0.30	1	1	0.20	1	1	0.10			0.10	4	3	2.10
203	203			0.22	1	1	0.64			0.64	1	1	0.59	1	1	0.37			0.37			0.24			0.16	3	3	3.14
204,0	204.1,9			0.13	1	1	0.36	3	3	0.37	1	1	0.35	1	1	0.30			0.22	3	3	0.14			0.06	3	3	1.80
204,1-4	204,0,5-7			0.50	1	1	1.10	3	3	1.10	1	1	1.00	1	1	0.70	1		0.50			0.30			0.20	6	6	4.90
204	204-207			0.60	1	1	1.50	3	3	1.50	2	2	1.30	3	2	1.00	2	1	0.70			0.40			0.30	9	8	6.70
TOTAL		28	22	25.81	95	79	68.89	88	74	64.07	87	81	52.33	55	46	39.67	37	29	26.83	17	16	14.98	20	19	9.52	399	344	276.29

O : All tumours
O': Histologically confirmed
E : Expected.

B. Cases of invasive cervical cancer not treated by radiotherapy

TIME SINCE DIAGNOSIS OF PRIMARY CERVICAL CANCER (IN YEARS)

Number of women starting intervals		<1 1130			1–4 998			5–9 670			10–14 442			15–19 313			20–24 189			25–29 83			30+ 24			Total (excl. <1)		
ICD7	ICD8	O	O'	E	O	O'	E	O	O'	E	O	O'	E	O	O'	E	O	O'	E	O	O'	E	O	O'	E	O	O'	E :
140	140			0.00			0.02			0.01			0.01			0.01			0.01			0.00			0.00			0.06
141	141			0.01			0.05	1		0.05			0.05			0.05			0.03			0.01			0.01	1	1	0.25
142	142			0.01			0.04			0.03			0.03			0.02			0.02			0.01			0.00			0.15
143–4	143–5			0.02			0.07			0.08			0.07			0.07	1	1	0.04			0.02			0.01	1	1	0.36
145,7–8	146,8–9			0.02			0.05			0.06	1	1	0.06			0.04			0.03			0.01			0.00	1	1	0.25
146	147			0.00			0.01			0.01	1	1	0.01			0.01			0.00			0.00			0.00	1	1	0.04
150	150			0.02			0.10	1	1	0.10			0.10			0.10			0.04			0.02			0.01			0.47
151	151			0.10			0.50	1		0.40			0.40	1	1	0.30			0.20			0.10			0.10	2	2	2.00
152	152			0.01			0.03			0.03			0.03	2	2	0.03			0.02			0.01			0.00	1	1	0.15
153	153			0.40	1	1	1.40	3	3	1.50	1		1.50			1.40	1	1	1.00			0.50			0.20	9	7	7.50
154	154			0.20	3	3	0.60	1	1	0.70			0.60			0.50	1	1	0.40			0.20			0.10	5	3	3.10
155.0	155			0.02	2	1	0.05	1	1	0.05			0.04			0.04	1	1	0.03			0.01			0.01	1	1	0.23
155.1	156			0.04			0.15			0.16			0.15			0.14			0.10			0.05			0.02	1	1	0.77
157	157			0.10			0.30			0.30			0.30			0.30			0.20			0.10			0.04			1.54
160	160			0.01			0.03			0.03			0.02			0.02			0.01			0.01			0.00			0.12
161	161	1	1	0.01			0.05			0.05	1	1	0.05			0.04			0.03			0.01			0.00	2	2	0.23
162–3	162–3	1	1	0.10	12	12	0.50	3	3	0.50	1	1	0.60	1	1	0.50			0.40			0.20			0.10	2	1	2.80
170	174			1.20			4.20	3	3	4.20	5	5	3.50	2	2	2.80	5	5	1.70			0.70			0.20	26	26	17.30
172	182.0,			0.26			0.95			1.03			0.96			0.85			0.53			0.21	1	1	0.07			4.60
173–4	181,2.9			0.04	4	4	0.25			0.17			0.14			0.05			0.07			0.01			0.03			0.72
175	183			0.20			0.80	1	1	0.80			0.60			0.50			0.30			0.10			0.10	2	2	3.20
176	184	2	2	0.10			0.50	1	1	0.40			0.30	1	1	0.20			0.10			0.10			0.10	6	6	1.70
180	189.0–.1			0.05			0.17			0.19			0.17			0.16			0.11			0.05			0.04	2	2	0.87
181	188			0.10			0.20			0.30			0.30			0.30			0.20			0.10			0.02			1.44
190	172			0.10			0.20	1	1	0.20			0.10			0.10	1	1	0.10			0.03			0.01	2	2	0.74
191	173																											0.12
192	190																											0.72
193	191–2			0.05	1	1	0.17			0.17			0.15			0.12			0.07			0.03	1	1	0.01	1	1	0.54
194	193			0.05			0.15			0.14			0.10			0.08			0.04			0.02			0.01			0.04
195	194			0.00			0.01			0.01			0.01			0.01			0.00			0.00			0.00			0.04
196	170			0.01			0.03			0.03			0.02			0.02			0.01			0.01			0.00			0.11
197	171			0.02	1	1	0.08	1		0.07			0.05			0.04			0.02			0.01			0.00	1	1	0.27
200,202	200,202			0.10			0.20			0.20			0.20			0.20			0.10			0.10			0.10	1	2	1.10
201	201			0.04	1	1	0.10			0.10			0.10			0.10			0.10			0.02			0.01	2	2	0.53
203	203			0.03			0.10			0.10			0.10			0.10			0.10			0.10			0.03			0.63
204.0	204.1,.9			0.02			0.06			0.06			0.06			0.06			0.05			0.02			0.01			0.32
204.1–4	204.0,5–7			0.08	1	1	0.24			0.24			0.14			0.14			0.15			0.08			0.03	1	1	1.02
204	204–207			0.10	1	1	0.30			0.30			0.20			0.20			0.20			0.10			0.04	1	1	1.34
TOTAL		4	4	3.53	26	25	12.39	15	12	12.50	10	9	11.04	5	5	9.42	10	10	6.32			2.95	2	2	1.37	68	63	55.99

O : All tumours
O' : Histologically confirmed
E : Expected

C. Cases of carcinoma in situ not treated by radiotherapy

TIME SINCE DIAGNOSIS OF PRIMARY CERVICAL CANCER (IN YEARS)

		<1 (7260)			1-4 (6553)			5-9 (4131)			10-14 (2058)			15-19 (944)			20-24 (335)			25-29 (92)			30+ (12)			Total (excl. <1)		
ICD7	ICD8	O	O'	E	O	O'	E	O	O'	E	O	O'	E	O	O'	E	O	O'	E	O	O'	E	O	O'	E	O	O'	E
140	140			0.01			0.05	1		0.03			0.03			0.02			0.01			0.01			0.00			0.15
141	141			0.05	1		0.22	1		0.24	1	1	0.17			0.10			0.04			0.00			0.00	2	2	0.78
142	142			0.05	1	1	0.18			0.16			0.10			0.05			0.02			0.01			0.00	1	1	0.51
143-4	143-5			0.07	1		0.29	2	2	0.34			0.26			0.14	1	1	0.06			0.01			0.01	4	4	1.10
145,7-8	146,8-9			0.05	3	3	0.21			0.25			0.20	1	1	0.11			0.04			0.00			0.00	4	4	0.82
146	147			0.01			0.04			0.04			0.03			0.02			0.01			0.00			0.00			0.14
150	150			0.01	4	4	0.20	2	2	0.30	2	2	0.20			0.10			0.10			0.10			0.01	1	1	0.90
151	151			0.30			1.10			1.10	5	5	0.80	1	1	0.50			0.20			0.01			0.10	9	9	3.81
152	152			0.04	6	6	0.13	3	3	0.14	2	2	0.10			0.05			0.02			0.30			0.01			0.45
153	153			1.10	7	7	4.50	4	4	4.90			3.90	4	4	2.30	2	2	1.10	1	1	1.10			0.30	20	19	17.10
154	154			0.50	3	3	1.90	1	1	2.10			1.60	1	1	0.90	2	2	0.40			0.40			0.10	10	10	7.02
155.0	155			0.04			0.40			0.20			0.10			0.10			0.03			0.03			0.01	1	1	0.64
155.1	156			0.10			0.10			0.40			0.30			0.20			0.10			0.10			0.03	1	1	1.44
157	157	1		0.20			0.80			1.00	1	1	0.80			0.50			0.30			0.10			0.10	1	1	3.51
160	160			0.03			0.11			0.11			0.07			0.04			0.02			0.00			0.00	1	1	0.35
161	161			0.06			0.31			0.27			0.19	1	1	0.10			0.04			0.10			0.01	1	1	0.93
162-3	162-3	5	5	0.60	8	8	2.50	8	7	3.00	6	6	2.30	2	2	1.30			0.50			0.60			0.10	26	23	9.71
170	174			5.10	18	18	20.00	21	21	20.40	10	10	13.20	5	5	6.30			2.30	1	1	0.18			0.00	57	57	62.80
172	182.0,			0.79			3.38			3.90			3.03			1.72			0.87			0.02			0.02			13.10
173-4	181,2.9			0.32			1.14			1.11			0.67			0.28			0.13			0.10			0.00			3.35
175	183	2	2	0.90	8	8	3.30	2	2	3.20	2	2	2.10	3	3	1.00			0.40			0.03			0.10	4	4	10.11
176	184	3	3	1.20	1	1	1.20	12	12	1.10	5	5	0.60			0.60			0.10			0.04			0.02	28	28	3.35
180	189.0—1	2	2	0.20	2	1	0.70	4	4	0.70	5	5	0.50			0.30			0.10			0.06	1	1	0.00	8	8	2.34
181	188	2	2	0.20	2	2	0.83			0.89	2	2	0.69			0.43			0.20			0.02			0.01	4	4	3.11
190	172	1	1	0.40	2	2	1.30	2	2	1.10	3	3	0.60			0.30	1	1	0.01			0.20			0.00	7	7	3.33
191	173																											
192	190	1	1	0.03			0.09			0.09			0.06			0.04			0.02			0.02			0.00	4	4	0.30
193	191-2	1	1	0.20	2	2	0.80	1	1	0.70			0.50			0.20	1	1	0.10			0.01			0.00	4	4	2.32
194	193			0.30	3	3	1.00			1.00			0.40			0.20			0.10			0.00			0.00	4	4	2.71
195	194			0.01			0.05			0.10			0.03			0.03			0.01			0.00			0.00			0.14
196	170			0.04			0.12			0.30			0.06			0.09			0.01			0.01			0.00			0.32
197	171			0.11	4	4	0.37	1	1	0.60			0.18			0.20			0.03			0.00			0.01	1	1	0.99
200,202	200,202			0.10	2	2	0.40	1	2	0.65	2	2	0.40	1	1	0.18			0.00	1		0.02			0.00	7	7	1.60
201	201			0.28	1	1	0.85	1	1	0.40	1	1	0.38	1	1	0.20			0.07			0.03			0.01	5	5	2.15
203	203			0.10			0.40	1	1	0.40			0.40			0.11			0.10			0.02			0.00	5	5	1.54
204.0	204.1,.9			0.05			0.18	1	1	0.21			0.17			0.29			0.05			0.03			0.00	1	1	0.74
204.1-4	204.0,5-7			0.25			0.82	2	2	0.79	1	1	0.43	1	1	0.40			0.15			0.05			0.01	3	3	2.52
204	204-207			0.30			1.00	2	2	1.00	1	1	0.60	1	1	0.60			0.20							4	4	3.26
TOTAL		16	16	13.80	70	67	50.07	71	70	51.87	45	45	35.55	22	22	18.71	7	7	7.73	3	2	1.99	1	1	0.26	219	214	166.18

Number of women starting intervals

O : All tumours
O' : Histologically confirmed
E : Expected

Table 3. Breast cancer in women in Connecticut by age at diagnosis of cervical cancer, stage and treatment

TIME SINCE DIAGNOSIS OF PRIMARY CERVICAL CANCER (IN YEARS)

(O' = Histologically confirmed; O = All tumours; E = Expected)

INVASIVE — RADIOTHERAPY

Age	<1 O'	<1 O	<1 E	1–4 O'	1–4 O	1–4 E	5–9 O'	5–9 O	5–9 E	10–14 O'	10–14 O	10–14 E	15–19 O'	15–19 O	15–19 E	20–24 O'	20–24 O	20–24 E	25–29 O'	25–29 O	25–29 E	30+ O'	30+ O	30+ E	Total O'	Total O	Total E
<30			0.01			0.04	1	1	0.10			0.10			0.20			0.20			0.10			0.10			0.84
30–39	3	3	0.30			1.30	2	2	2.10	2	2	2.30	1	1	1.90			1.30			0.80	1	1	0.70	6	6	10.40
40–49	2	2	1.60	2	2	4.80	2	2	5.10			4.50	2	2	3.60	1	3	2.70			1.80	3	3	1.10	10	12	23.60
50–59	1	1	2.30	8	8	6.30	6	6	5.70	6	6	4.30	1	1	3.20	3	3	2.00	1	1	0.90	3	3	0.30	24	25	22.70
60–69	1	1	2.10	3	3	5.30	1	1	4.40	3	3	3.10	1	1	1.70			0.70			0.20			0.10	8	8	15.50
70+		1	1.50		1	3.00	2	2	1.60	1	1	0.60			0.20			0.10			0.00			0.00	3	4	5.50

INVASIVE — NO RADIOTHERAPY

Age	<1 O'	<1 O	<1 E	1–4 O'	1–4 O	1–4 E	5–9 O'	5–9 O	5–9 E	10–14 O'	10–14 O	10–14 E	15–19 O'	15–19 O	15–19 E	20–24 O'	20–24 O	20–24 E	25–29 O'	25–29 O	25–29 E	30+ O'	30+ O	30+ E	Total O'	Total O	Total E
<30			0.01			0.04	1	1	0.10			0.10			0.10			0.10			0.03			0.01	1	1	0.48
30–39			0.01	2	2	0.60	2	2	0.90	1	1	0.90			0.70			0.40			0.20			0.10	5	5	3.80
40–49	4	4	0.40	4	4	1.50	2	2	1.60	2	2	1.30	1	1	1.20			0.90			0.40			0.20	9	9	7.10
50–59	1	1	0.30	3	3	1.40	4	4	1.00			0.80			0.60			0.40			0.10			0.00	7	7	4.30
60–69	2	2	0.20	1	1	0.60	1	1	0.50			0.30			0.20			0.10			0.04			0.00	2	2	1.74
70+	1	1	0.10	1	1	0.30	1	1	0.20			0.10			0.03			0.00			0.00			0.00	2	2	0.63

IN SITU

Age	<1 O'	<1 O	<1 E	1–4 O'	1–4 O	1–4 E	5–9 O'	5–9 O	5–9 E	10–14 O'	10–14 O	10–14 E	15–19 O'	15–19 O	15–19 E	20–24 O'	20–24 O	20–24 E	25–29 O'	25–29 O	25–29 E	30+ O'	30+ O	30+ E	Total O'	Total O	Total E
<30			0.10	1	1	0.60	1	1	0.80	1	1	0.70	1	1	0.40			0.20			0.04			0.00	4	4	2.74
30–39	1	1	1.00	6	6	5.00	8	8	6.70	3	3	5.00	3	3	2.50	1	1	0.80	1	1	0.10			0.01	22	22	20.11
40–49	3	3	2.20	4	4	8.60	8	8	8.40	3	3	5.00	1	1	2.20	1	1	0.90	1	1	0.10			0.04	18	18	25.20
50–59	3	3	1.00	4	4	3.50	4	4	2.90	1	1	1.70	1	1	1.00			0.30			0.10			0.00	10	10	9.51
60–69	2	2	0.50	2	2	1.60			1.30			0.70			0.30			0.10			0.00			0.00	2	2	4.00
70+	1	1	0.20			0.70	1	1	0.40			0.20			0.04			0.00			0.00			0.00	1	1	1.34

O : All tumours
O': Histologically confirmed
E : Expected

SECOND PRIMARY CANCERS AMONG 5446 WOMEN TREATED FOR CANCER OR CARCINOMA *IN SITU* OF THE CERVIX UTERI IN SLOVENIA 1950-1969

V. Pompe-Kirn, B. Ravnihar, M. Sok & M. Primic-Žakelj

Cancer Registry of Slovenia
Institute of Oncology
Ljubljana, Yugoslavia

Introduction

The Cancer Registry of Slovenia was founded in 1950 to provide continuing information on cancer incidence and on survival of cancer patients, to serve as a basis for planning and evaluating cancer control services and for epidemiological and clinical studies.

The main data sources are reports from hospital in- and out-patient departments; additional sources are autopsy protocols and death certificates. For cases brought to the attention of the Registry by death certificate only, additional information is required from the certifying physician. Registration is compulsory; reports are required for each admission or out-patient attendance. The follow-up is annual, for life and is an active one. If no follow-up information has been received, the Registry contacts the relevant regional health homes. When a patient has migrated, the Registry tends to trace him. The items coded for each cancer case are: date of diagnosis, primary site, histological diagnosis, stage of disease, methods of diagnosis, methods of treatment and status at discharge.

All reports for an individual are kept in folders which, labelled with a serial number, are filed by year of diagnosis, site and sex. Duplication, error and consistency are checked by procedures which include matching against an alphabetical index file and against a case folder file that contains information on patients already registered. Cancers and not patients count as units in the Registry, except multiple skin, colon and bladder carcinomas, which are counted as one case.

Cytology as a method of confirmation is widely used in Slovenia, especially for certain cancer sites, e.g., breast, lung and prostate. Thus, a great proportion of cases without histology are confirmed by cytology.

Second primary cancers are recorded only after a thorough review and check of all the available data on the first primary cancer, and by strictly respecting the relevant criteria. When there is any doubt, a case is not registered as a second cancer.

Information on first and subsequent cancer treatments is kept in the Registry's data bank. Since in Slovenia radiotherapy is almost completely centralized at the Institute of Oncology, Ljubljana, all the relevant records are available there.

The population of Slovenia was 1 514 971 in 1953, 1 619 300 in 1961 and 1 727 137 in 1971.

The incidence of cervix uterine cancer increased to 34/100 000 in the year 1962 and then began to decrease, reaching a rate of 17/100 000 in 1978. The incidence of in-situ cervical cancer reached its first peak in the period 1960-1964, with a rate of 14/100 000 and then declined; from 1972 it increased again, up to a rate of 18/100 000 in 1978.

Material and methods

As seen in Table 1, a total of 5446 women were included in the study - 4332 with invasive and 1114 with in-situ cervical cancer. They were diagnosed in the period 1950-1969 and were followed until the end of 1977. They accrued 56 892.83 woman-years at risk.

Table 1. Slovenia Cancer Registry: Characteristics of the population under study

	Invasive tumours			In situ (no radiotherapy)	Total
	Radiotherapy	No radiotherapy	Total invasive		
Number of women	2 942	1 390	4 332	1 114	5 446
Woman-years at risk by time since first treatment:					
<1 year	2 668.67	1 217.75	3 886.42	1 108.17	4 994.59
1-4 years	6 847.33	4 348.92	11 196.25	4 405.58	15 601.83
5-9 years	6 276.75	4 985.83	11 262.58	5 322.83	16 585.41
10-14 years	4 424.08	3 556.50	7 980.58	3 743.50	11 724.08
15-19 years	2 722.50	1 731.08	4 453.58	1 336.42	5 790.00
20-24 years	1 372.92	475.00	1 847.92	87.17	1 935.09
25-29 years	241.33	19.08	260.41	1.42	261.83
30+ years	-	-	-	-	-
All years	24 553.58	16 334.16	40 887.74	16 005.09	56 892.83
Number of women by age at diagnosis:					
<30	51	67	118	156	274
30-39	384	398	782	527	1 309
40-49	813	423	1 236	320	1 556
50-59	883	283	1 166	102	1 268
60-69	589	147	736	8	744
70+	222	72	294	1	295

All cervical cancer cases first diagnosed at autopsy or registered from a death certificate only were excluded; all patients who had had a malignancy prior to diagnosis of cervical cancer and all patients irradiated for in-situ cancer were also excluded.

There was no difficulty in classifying cases according to stage.

Histological confirmation was available for 90% of the invasive cervical cancer cases and for 100% of the in-situ cases. Of the total of 155 second primaries, 86% were histologically confirmed; and half of the cases not examined histologically were confirmed cytologically.

Of the patients with invasive cancer, 68% were irradiated during their first treatment, i.e., within four months after diagnosis. In accordance with the general rules accepted at the beginning of the study, these were the only patients who were considered to have had radiotherapy.

Radiation treatment techniques used at the Institute of Oncology in the study period 1950-1969 were as follows. Until 1962, the six-field X-ray technique was used, in addition to intracavitary treatment with radium; two anterior-posterior and posterior-anterior fields, with a 3-cm gap in the middle, and lateral fields, were used. From 1962 onwards, Co^{60} was used for most gynaecological treatments: source-skin distance, 60 or 70 cm; four fields; two anterior-posterior and two posterior-anterior fields 2 cm apart, as measured on the skin.

The expected number of second primaries was calculated at IARC, Lyon on the basis of age-specific cancer incidence rates for Slovenia, published in *Cancer Incidence in Five Continents* (Volumes I, II and III).

Results

The observed total incidence of second primary cancers was lower than expected in exposed and non-exposed patients with invasive cervical cancer and in those with in-situ cervical cancer.

For lung cancer, however, the relative risk was significantly higher in all three groups. In the group of exposed women with invasive cervical cancer, the relative risk was also higher for bladder cancer and myeloid leukaemia in the first ten years after diagnosis of cervical cancer.

The observed incidences of stomach and rectal cancer were lower in all three groups.

Discussion

The incidence of all second primaries was lower than expected in Slovenia. This phenomenon could be explained by the fact that the criteria for recording a malignancy as a second primary in the Cancer Registry of Slovenia are rather strict. As already mentioned, a case is recorded as a second primary only after thorough review and checking of all the available data on the first primary cancer, and respecting the relevant criteria. This may be the reason for the deficit of second primary cancers of the stomach, rectum and other genital organs (ICD8 184) in our material as compared with the incidence observed in the pooled data from all registries. As to the excess of lung cancers and the deficits of breast, ovary and corpus uteri cancers, we agree with the general comments given in the Summary Chapter.

Table 2. Observed and expected numbers of second primary cancers in women diagnosed with primary cervical cancer in Slovenia

A. Cases of invasive cervical cancer treated by radiotherapy

TIME SINCE DIAGNOSIS OF PRIMARY CERVICAL CANCER (IN YEARS)

ICD7	ICD8	<1 (2942) O	O'	E	1-4 (2352) O	O'	E	5-9 (1412) O	O'	E	10-14 (1065) O	O'	E	15-19 (700) O	O'	E	20-24 (412) O	O'	E	25-29 (153) O	O'	E	30+ O	O'	E	Total (excl. <1) O	O'	E
140	140			0.00			0.13			0.15			0.12			0.00			0.00			0.00			0.00			0.40
141	141			0.00			0.00			0.00			0.00			0.00			0.00			0.00			0.00			0.00
142	142			0.00			0.00			0.00			0.00			0.00			0.00			0.00			0.00			0.00
143-4	143-5																											
145,7-8	146,8-9																											
146	147																											
150	150			0.00	2		0.22	2		0.24	2	2	0.19	3	3	0.13									0.00	10	9	0.78
151	151			1.59	1		4.41	2	2	4.79	2	2	3.87	3	3	2.72	1	1	1.65	1	1	0.35			0.00			17.79
152	152			0.33	1		0.98			1.16			1.01	1		0.77			0.48			0.10			0.00	4	4	4.50
153	153			0.38	1		1.11			1.30			1.13			0.86			0.51			0.10			0.00	2	2	5.01
154	154			0.00	1		0.21			0.22			0.16			0.11			0.00			0.00			0.00			0.70
155,7-0	155			0.48			1.30	1		1.35			1.05	2	2	0.69			0.40			0.00			0.00	3	3	4.79
155,1	156			0.16			0.48			0.58			0.51			0.39			0.24			0.00			0.00			2.20
157	157			0.00	1		0.00			0.00			0.00			0.00			0.00			0.00			0.00	1		0.00
160	160																											
161	161			0.00																								
162-3	162-3	1	1	0.30	8	4	0.86	8	6	0.97	4	3	0.82	5	4	0.60	1		0.36			0.00			0.00	21	14	3.61
170	174	2	1	1.53	2	1	4.21	3	2	4.43	2	2	3.48			2.39	1		1.28			0.23			0.00	12	9	16.02
172,0	182.0	1	1	0.50	1		1.43			1.57			1.29			0.93			0.49			0.00			0.00			5.71
173-4	181,2.9																											
175	183			0.58	2		1.61			1.66			1.30	1	1	0.87			0.45			0.00			0.00	3	3	5.89
176	184			0.14			0.39	1		0.44	1		0.37			0.27			0.16			0.00			0.00	1	1	1.63
180	189,0-.1			0.00	2		0.27			0.30			0.25			0.19			0.11			0.00			0.00			1.12
181	188			0.00	2		0.22	1		0.29	1		0.27	1		0.21			0.13			0.00			0.00	3	3	1.12
190	172			0.00	1		0.24	1		0.27	1	1	0.21			0.14			0.00	1		0.00			0.00	3	1	0.86
191	173	4		1.16	3		3.19	3		3.38	3	3	2.69	1	1	1.98	1	1	1.21			0.25			0.00	12	11	12.70
192	190			0.14			0.35			0.31			0.21			0.13			0.00			0.00			0.00			1.00
193	191-2			0.14	1		0.39	1		0.41			0.32			0.23	1		0.14			0.00			0.00	1	1	1.49
194	193																											
195	194																											
196	170			0.00	1		0.10			0.10			0.00			0.00			0.00			0.00			0.00			0.10
197	171			0.00			0.16			0.16			0.13			0.00			0.00			0.00			0.00			0.45
200,202	200,202			0.00			0.20			0.21			0.16			0.12			0.00			0.00			0.00	2	2	0.69
201	201			0.00	1		0.16	1		0.16			0.12			0.00	1		0.00			0.00			0.00	1	1	0.44
203	203			0.00			0.17			0.20			0.17			0.14			0.00			0.00			0.00	1	1	0.68
204,0	204,1,9			0.17	1		0.43	1		0.41	1	1	0.30			0.18	1	1	0.18			0.00			0.00	1	1	1.32
204,1-4	204,0,5-7			0.00	1		0.00	1		0.13	1		0.15			0.15	1		0.00			0.00			0.00	2	2	0.43
204	204-207			0.17	1		0.43	1		0.54			0.45	1		0.33	1		0.00			0.00			0.00	3	3	1.75
TOTAL		8	7	7.60	24	16	23.22	23	20	25.09	15	14	20.28	13	12	14.20	3	3	7.61	3	2	1.03	0	0	0.00	81	67	91.43

O : All tumours
O': Histologically confirmed (all leukaemias were confirmed histologically)
E : Expected

B. Cases of invasive cervical cancer not treated by radiotherapy

TIME SINCE DIAGNOSIS OF PRIMARY CERVICAL CANCER (IN YEARS)

		<1 (1390)			1-4 (1163)			5-9 (1046)			10-14 (895)			15-19 (528)			20-24 (184)			25-29 (23)			30+			Total (excl. <1)		
ICD7	ICD8	O	O'	E	O	O'	E	O	O'	E	O	O'	E	O	O'	E	O	O'	E	O	O'	E	O	O'	E	O	O'	E
140	140																											
141	141																											
142	142																											
143-4	143-5																											
145,7-8	146,8-9			0.00			0.00			0.00			0.00			0.00			0.00			0.00			0.00	1	1	0.00
146	147																											
150	150																											
151	151	1	1	0.36	1	1	1.24	1		1.86			1.76			1.22			0.47			0.00			0.00	2	1	6.55
152	152			0.00			0.33			0.53			0.53			0.37			0.14			0.00			0.00	1	1	1.90
153	153	1	1	0.10			0.41			0.65			0.63			0.43			0.15			0.00			0.00	1	1	2.27
154	154																											
155.0	155			0.10			0.34			0.49			0.45			0.31			0.12			0.00			0.00	3	3	1.71
155.1	156			0.00			0.15			0.26			0.27			0.19			0.00			0.00			0.00	1	1	0.87
157	157																											
160	160																											
161	161																											
162-3	162-3			0.00	3	3	0.30	2		0.49	1		0.48	1		0.33			0.11			0.00			0.00	6	4	1.71
170	174			0.54	2	2	2.19	5		3.18			2.68			1.44			0.43			0.00			0.00	8	7	9.92
172	182.0			0.16			0.66			1.04			0.98			0.59			0.17			0.00			0.00			3.44
173-4	181.2.9																											
175	183	1	1	0.20	1	1	0.80			1.16			0.99			0.55			0.16			0.00			0.00			3.66
176	184			0.00	1	1	0.15			0.23			0.21			0.14			0.00			0.00			0.00	1	2	0.73
180	189.0--1			0.00			0.00			0.16			0.16			0.11			0.00			0.00			0.00	1	2	0.43
181	188			0.00			0.16			0.11			0.12	1	1	0.00			0.00			0.00			0.00			0.23
190	172			0.00	1	1	0.16			0.23			0.17			0.00			0.00			0.00			0.00	1	1	0.56
191	173	2	2	0.28	2	2	0.99	1	1	1.46	1	1	1.37	1	1	0.93			0.34			0.00			0.00	5	5	5.09
192	190																											
193	191-2			0.00			0.18	1	1	0.22			0.18			0.00	1	1	0.00		1	0.00			0.00	2	2	0.58
194	193			0.00			0.14	1	1	0.20			0.18			0.11			0.11			0.00			0.00	2	1	0.63
195	194																											
196	170																											
197	171																											
200,202	200,202			0.00			0.00			0.11			0.00			0.00			0.00			0.00			0.00			0.11
201	201			0.00			0.00			0.11			0.00			0.00			0.00			0.00			0.00			0.11
203	203			0.00			0.00	2	2	0.11	1	1	0.11			0.11			0.00			0.00			0.00	2	2	0.22
204.0	204.1,.9			0.00			0.18			0.20			0.15			0.15			0.00			0.00			0.00	2	2	0.53
204.1-4	204.0,5-7			0.00			0.00			0.11			0.13			0.13			0.00			0.00			0.00	1	1	0.24
204	204-207			0.00	2	2	0.18	2	2	0.31	1	1	0.28			0.28			0.00			0.00			0.00	3	3	0.77
TOTAL		5	5	1.74	11	11	8.22	14	12	12.91	5		11.55	4	2	6.72	1	1	2.09		1	0.00			0.00	37	31	41.49

O : All tumours
O': Histologically confirmed
E : Expected

C. Cases of carcinoma in situ not treated by radiotherapy

TIME SINCE DIAGNOSIS OF PRIMARY CERVICAL CANCER (IN YEARS)

		<1			1–4			5–9			10–14			15–19			20–24			25–29			30+			Total (exel. <1)		
Number of women starting		1114			1107			1099			947			523			61			2								
ICD7	**ICD8**	O	O'	E	O	O'	E	O	O'	E	O	O'	E	O	O'	E	O	O'	E	O	O'	E	O	O'	E	O	O'	E
140	140																											
141	141																											
142	142																											
143–4	143–5																											
145,7–8	146,8–9																											
146	147																											
150	150																											
150	151			0.13	1		0.64	1	1	1.09			1.13			0.62			0.00			0.00			0.00	2	2	3.48
151																											
152	152			0.00			0.20			0.36			0.38			0.20			0.00			0.00			0.00			1.14
153	153			0.00			0.24			0.43			0.45			0.24			0.00			0.00			0.00			1.36
154	154																											
155.0	155			0.00			0.13	1	1	0.24			0.26			0.15			0.00			0.00			0.00	1	1	0.78
155.1	156			0.00			0.00			0.16	1	1	0.19			0.11			0.00			0.00			0.00	1	1	0.46
157	157			0.00			0.00	1	1	0.00			0.00			0.00			0.00			0.00			0.00	1	1	0.00
160	160			0.00			0.00			0.00			0.00			0.00			0.00			0.00			0.00	1	1	0.00
161	161			0.00			0.17			0.34			0.37			0.19			0.00			0.00			0.00			1.07
162–3	162–3			0.34			1.73	2	2	2.99	4	4	2.66	1		1.07			0.00			0.00			0.00	7	7	8.45
170	174				1		0.41	2	2	0.82	2	2	0.88			0.42			0.00			0.00			0.00	5	5	2.53
172	182.0			0.00			0.00																					
173–4	181,2.9			0.12			0.60			1.02			0.96			0.40			0.00			0.00			0.00			2.98
175	183			0.00			0.10			0.17			0.17			0.00			0.00			0.00			0.00			0.44
176	184			0.00			0.00			0.11			0.12	1		0.00			0.00			0.00			0.00	1	1	0.23
180	189.0–1																											
181	188			0.00			0.15	2	2	0.25	1		0.19						0.00			0.00			0.00	3	3	0.59
190	172			0.11			0.54			0.95			0.99			0.52			0.00			0.00			0.00	1	1	3.00
191	173						0.14			0.21	1		0.18						0.00			0.00			0.00			0.53
192	190									0.14			0.13						0.00			0.00			0.00			0.27
193	191–2																											
194	193																											
195	194																		0.00			0.00			0.00	1	1	0.00
196	170			0.00			0.00			0.10	1		0.00						0.00			0.00			0.00	1		0.10
197	171																											
200,202	200,202																											
201	201																											
203	203																											
204,0	204,1.,9			0.00			0.14			0.14			0.14			0.00			0.00			0.00			0.00	1	1	0.28
204,1–4	204,0.5–7			0.00	1	1	0.00			0.00			0.12			0.14			0.00			0.00			0.00	1	1	0.26
204	204–207			0.00	1	1	0.14			0.26			0.14			0.00			0.00			0.00			0.00	1	1	0.54
TOTAL				0.70	3	3	5.19	9	9	9.64	10	10	9.20	2	2	3.92			0.00			0.00			0.00	24	24	27.95

O : All tumours
O' : Histologically confirmed
E : Expected

Table 3. Breast cancer in women in Slovenia by age at diagnosis of cervical cancer, stage and treatment

TIME SINCE DIAGNOSIS OF PRIMARY CERVICAL CANCER (IN YEARS)

Stage / Treatment	Age	<1 O	<1 E	1–4 O	1–4 E	5–9 O	5–9 E	10–14 O	10–14 E	15–19 O	15–19 E	20–24 O	20–24 E	25–29 O	25–29 E	30+ O	30+ E	Total (excl. <1) O	Total (excl. <1) E
INVASIVE RADIOTHERAPY	<30		0.01		0.01		0.03		0.05		0.05		0.04		0.00				0.18
	30–39		0.07		0.30	1	0.55		0.62		0.48		0.26		0.05			1	2.26
	40–49	1	0.41	2	1.21	1	1.35	4	1.15		0.90		0.56		0.11			8	5.28
	50–59	1	0.50	1	1.31		1.30	1	1.01		0.66		0.30		0.05			3	4.63
	60–69		0.39		1.07		1.00		0.59		0.29		0.12		0.02				3.09
	70+		0.15		0.32		0.21		0.06		0.00		0.00		0.00				0.59
INVASIVE NO RADIOTHERAPY	<30				0.01		0.05		0.11		0.08		0.02		0.00				0.27
	30–39		0.08	1	0.46	1	0.96		0.94		0.44		0.12		0.00			2	2.92
	40–49		0.22	1	0.89		1.19		0.90		0.53		0.17		0.00			1	3.72
	50–59	1	0.15	3	0.59		0.71		0.54		0.33		0.09		0.00			4	2.26
	60–69	1	0.07	1	0.22		0.40		0.14		0.05		0.01		0.00			1	0.66
	70+		0.02		0.02		0.02		0.00		0.00		0.00		0.00				0.04
IN SITU NO RADIOTHERAPY	<30				0.03	1	0.13	1	0.19		0.09		0.00		0.00			2	0.44
	30–39		0.10	2	0.62	2	1.34		1.34		0.53		0.02		0.00			4	3.85
	40–49		0.17		0.77		1.12		0.85		0.34		0.04		0.00				3.12
	50–59		0.06		0.28	1	0.37		0.27		0.11		0.01		0.00			1	1.04
	60–69				0.03		0.03		0.01		0.00		0.00		0.00				0.07

O : All tumours
O': Histologically confirmed
E : Expected

ORGAN DOSES FROM RADIOTHERAPY OF CANCER OF THE UTERINE CERVIX[1]

M. Stovall

Department of Physics
University of Texas System Cancer Center
M.D. Anderson Hospital
Houston, TX 77030, USA

This chapter summarizes the results of a preliminary investigation of the radiation dose delivered to various organs from radiotherapy of cancer of the uterine cervix. The organs considered are the bladder, rectum, ovaries, kidneys, stomach, lungs, pancreas, breasts, thyroid, salivary glands and brain. The data presented were derived to test the feasibility of a study of radiation-induced second tumours and should not be considered as definitive organ doses.

The work reported is part of an extensive investigation of organ doses from radiotherapy of cancer of the cervix by the Dosimetry Subcommittee[2]; this work is in progress.

Radiation therapy techniques

Most techniques for radiotherapy of cancer of the cervix are variations on two classical methods developed in the early 1930s: the Manchester system (Tod, 1947; Paterson, 1949), which was based on the Paris technique (Regaud, 1929), and the Stockholm system (Kottmeier, 1954, 1958). These techniques prescribe external beam and/or intracavitary dose levels appropriate for the stage of the disease. The essential difference between the two techniques is in the intracavitary treatment: the Stockholm technique utilizes applicators loaded with sources of higher activity, with shorter treatment time. A widely used modification of the Manchester system is the Fletcher technique (Fletcher, 1973). Typical dosages prescribed by the Manchester, Stockholm, and Fletcher systems are outlined briefly in Table 1.

There are numerous applicators which are designed for intracavitary therapy of cervical cancer, based on the above techniques. The dose to the organs in the pelvis, particularly the bladder and rectum, is dependent upon the particular applicator design and size. However, for organs outside the pelvis, the applicator design is of small importance and can be ignored for the purpose of this investigation.

---

[1] This work was partially supported by contract N01-CP-01047 with the National Cancer Institute, USA

[2] Dosimetry Subcommittee: Marilyn Stovall, University of Texas System Cancer Center, M.D. Anderson Hospital, Houston, TX, USA; Marvin Rosenstein, Bureau of Radiological Health, Food and Drug Administration, US Department of Health and Human Services, Rockville, MD, USA; Goran Svensson, Harvard Medical School, Boston, MA, USA

Table 1. Commonly used systems of radiotherapy for cancer of the uterine cervix

	Stockholm system		Manchester system		Fletcher system	
	External beam[a]	Intracavitary[b]	External beam[a]	Intracavitary[b]	External beam[a]	Intracavitary[b]
Stage I	None	7000 mgh	None	9800 mgh	None	10 000 mgh
Stage II	3000 (Co-60) or 2000 (Ortho)	7000 mgh	None	9800 mgh	3000 (Betatron) or 3500 (Ortho)	7500 mgh
Stage III	4000 (Co-60) or 2400 (Ortho)	7000 mgh	3000 (Co-60) or 2500 (Ortho)	8500 mgh	5500 (Betatron) or 5500 (Ortho)	5000 mgh
Stage IV	4500 (Co-60) or 2400 (Ortho)	None	5000 (Co-60)	3000 mgh	7000 (Betatron) or 6000 (Ortho)	None

[a] Dose (rad) to midline pelvis
[b] Expressed as milligram-hours

The external beam pelvic fields, for the most part, are parallel-opposed anterior and posterior fields, typically 15 × 15 cm², sometimes with midline blocking of approximately 3 cm if the patient also received intracavitary irradiation. Other commonly used field arrangements are the four-field box technique (anterior, posterior and lateral fields), six-field technique (right and left anterior, sacral and gluteal fields), and arc therapy, usually 360° rotation. Most patients in this study were treated with orthovoltage machines (200-400 keVp) with half-value layers of 1.5-4.0 mm Cu, although some patients were treated with cobalt-60 units or betatrons with photon beams of approximately 25 MV.

For the last several decades, the radiotherapy of cervical cancer has been highly stylized; major changes in dose prescriptions occurred only with the advent of high-energy machines.

Organ doses

In order to estimate organ doses, measurements were made in an Alderson Rando phantom during simulation of typical teletherapy and intracavitary treatment. The phantom is representative of a typical adult female, including a skeleton, lungs and other soft tissue, with a height of 160 cm and an antero-posterior pelvic diameter of 20 cm. Thermoluminescent dosimeters (TLD) containing lithium fluoride powder were placed in the phantom at several locations within each organ; the locations were selected to determine the range of dose within the organ, as well as the average dose.

The external beam treatments were delivered using two pelvic fields: parallel-opposed, anterior and posterior, 15 × 15 cm². Three typical teletherapy machines were used, with machine parameters suitable for treatment of cancer of the cervix:

(1) 250 kVp, Philips 250, Th III filter, 3.0 mm Cu HVL, 70 cm F.S.D.
(2) Cobalt-60, AECL Theratron-80, 80 cm S.S.D.
(3) 25 MV X-rays, Allis-Chalmers Betatron, 100 cm T.S.D.

Organ doses from intracavitary therapy were measured by placing a single radium tube in the Alderson phantom at the position of the uterine cervix. With the exception of the bladder, rectum and ovaries, all organs were sufficiently far from the radium that a single source could simulate tandem and ovoids. The dose to the bladder, rectum and ovaries was calculated using a computer program in routine clinical use, assuming a tandem and ovoids of typical size and loading.

The results of the teletherapy measurements are presented in Table 2 as organ dose (rad) per 1000 rad midline dose on the central axes of the pelvic fields, for each of the three machines. The organ doses from intracavitary radium are shown in Table 3, expressed as rad per 1000 milligram-hours (mgh).

Table 2. Organ dose (rad) from external beam therapy per 1000 rad midline dose on central axis

	250 kVp, Philips 250 Th III filter 3.0 mm Cu HVL 70 cm F.S.D.	Cobalt-60 AECL Theratron-80 80 cm S.S.D.	25 MV X-rays Allis-Chalmers Betatro 100 cm T.S.D.
Given dose[a] to each field (rad)	1 120	855	585

	250 kVp, Philips 250 Th III filter 3.0 mm Cu HVL 70 cm F.S.D.	Cobalt-60 AECL Theratron-80 80 cm S.S.D.	25 MV X-rays Allis-Chalmers Betatron 100 cm T.S.D.
Given dose[a] to each field (rad)	1120	855	585
D_{max}(cm)	0	0.5	4.5
Bladder	â 1000 +	â 1000 +	â 1000 +
Rectum	â 1000 +	â 1000 +	â 1000 +
Ovaries	710 (620-800)	1020 (1015-1030)	1030 (1030-1030)
Kidneys	62.6 (25.5-115)	24.5 (13.5-41.0)	13.3 (6.8-24.0)
Stomach	55.7 (16.2-120)	23.1 (10.7-41.6)	13.0 (5.3-27.7)
Pancreas	49.1 (48.8-49.4)	20.2 (19.5-20.9)	9.2 (9.2-9.3)
Lungs	6.2 (2.8-12.3)	6.1 (3.7-9.6)	3.4 (2.4-5.1)
Breasts	6.4 (3.4-10.8)	6.4 (2.4-8.9)	3.5 (2.4-6.6)
Thyroid	2.5 (2.3-2.6)	3.1 (2.9-3.6)	2.5 (2.3-2.9)
Salivary glands	1.9 (1.7-2.2)	2.0 (1.8-2.2)	2.2 (2.0-2.3)
Brain	1.8 (1.1-2.3)	1.3 (1.1-1.5)	2.2 (2.1-2.5)
Active bone-marrow			
Total	—	212 (1.3-480)	—
Total, excl. pelvis	—	60 (I.3-310)	—

[a] Dose at D_{max} in phantom, including backscatter

Table 3. Organ dose (rad) from intracavitary therapy per 1000 milligram-hours of radium

	Dose (rad) Mean (minimum-maximum within organ)
Bladder [a]	~ 600 +
Rectum [a]	~ 600 +
Ovaries [b]	155 (117-187)
Kidneys	13.2 (7.2-21.0)
Stomach	11.0 (4.7-20.8)
Pancreas	12.5 (11.2-13.8)
Lungs	2.1 (1.1-4.0)
Breasts	1.7 (1.2-2.5)
Thyroid	0.7 (0.6-0.8)
Salivary glands	0.4 (0.3-0.4)
Brain	0.3 (0.2-0.3)
Active bone marrow	
Total	36.0 (1.3-80)
Total, excluding pelvis	11.0 (1.3-40)

[a] Highly dependent upon application design and placement
[b] Calculated from three-source tandem (15+10+10 mg) and ovoids (15+15 mg)

The three radiotherapy systems described above were similar. A typical treatment technique was therefore chosen for each disease stage to represent these systems. The data from Tables 2 and 3 were then used to estimate total mean organ doses for the typical treatments, summarized in Table 4. The treatment techniques selected as typical are described in terms of midline dose on the central axis for the teletherapy and number of milligram-hours for the intracavitary therapy.

Table 4. Mean organ dose (rad) for typical radiotherapy

		Stage I	II	III	IV
Intracavitary (radium)		9 000 mgh[a]	8 000 mgh	7 000 mgh	—
External beam 250 kVp X-rays Cobalt-60 25 MV X-rays		—	3 000 rad[b]	4 000 rad[b]	6 000 rad[b]
Cobalt-60		—	3 000 rad[b]	4 000 rad[b]	5 000 rad[b]
25 MV X-rays		—	4 000 rad[b]	5 000 rad[b]	7 000 rad[b]
Bladder	250 kVp	5400 +	7800 +	8200 +	6000
	Co-60	5400 +	7800 +	8200 +	5000
	25 MV	5400 +	8800 +	9200 +	7000
Rectum	250 kVp	5400 +	7800 +	8200 +	6000
	Co-60	5400 +	7800 +	8200 +	5000
	25 MV	5400 +	8800 +	9200 +	7000
Ovaries	250 kVp	1400	3370	3920	4260
	Co-60	1400	4300	5160	5100
	25 MV	1400	5360	6240	7210
Kidneys	250 kVp	199	294	343	376
	Co-60	199	180	190	122
	25 MV	199	159	159	93
Stomach	250 kVp	99	255	300	334
	Co-60	99	157	169	115
	25 MV	99	140	142	91
Pancreas	250 kVp	113	247	284	295
	Co-60	113	161	168	101
	25 MV	113	137	134	64
Lungs	250 kVp	19	35	39	37
	Co-60	19	35	39	31
	25 MV	19	30	32	24
Breasts	250 kVp	15	33	37	38
	Co-60	15	33	37	32
	25 MV	15	28	29	25
Thyroid	250 kVp	6	13	15	15
	Co-60	6	15	17	16
	25 MV	6	16	17	18
Salivary glands	250 kVp	4	9	10	11
	Co-60	4	9	11	10
	25 MV	4	12	14	15
Brain	250 kVp	3	8	9	11
	Co-60	3	6	7	6
	25 MV	3	11	13	15
Active bone marrow Total	Co-60	325	924	1100	1060
Total, excl. pelvis	Co-60	100	268	317	300

[a] mgh, milligram-hours

[b] Absorbed dose at midline on central axis

Discussion

The following limitations apply to the estimation of organ doses for individual patients in the entire study on the basis of the doses reported here:

(1) The dose to tissues outside the teletherapy treatment beam is composed of (a) scatter within the patient from the treatment beam, and (b) leakage through the head of the unit and collimator scatter. For the measurements reported here, no attempt was made to separate the organ doses into these components. It is reasonable to expect that the scatter from the treatment beam is a function of the energy of the incident beam and does not vary with the particular model of machine. However, the leakage through the head may vary with machine design. Measurements on several types of machine indicate that at approximately 40 cm from the central axis the doses from the two components are equal; at approximately 60 cm almost all of the organ dose is due to head leakage. Therefore, a more accurate estimate of organ dose, particularly for distant organs, requires data on the type of machine used for treatment.

(2) Irradiation with a betatron results in some organ dose, due to incidental neutrons (Swanson, 1979), although neutron dose was not measured as part of this study. The neutron dose is small - approximately 10% of the local photon dose outside the therapy beam. However, neutrons may be important, since they have a high Relative Biological Effectiveness (RBE) for late effects.

(3) The measurements reported here were made in an Alderson Rando phantom, which simulates a typical adult female. Organ doses will differ to some extent for patients of other sizes.

(4) The external beam fields used for these measurements were parallel-opposed, anterior and posterior fields, 15×15 cm^2. As noted in Section 1, some treatment techniques involve other field arrangements. Dose to organs in or near the pelvis is highly dependent upon the field arrangement.

(5) Radium was the intracavitary source most commonly used to treat patients included in this study. However, some patients were treated with other sources, such as radon, caesium-137, cobalt-60, and iridium-192. The organ doses from these isotopes would be somewhat less than those from radium sources. (All radium doses are due to gamma rays only, the alpha and beta particles being filtered out by the walls of the sources and applicators.)

It is emphasized that the organ doses presented here are preliminary results. They are suitable for testing the feasibility of the epidemiological study and to serve as a guide for further planning. As the work of the Dosimetry Subcommittee progresses, these data will be refined and expanded in order to take into account all of the variables which influence organ dose, with the accuracy and precision consistent with the design of the overall study.

References

Fletcher, G. H. (1973) *Textbook of Radiotherapy*, 2nd ed., Philadelphia, Lea & Fibiger

Kottmeier, H. L. (1954) Modern trends in the treatment of cancer of the cervix. *Acta Radiol.*, *Suppl. 116*, 405-414

Kottmeier, H. L. (1958) Current treatment of the cervix. *Am J. Obstet. Gynecol.*, *76*, 243-281

Paterson, R. (1949) *Treatment of Malignant Disease by Radium and X-rays; Being a Practice of Radiotherapy*, Baltimore, William & Wilkins Co.

Regaud, C. (1929) Radium therapy of cancer at the Radium Institute of Paris. *Am. J. Roentgenol.*, *21*, 1-24

Swanson, W. P. (1979) *An Estimate of the Risk in Radiation Therapy Due to Unwanted Neutrons (Working Paper)*, (NBS-BRH Conference on Neutrons from Electron Medical Accelerators, Gaithersburg, MD, 9-10 April, 1979)

Tod, M. C. (1947) Optimum dosage in the treatment of cancer of the cervix by radiation. *Acta Radiol.*, *28*, 564-575

SUMMARY CHAPTER

N.E. Day, J.D. Boice, A. Andersen, L.A. Brinton, R. Brown, N.W. Choi, E.A. Clarke, M.P. Coleman, R.E. Curtis, J.T. Flannery, M. Hakama, T. Hakulinen, G.R. Howe, O.M. Jensen, R.A. Kleinerman, D. Magnin, K. Magnus, K. Makela, B. Malker, A.B. Miller, N. Nelson, C.C. Patterson, F. Pettersson, V. Pompe-Kirn, M. Primic-Žakelj, P. Prior, P. Ravnihar, R.G. Skeet, J.E. Skjerven, P.G. Smith, M. Sok, R.F. Spengler, H.H. Storm, G.W.O. Tomkins & C. Wall (for affiliations, see page 3)

CONTENTS

1. Introduction

This chapter comprises an examination of the extent to which results from fifteen cancer registries can be analysed in a unified way to yield information on radiation carcinogenesis. Several points must be stressed at the outset.

First, these results represent an intermediate step in the overall series of studies described in the introductory chapter. Much of the data needed to establish quantitative associations between risk and dose will be available only when the detailed case-control and dosimetry studies are complete and supplemented by review of pathology (see Introductory Chapter, especially Figure 1).

Second, the study of second primary cancers involves special problems that are of little concern in most epidemiological studies. There is the difficulty of deciding whether a second cancer is a genuine second primary or a metastatic lesion, or local recurrence, of the original primary. There is also the problem that treatment of the primary cancer may affect the risk of a subsequent cancer for some organs in a way unrelated to a direct radiogenic effect; the organ, for example, may be removed.

Third, there is considerable variation among the results from the different registries. Such variation may be due to differences between countries or areas in diagnostic and cancer registration practices which determine the completeness and validity of the data to be analysed, in the practice of radiation therapy, and in host and environmental factors.

Fourth, patients with cancer of the cervix are not representative of the general population in many respects, so that comparisons with the general population must be interpreted with caution.

Bearing in mind these caveats, the extent to which the overall data suggest that radiation exposure alters risk, and by how much, will be examined for each site. Using the average organ doses estimated from the preliminary dosimetry studies, the compatibility will be examined between the results obtained for each site and the recently proposed risk estimates (Advisory Committee on the Biological Effects of Ionizing Radiations, 1980). These latter are based mainly on a single brief exposure, and not on the protracted exposures characteristic of radiotherapy.

2. Evidence to support a radiation effect

An excess incidence of cancer is the basic evidence required to support a causal relationship between radiation exposure and occurrence of cancer at a particular site. Excesses of cancer can occur, however, for reasons other than radiation exposure, and the characteristics of the excess, and of the comparison group against which it is measured, have to be examined. Support for an association with radiation is in large part related to the consistency of findings with those of other large studies of populations exposed to radiation, especially the atomic bomb survivors (Kato & Schull, 1982) and British patients treated with radiotherapy for ankylosing spondylitis (Smith & Doll, 1982). Consideration has therefore been given to the variation in risk of having a second primary cancer at different times after radiotherapy; the variation in risk by age at exposure; the risk to heavily irradiated organs close to the pelvis; and the comparison of the risk among irradiated patients with that of patients who were not treated by radiotherapy.

In the studies of atomic bomb survivors and British patients with ankylosing spondylitis treated by radiotherapy, most cancers, except leukaemia, did not show increased rates until ten or more years after the radiation exposure (Advisory Committee on the Biological Effects of Ionizing Radiations, 1980). Among the atomic bomb survivors (Kato & Schull, 1982) and most medically irradiated populations (Boice, 1981), no diminution of the excess cancer risk has been observed even after 35 years of observation. In fact, for most solid tumours, the temporal pattern of incidence of radiogenic cancer appears to follow the natural incidence. Excess cancers do not occur before the ages normally associated with increased incidence, i.e., later life. For leukaemia, however, a wave-like pattern of excess incidence over time is frequently observed, the excess beginning within two to four years after exposure, peaking after about six to eight years, and then decreasing towards normal levels. In this study, evidence of similar variation in the excess risks of leukaemia and other second cancers has been sought among women irradiated for cervical cancer.

Perhaps the most powerful way of establishing the presence of a radiation effect is to demonstrate a dose-response relationship for the induction of second cancers. Individual organ doses for the patients in this study were not available but will be the focus of subsequent reports. A simple comparison can be made, however, between the excess cancer risk among patients treated by radiation and the two groups of cervical cancer patients (invasive and in-situ) treated in other ways, although the non-exposed women may differ to some extent from exposed women by factors other than radiation which might affect their risks of second cancers (e.g., social class, smoking habits). A caveat, however, is that some of the women in the two comparison groups may have received radiotherapy (see section 5.1 (d)).

Another way of studying the possible carcinogenic effects of radiation treatment would be to examine the excess cancer risk in organs at different distances from the cervix. Although organs vary appreciably with regard to their carcinogenic response to radiation (Advisory Committee on the Biological Effects of Ionizing Radiations, 1980), it is likely that organs close to the pelvis would show an increased risk of cancer development. It would be surprising, however, if the risk to organs remote from the uterine cervix were substantially increased over expectation.

Some cancers seem rarely, if ever, to be found in excess in irradiated populations. Chronic lymphocytic leukaemia and Hodgkin's disease are two examples. In contrast the breast, thyroid and bone marrow are thought to have a relatively high sensitivity to cancer induction by radiation, whereas the kidney, bladder, brain, salivary gland, bone, skin, larynx, ovary, uterus and connective tissue have been classified as having a relatively low sensitivity (Advisory Committee on the Biological Effects of Ionizing Radiations, 1980). General consistency with the experience gained from other radiation studies in this respect would strengthen interpretations of the findings in this study.

Little precise knowledge is available about the variation in risk of induced cancer for persons exposed to radiation at different ages. It would seem, however, from the available data that for most, but not all, cancers the relative risk of induction following exposure does not vary appreciably by age at exposure, for persons exposed when older than about 20 years (Boice, 1981; Kato & Schull, 1982; Smith & Doll, 1982). For a fixed period of follow-up, however, the risk difference (i.e., absolute excess risk) increases appreciably with age at exposure.

3. Subjects and methods

Over 180 000 women with cervical neoplasia were studied (Table 1A). Approximately 97 000 women had invasive cervical cancer, of whom 82 000 were known to have received radiation therapy; 84 000 had in-situ cancer. More details on the eligibility of women for inclusion and on classification procedures are given in the Introductory Chapter and in the individual cancer registry chapters. Women known to have received radiation therapy accrued approximately 625 000 woman-years of observation; approximately 180 000 woman-years were accumulated ten and more years after diagnosis (Table 1B). The average period of observation was 7.1 years.

Table 1A. Numbers of women by registry, stage of cervical cancer and treatment status

Registry	Invasive cervical cancer		In-situ cancer
	Radiotherapy	No radiotherapy	
Canada			
Alberta	2 096	411	-
British Columbia	2 232	81	230
Manitoba	1 337	1 035	4 832
New Brunswick	1 449	-	-
Nova Scotia	695	84	-
Ontario	7 322	717	-
Saskatchewan	1 277	232	-
Denmark	20 024	5 127	15 367
Finland	7 285	1 206	3 290
Norway	5 282	724	2 130
Sweden	14 760	-	43 971
United Kingdom			
Birmingham	3 808	819	2 034
South Thames	6 110	1 217	3 774
USA			
Connecticut	5 997	1 130	7 260
Yugoslavia			
Slovenia	2 942	1 390	1 114
Total	82 616	14 173	84 002

Table 1B. Woman-years at risk for developing a second primary cancer by stage, treatment and time since diagnosis of cervical cancer

Time since diagnosis (years)	Invasive cervical cancer		In-situ cancer
	Radiotherapy	No radiotherapy	
< 1	76 565	20 892	79 945
1-4	204 507	36 255	249 594
5-9	164 918	32 572	155 487
10-14	100 638	19 002	43 020
15-19	49 134	8 943	10 601
20-24	21 005	3 073	1 958
25-29	6 975	727	283
30+	1 696	161	24
Total	625 438	121 625	540 912
Mean years of follow-up	7.57	8.58	6.43

Table 2A. Observed (O) and expected (E) numbers of second primary cancers by stage of cervical cancer and treatment status

Second primary cancer (ICD7)	Invasive cervical cancer						In-situ cancer		
	Radiotherapy			No radiotherapy					
	O	E	O/E	O	E	O/E	O	E	O/E
Buccal cavity and naso-pharynx (140-148)	60	46.61	1.3*	8	5.30	1.5	29	16.93	1.7**
Oesophagus (150)	40	27.32	1.5*	3	2.93	1.0	3	5.55	0.5
Stomach (151)	200	210.37	1.0	23	26.11	0.9	42	45.49	0.9
Small intestine (152)	21	9.46	2.2**	4	0.94	4.3*	3	3.70	0.8
Colon (153)	314	301.53	1.0	42	38.46	1.1	85	84.09	1.0
Rectum (154)	197	157.38	1.3**	29	21.78	1.3	48	43.00	1.1
Liver (155.0)	19	19.88	1.0	2	2.28	0.9	6	5.45	1.1
Gallbladder (155.1)	45	55.69	0.8	7	7.22	1.0	10	12.25	0.8
Pancreas (157)	120	95.88	1.3*	10	11.66	0.9	34	24.82	1.4
Nose (160)	13	7.12	1.8	2	0.72	2.8	6	2.21	2.7
Larynx (161)	16	7.21	2.2	4	1.10	3.6	5	3.33	1.5
Lung (162-163)	491	134.94	3.6***	60	20.96	2.9***	106	48.91	2.2***
Breast (170)	569	804.41	0.7***	118	124.91	0.9	409	426.59	1.0
Corpus uteri (172)	126	209.13	0.6***	2	31.44	0.1***	48	91.83	0.5***
Other uterus (173)	21	18.11	1.2	0	1.72	0.0	6	11.52	0.5
Ovary (175)	136	198.31	0.7***	16	30.95	0.5**	91	102.25	0.9
Other genital (176)	101	43.00	2.4***	17	5.94	2.9***	95	12.44	7.6***
Kidney (180)	69	66.50	1.0	18	8.41	2.1**	27	25.34	1.1
Bladder (181)	194	73.74	2.6***	16	9.26	1.7*	31	20.49	1.5*
Melanoma (190)	36	47.08	0.8	8	7.99	1.0	44	39.69	1.1
Other skin (191)	206	219.76	0.9	40	34.48	1.2	43	49.49	0.9
Eye (192)	7	8.47	0.8	2	1.04	1.9	4	3.84	1.0
Brain (193)	51	67.54	0.8*	16	10.34	1.6	39	42.33	0.9
Thyroid (194)	36	31.47	1.1	1	4.23	0.2	19	22.07	0.9
Bone (196)	11	5.72	1.9	0	0.69	0.0	2	3.08	0.7
Connective tissue (197)	27	14.57	1.9***	5	1.85	2.7	6	8.39	0.7
Lymphoma (200,202)	61	53.77	1.1	8	6.99	1.1	28	20.71	1.4
Hodgkin's disease (201)	14	16.87	0.8	3	2.46	1.2	14	11.21	1.3
Multiple myeloma (203)	33	33.92	1.0	1	4.02	0.3	12	10.56	1.1
All leukaemia (204)	77	65.83	1.2	13	8.76	1.5	39	24.95	1.6*
Chronic and unspecified lymphatic leukaemia (204.0)	18	22.64	0.8	6	3.04	2.0	7	6.07	1.2
Myeloid and acute leu-kaemia (204.1-4)	58	40.94	1.4*	6	5.41	1.1	31	18.25	1.7*
Close and intermediate sites[b]	1601	1479.27	1.1***	191	198.71	1.0	534	494.14	1.1
Close and intermediate sites excluding genital cancers (172-176)	1217	1010.72	1.2***	156	128.66	1.2*	294	276.10	1.1
Total (all sites except cervix)	3324	3062.54	1.1***	479	435.40	1.1*	1346	1238.05	1.1***

[a] Numbers exclude the first year of observation

[b] Stomach (151), Small intestine (152), Colon (153), Rectum (154), Liver (155.0), Gallbladder (155.1), Pancreas (157), Corpus uteri (172), Other uterus (173), Ovary (175), Other genital (176), Kidney (180), Bladder (181), Bone (196) and Connective tissue (197).

* $0.01 < p < 0.05$ ** $0.001 < p < 0.01$ *** $p < 0.001$

Table 2B. Observed (O) and expected (E) numbers of second primary cancers by stage of cervical cancer and treatment status for ten-year survivors

Second primary cancer (ICD7)	Invasive cervical cancer						In-situ cancer		
	Radiotherapy			No radiotherapy					
	O	E	O/E	O	E	O/E	O	E	O/E
Buccal cavity and naso-pharynx (140-148)	30	18.01	1.7*	4	2.31	1.7	7	3.69	1.9
Oesophagus (150)	12	11.21	1.1	-	1.22	0.0	3	1.43	2.1
Stomach (151)	86	86.05	1.0	7	11.32	0.6	12	11.17	1.1
Small intestine (152)	9	3.78	2.4*	2	0.40	5.0	-	0.73	0.0
Colon (153)	145	133.11	1.1	23	17.71	1.3	21	22.38	0.9
Rectum (154)	118	68.59	1.7***	14	9.84	1.4	11	11.03	1.0
Liver (155.0)	8	8.76	1.0	1	1.03	1.0	-	1.04	0.0
Gallbladder (155.1)	21	25.32	0.8	5	3.44	1.5	1	3.16	0.3
Pancreas (157)	50	42.72	1.2	5	5.38	0.9	11	6.77	1.6
Nose (160)	7	3.24	2.2	2	0.29	6.9	2	0.47	4.3
Larynx (161)	6	2.96	2.0	2	0.47	4.3	1	0.71	1.4
Lung (162-163)	134	57.83	2.3***	21	9.53	2.2**	30	12.04	2.5***
Breast (170)	203	304.63	0.7***	43	48.18	0.9	82	83.65	1.0
Corpus uteri (172)	78	83.40	0.9	2	13.59	0.2**	10	22.23	0.5**
Other uterus (173)	9	5.85	1.5	0	0.61	0.0	1	1.96	0.5
Ovary (175)	69	76.09	0.9	6	12.26	0.5	14	19.30	0.7
Other genital (176)	47	19.23	2.4***	7	2.50	2.8*	16	2.92	5.5***
Kidney (180)	23	28.41	0.8	8	3.77	2.1	7	5.36	1.3
Bladder (181)	112	33.14	3.4***	5	4.33	1.2	11	5.03	2.2*
Melanoma (190)	14	18.14	0.8	3	2.85	1.1	8	5.77	1.4
Other skin (191)	88	99.65	0.9	14	15.02	0.9	10	13.07	0.8
Eye (192)	3	3.26	0.9	0	0.41	0.0	2	0.66	3.0
Brain (193)	15	25.41	0.6*	8	3.93	2.0	3	5.92	0.5
Thyroid (194)	16	11.71	1.4	1	1.55	0.7	4	3.51	1.1
Bone (196)	4	2.06	1.9	-	0.21	0.0	1	0.42	2.4
Connective tissue (197)	12	5.29	2.3*	2	0.58	3.5	1	1.42	0.7
Lymphoma (200,202)	28	23.11	1.2	1	2.99	0.3	7	4.24	1.7
Hodgkin's disease (201)	6	6.20	1.0	1	0.88	1.1	2	1.70	1.2
Multiple myeloma (203)	22	14.84	1.5	1	1.84	0.5	3	2.84	1.1
All leukaemia (204)	22	27.37	0.8	2	3.55	0.6	6	4.96	1.2
Chronic and unspecified lymphatic leukaemia (204.0)	9	9.78	0.9	-	1.21	0.0	1	1.48	0.7
Myeloid and acute leu-kaemia (204.1-4)	13	16.72	0.8	2	2.21	0.9	5	3.41	1.5
Close and intermediate sites[a]	785	621.80	1.3***	87	86.97	I.0	117	114.92	1.0
Close and intermediate sites excluding genital cancers (172-176)	588	437.23	1.3***	72	58.01	1.2	76	68.51	1.1
Total (all sites except cervix)	1401	1251.95	1.1***	190	181.89	1.0	290	261.51	1.1

[a] Stomach (151), Small intestine (152), Colon (153), Rectum (154), Liver (155.0), Gallbladder (155.1), Pancreas (157), Corpus uteri (172), Other uterus (173), Ovary (175), Other genital (176), Kidney (180), Bladder (181), Bone (196) and Connective tissue (197).

* $0.01 < p < 0.05$ ** $0.001 < p < 0.01$ *** $p < 0.001$

The observed and expected second cancers from all registries were combined and evaluated by stage of primary cervical cancer (invasive, in-situ), type of treatment (known to have had radiotherapy, other), time since diagnosis of cervical cancer, age at diagnosis, and histologic confirmation of second cancers (Tables 2A and 2B, Appendices A-B). The expected numbers of second cancers were estimated by applying cancer incidence rates for the general population from each registry to the appropriate woman-years of observation. The relative risk was taken as the ratio of observed to expected incident cancers.

For all analyses, the first year of observation was excluded to reduce the effect of incorrectly included metastatic cancers or indolent cancers present at the diagnosis of cervical cancer and detected soon after the diagnosis because of close medical surveillance of the patient.

The basis for the statistical methods used was the assumption that the observed number of second cancers in any specific category followed a Poisson distribution. The Poisson parameter was expressed as the product of the expected number of cases in each category and the relative risk for that category (relative to the population on which the expected numbers were based). Tests of significance and confidence intervals for the relative risk were calculated using the exact Poisson probabilities when the observed number of cases was small; otherwise an accurate asymptotic approximation was used (Rothman & Boice, 1979).

For most cancers, radiation-related excess risks can be expected to become apparent 10 to 15 years after exposure, taken as the time of diagnosis of the cervical cancer. This effect was tested for in two main ways: (a) for whether the relative risk ten or more years after exposure was greater than unity (Table 2B); and (b) for linear trend of increasing relative risk with increasing time since exposure (Mantel, 1963).

Testing for differences between the radiation-treated group and the non-irradiated group in the relative risk after ten or more years of follow-up lacks power, since the expected numbers in the latter group are small. In addition, and for the same reason, trend tests for the non-irradiated groups were not informative for individual sites.

Statistical tests were based on a straightforward multiplicative parameterization of the Poisson variable, using likelihood ratio tests. The computer package GLIM (Baker & Nelder, 1978) is very convenient for this purpose. For example, testing for trend, the logarithm of the Poisson parameter μ is written

$$\log \mu = \log E + \alpha + \beta t \text{ (that is, } \mu = E \exp[\alpha + \beta t]),$$

where E is the expected number of cases in that category, t is the time since exposure (categorized into 1-4, 5-9,...,30+), α is a parameter giving the overall relative risk and β is the trend parameter. The null hypothesis is $\beta = 0$.

For assessing heterogeneity among cancer registries, the relative risk component of the Poisson parameter can be modelled as the product of a registry effect and a time period of follow-up effect:

$$\log \mu_{ij} = \log E_{ij} + \alpha_i + \beta_j,$$

where E_{ij} is the expected number of cases for registry i, with parameter α_i, and time period of follow-up j, with parameter β_j. If the registries do not differ, then all the α_i are equal. The registries may differ, however, in the way the relative risk evolves with time period of follow-up.

In this case, the β_j would differ among registries, and one would model the Poisson parameter as

$$\log \mu_{ij} = \log E_{ij} + \beta_{ij}.$$

In a similar manner, to evaluate the joint effect of time period of follow-up and age at start of follow-up, the relative risk is modelled as the product of the two effects

$$\log \mu_{jk} = \log E_{jk} + \beta_j + \gamma_k,$$

where E_{jk} is the expected number of cases for time period j, with parameters β_j as before, and age at start of follow-up k, with parameter γ_k.

These methods are derived from the multiplicative models described by Breslow and Day (1975), and developed by Gail (1978), Land (see Beebe et al., 1970) and Breslow et al. (1983).

Throughout the chapter, statistical significance is at the 5% level, unless otherwise stated.

4. Results and discussion

The observed and expected numbers, pooled for all registries, are given in Appendix A by site and time since diagnosis of the cervical cancer for each of the three main groups. In Appendix B, the data for a number of sites are further categorized by age at diagnosis of cervical cancer. Tables 2A and 2B give a summary of the data given in Appendix A. It is seen that the ratios of the total numbers of observed to expected second cancers are remarkably similar for the three groups of women: invasive irradiated, invasive non-irradiated and in-situ. Each group experienced an approximately 10% excess over expectation (Table 2A). Table 2B gives the corresponding figures for women surviving more than ten years after treatment.

Among those treated with radiation, 3324 developed second cancers more than one year after diagnosis, compared with 3063 expected (p<0.001). The excess was concentrated among cancers of the lung (491 observed versus 135 expected), other genital organs (101 versus 43), bladder (194 versus 74) and rectum (197 versus 157). Statistically significant excesses were also observed for cancers of the buccal cavity, oesophagus, small intestine, pancreas and connective tissue and for acute and non-lymphocytic leukaemia. Substantial and significant deficits of cancers of the breast (569 versus 804), uterine corpus (126 versus 209) and ovary (136 versus 198) were seen. A statistically significant deficit of brain cancer also occurred. The relative risk of developing any second primary cancer increased significantly with time after exposure (Table 2B and Figure 1). Risks of second cancers were noticeably higher in Connecticut and lower in Saskatchewan than in the other registries (Table 6).

Among women with invasive cervical cancer not treated with radiation, 479 cancers were observed and 435 expected (p=0.03). The excess was accounted for almost entirely by cancer of the lung (60 versus 21), although statistically significant elevated risks were also found for other genital cancers and cancers of the small intestine, kidney and bladder. Cancer of the uterine corpus occurred much less frequently than expected (2 versus 31) as did ovarian cancer (16 versus 31). In contrast to patients receiving radiotherapy, the relative risk of second cancer development at all sites combined decreased slightly with time after diagnosis (p=0.10, Figure 1).

For patients with in-situ cancer, 1346 second cancers were detected compared with 1238 expected (p=0.002). The excess was seen predominantly in the lung (106 *versus* 49) and 'other' genital organs (95 *versus* 12). Statistically significant excesses were also observed for cancers of the buccal cavity and the bladder and for leukaemia. A substantial deficit of uterine corpus cancer was found (48 *versus* 92).

4.1 *Sites at close and intermediate distance from the cervix, combined*

A technique used to evaluate possible radiation effects has been to combine and analyse groups of organs that receive similar radiation exposure (Court Brown & Doll, 1965; Smith & Doll, 1968). In the treatment of cervical cancer with radiation, it is likely that certain organs received substantial doses of radiation: these include the stomach, small intestine, colon, rectum, liver, gallbladder, pancreas, uterine corpus, ovary, other genital organs, kidney, bladder, bone and connective tissue. Observed and expected numbers of cancers at these heavily and moderately irradiated sites have been combined. The total observed:expected ratios for these sites are displayed in Figure 1 by time since the initial diagnosis of cervical cancer. Among patients treated by radiotherapy, no excess of cancer occurred within the first ten years following exposure. However, there was a substantially elevated risk after ten years, as was observed in studies of ankylosing spondylitis patients (Smith & Doll, 1982) and atomic bomb survivors (Kato & Schull, 1982), and a significant increase in the observed:expected ratio with time since treatment, which continued throughout the period of follow-up [χ_1^2(trend)=43.9; p<0.001]. Adjusting for registry did not reduce the significance of the trend. No increase or trend was observed for these sites in either group of non-exposed patients (Figure 1).

When genital organs are excluded from the analysis, the pattern of risk over time does not change appreciably (Figure 1), [χ_1^2(trend)=14.4; p<0.001]. These findings provide strong support for an overall carcinogenic effect of high and moderate doses of radiotherapy for cervical cancer in exposed women.

The pattern of risk over time is given by age at initial irradiation in Table 3. For women under age 30 at exposure, the observed:expected ratio is high (close to 4) throughout the period of follow-up and changes little with time. For women aged 30-39, an observed:expected ratio significantly greater than one is also not associated with an increasing trend over time.

Table 3. Invasive cancer - radiotherapy. Relative risks for cancer of heavily and moderately irradiated sites[a], by age at irradiation and time since initial diagnosis

Age at irradia-tion (years)	Time since diagnosis of cervical cancer (years)															
	< 1		1-4		5-9		10-14		15-19		20-24		25-29		30 +		Total
< 30	28.57	(2)	9.09	(4)	1.43	(1)	5.26	(5)	1.72	(2)	3.42	(4)	3.03	(2)	5.26	(1)	3.61 (19)
30-39	2.52	(7)	2.26	(26)	1.10	(21)	1.23	(29)	1.63	(33)	1.66	(23)	0.73	(5)	2.93	(11)	1.50 (148)
40-49	1.58	(26)	1.04	(63)	1.00	(80)	1.11	(80)	1.36	(66)	1.29	(40)	1.85	(28)	1.41	(7)	1.16 (364)
50-59	0.82	(30)	1.00	(115)	1.07	(125)	1.26	(112)	1.24	(66)	1.01	(28)	1.95	(19)	2.61	(4)	1.14 (469)
60-69	0.81	(35)	0.80	(100)	0.88	(97)	1.22	(86)	1.42	(45)	1.55	(15)	1.54	(2)	-		0.99 (345)
70+	0.72	(31)	0.68	(65)	0.81	(47)	1.05	(26)	1.09	(9)	1.36	(3)	-		-		0.80 (150)

[a] See footnote to Table 2A

Figure 1. Observed to expected ratios of all sites combined, and of sites at close and intermediate distance from the cervix, with and without uterine cancers, by time since diagnosis of cervical cancer for patients with invasive cervical cancer treated with radiotherapy, patients with invasive cervical cancer not treated with radiotherapy, and patients with in-situ cervical cancer not treated with radiotherapy. 80% confidence intervals presented.

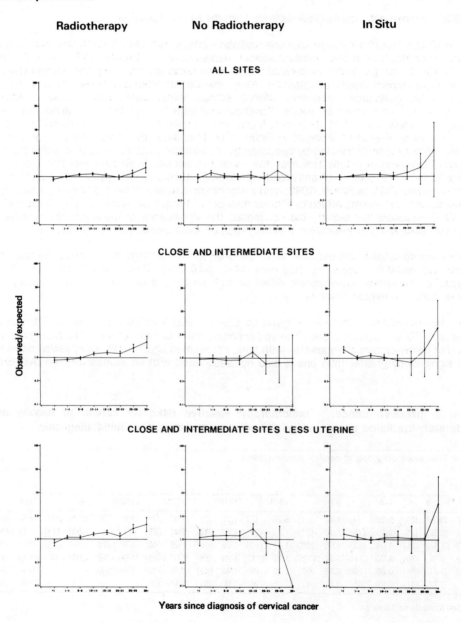

This apparently constant relative risk over time for those aged 20-39 might be due to two factors, namely misclassified metastases exerting an influence on risk during the early years of follow-up and radiation affecting risk among long-term survivors. As discussed in section 5.1(c), the effect of misclassification on the relative risk would be expected to be greater the younger the age of diagnosis of cervical cancer.

In the four ten-year age groups aged 40 years or more, both a significant excess after ten years or more of follow-up, and a significant trend with time are seen. The observed:expected ratios ten or more years after follow-up are similar in each of these ten-year age groups. Striking differences by age are seen, however, for the corpus uteri, bladder and colon; these are discussed in later sections where the results for each site are reviewed.

The high risk in the group aged 20-29 at exposure was not seen in studies of atomic bomb survivors (Kato & Schull, 1982) or ankylosing spondylitis radiotherapy patients (Smith & Doll, 1982), in whom an approximately constant relative risk with age at exposure was seen for persons irradiated after age 20.

4.2 Haematological malignancies

(a) Leukaemia (ICD7 204)

The average cumulative dose to active bone marrow among irradiated patients was probably between 300 and 1500 rad (Hutchison, 1968), which, in the absence of cell-killing, should have been sufficient to induce hundreds of radiogenic leukaemias if the leukaemia risk estimate given in the BEIR report (Advisory Committee on the Biological Effects of Ionizing Radiations, 1980) applied to these women. However, only 77 leukaemias were observed compared with 66 expected (RR=1.2; 95% CI=0.9-1.5). This finding confirms earlier reports that the radiation regimens used to treat cervical cancer are not as effective in inducing leukaemia as are other radiation exposures that have been studied (Boice & Hutchison, 1980). A possible explanation is that high doses to small volumes of bone marrow sterilize cells, as well as transform them, thereby reducing the number of surviving cells available for cancer induction (Hutchison, 1968; Smith, 1977; Major & Mole, 1978).

The excess of leukaemia in the irradiated group is confined to acute and myeloid leukaemia, with 58 observed and 41 expected (RR=1.4, 95% CI=1.1-1.8). The excess was most prominent 1-9 years after irradiation (Figure 2), and the pattern of risk over time is consistent with the induction periods associated with radiogenic leukaemia (Advisory Committee on the Biological Effects of Ionizing Radiations, 1980), although an increased risk beyond ten years would also have been expected. A radiation etiology for this excess is supported by the absence of an excess of chronic lymphocytic leukaemia (Figure 2). The increased risk of acute and myeloid leukaemia was found only in women under age 60 at exposure, although the age effect was not significant. The dose required to cause an excess of 17 leukaemias in the exposed group would be of the order of 15 to 30 rad to the relevant marrow cells, on the basis of currently accepted risk estimates (Advisory Committee on the Biological Effects of Ionizing Radiations, 1980). Much of the bone marrow outside the pelvis probably received less than 100 rad, a dose at which cell sterilization is thought not to be appreciable, and the leukaemia excess may be associated with such exposure.

The excess of acute and myeloid leukaemia among the in-situ patients is puzzling. It is confined entirely to Sweden; it may be due in part to limited radiotherapy given to some in-situ patients.

Figure 2. Observed to expected ratios of second cancers of each organ by time since diagnosis of cervical cancer for patients with invasive cervical cancer treated with radiotherapy, patients with invasive cervical cancer not treated with radiotherapy, and patients with in-situ cervical cancer not treated with radiotherapy. 80% confidence intervals presented. The sites are given in the order of the ICD, 7th Revision.

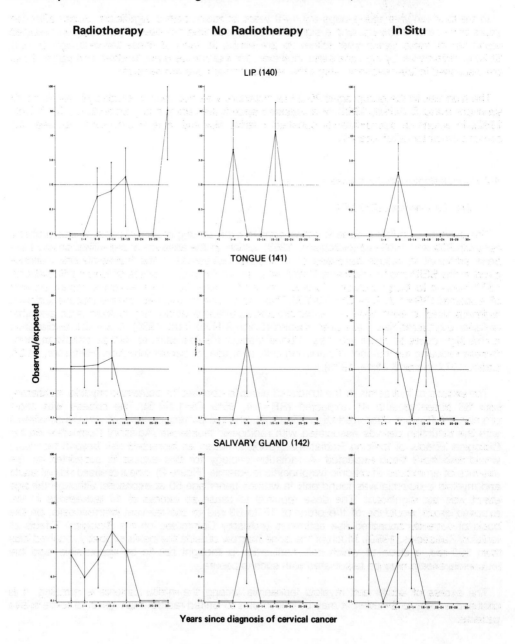

Radiotherapy   **No Radiotherapy**   **In Situ**

MOUTH (143-4)

OTHER PHARYNX (145, 7-8)

NASOPHARYNX (146)

Years since diagnosis of cervical cancer

Years since diagnosis of cervical cancer

Radiotherapy   **No Radiotherapy**   **In Situ**

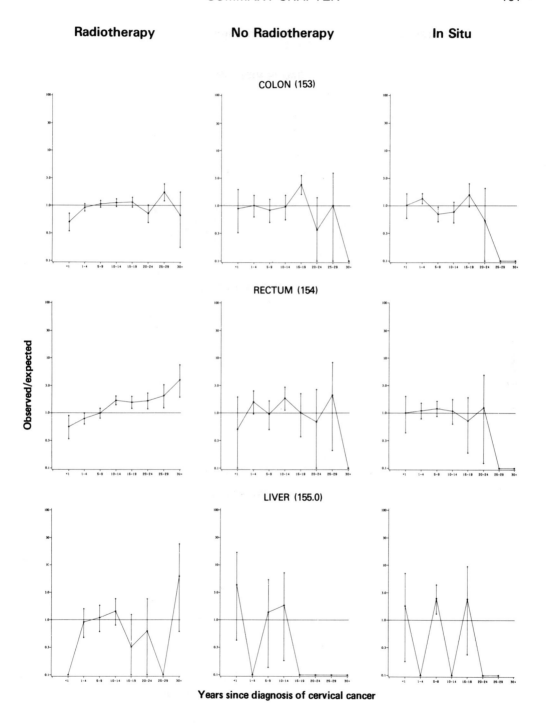

COLON (153)

RECTUM (154)

LIVER (155.0)

Observed/expected

Years since diagnosis of cervical cancer

DAY & BOICE

Radiotherapy   **No Radiotherapy**   **In Situ**

GALL BLADDER (155.1)

PANCREAS (157)

NOSE, SINUSES (160)

Years since diagnosis of cervical cancer

Radiotherapy   **No Radiotherapy**   **In Situ**

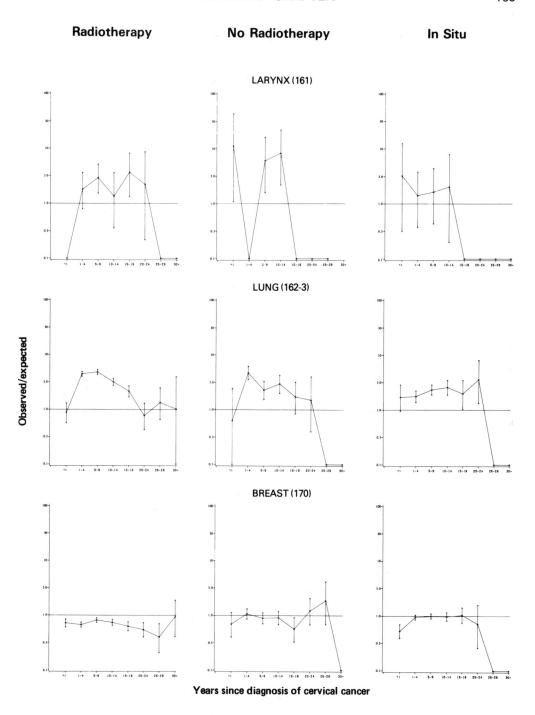

LARYNX (161)

LUNG (162-3)

BREAST (170)

Observed/expected

Years since diagnosis of cervical cancer

Radiotherapy   **No Radiotherapy**   **In Situ**

CORPUS UTERI (172)

OTHER UTERUS (173-4)

OVARY (175)

Observed/expected

Years since diagnosis of cervical cancer

Radiotherapy　　　**No Radiotherapy**　　　**In Situ**

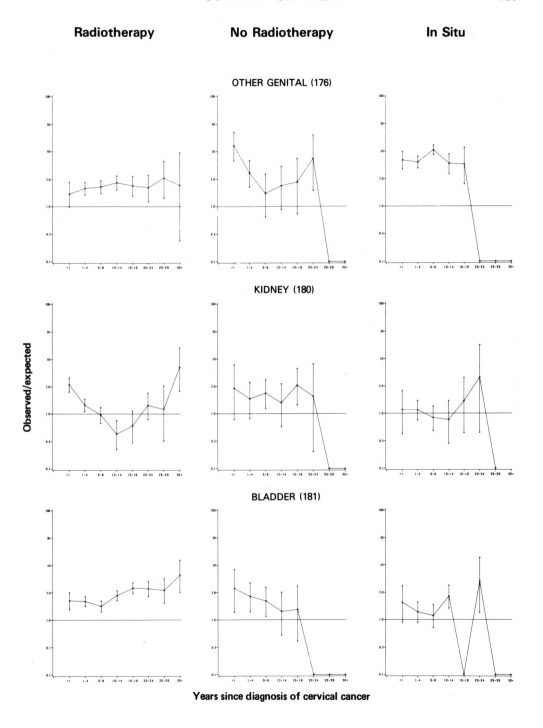

OTHER GENITAL (176)

KIDNEY (180)

BLADDER (181)

Observed/expected

Years since diagnosis of cervical cancer

Radiotherapy   **No Radiotherapy**   **In Situ**

MELANOMA (190)

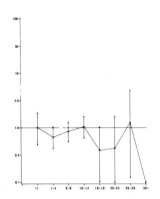
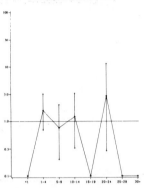
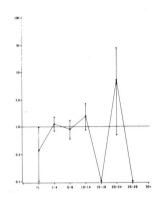

OTHER SKIN (191)

Observed/expected

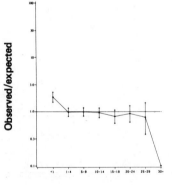
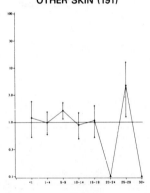
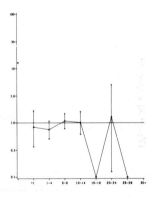

EYE (192)

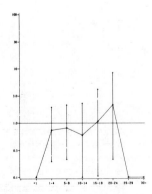
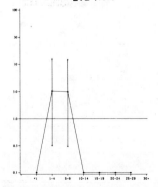
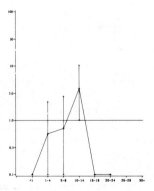

Years since diagnosis of cervical cancer

Radiotherapy   **No Radiotherapy**   **In Situ**

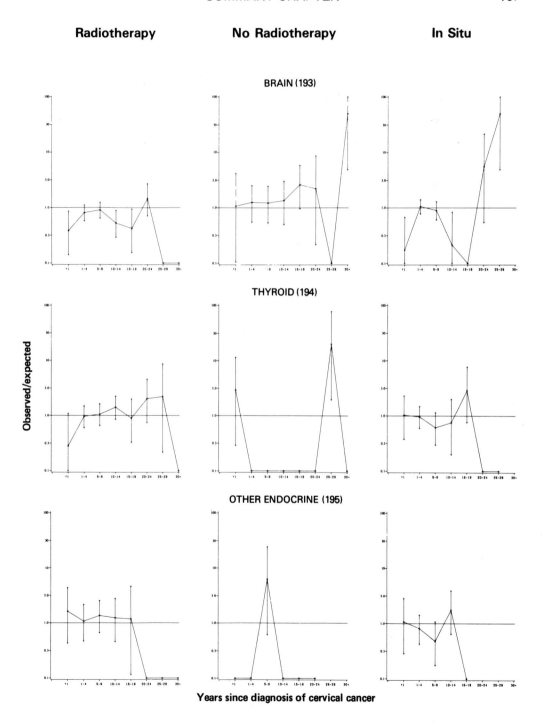

BRAIN (193)

THYROID (194)

OTHER ENDOCRINE (195)

Observed/expected

Years since diagnosis of cervical cancer

DAY & BOICE

Radiotherapy   **No Radiotherapy**   **In Situ**

BONE (196)

CONNECTIVE TISSUE (197)

LYMPHOMA (200, 202)

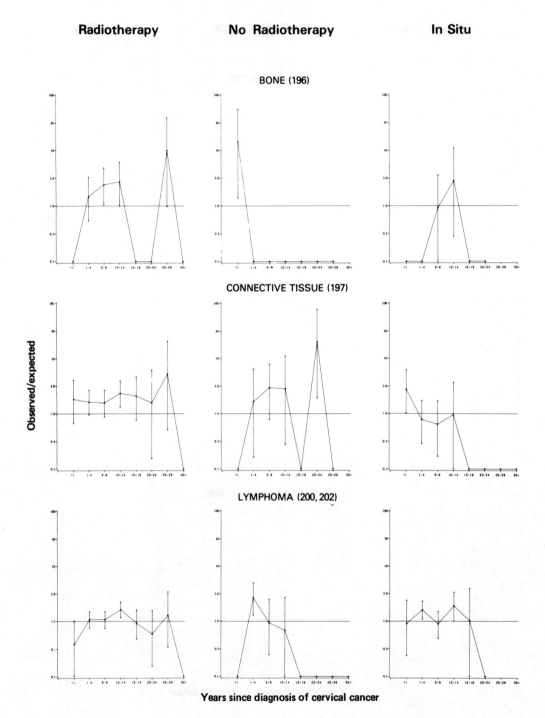

Observed/expected

Years since diagnosis of cervical cancer

Radiotherapy   **No Radiotherapy**   **In Situ**

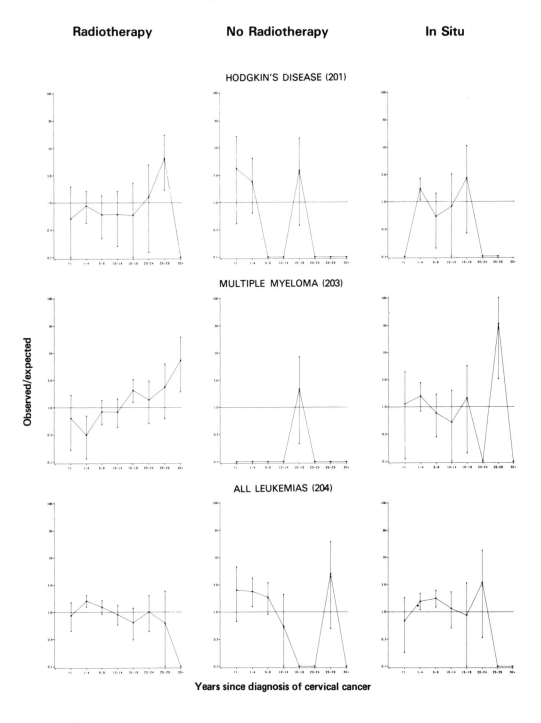

HODGKIN'S DISEASE (201)

MULTIPLE MYELOMA (203)

ALL LEUKEMIAS (204)

Observed/expected

Years since diagnosis of cervical cancer

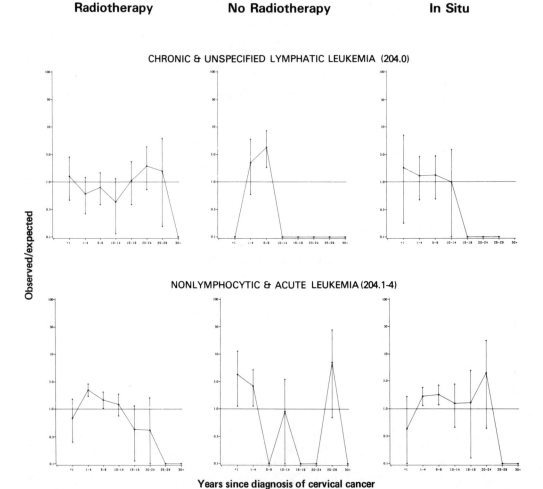

Radiotherapy   **No Radiotherapy**   **In Situ**

CHRONIC & UNSPECIFIED LYMPHATIC LEUKEMIA (204.0)

NONLYMPHOCYTIC & ACUTE LEUKEMIA (204.1-4)

Years since diagnosis of cervical cancer

(b) Lymphoma (200-202) and multiple myeloma (203)

No significant overall excess of Hodgkin's disease (14 *versus* 17), non-Hodgkin's lymphoma (61 *versus* 54) or multiple myeloma (33 *versus* 34) was found among the irradiated patients (Figure 2). Hodgkin's disease is not known to be associated with radiation, and non-Hodgkin's lymphomas (lymphosarcoma and reticulum-cell sarcoma) are only weakly associated (Advisory Committee on the Biological Effects of Ionizing Radiations, 1980). A statistically significant excess of non-Hodgkin's lymphoma occurred among ankylosing spondylitis patients treated with radiotherapy (Smith & Doll, 1982), but no effect has been shown clearly among atomic bomb survivors (Kato & Schull, 1982). The observed:expected ratios showed no variation with time since exposure for either Hodgkin's disease or non-Hodgkin's lymphoma.

The risk of multiple myeloma was decreased appreciably in the first ten years after radiotherapy (11 observed *versus* 19.1 expected; RR=0.6, 95% CI=0.3-1.0), as found in a previous large survey (Boice & Hutchison, 1980). However, the risk increased significantly with time after exposure, irrespective of age at exposure [χ^2_4(trend)=15.1; p<0.001]. The interpretation of the trend test is clouded, however, because the significance of the trend arises partly from the initial deficit, seen also in the non-radiotherapy group. This deficit might reflect a screening artefact, if multiple myeloma, which has a long prodromal phase, was diagnosed 'early' (at the time of diagnosis of the cervical cancer) and was thus removed from this analysis, which excluded all women with simultaneous cancers. However, 15 years or more after exposure multiple myeloma is in significant excess, with 16 observed and 7.6 expected (RR=2.0, 95% CI=1.2-3.4). Thus, these data provide additional evidence that multiple myeloma may be associated with radiation, with a long induction period (Kato & Schull, 1982).

4.3 *Sites close to the cervix*

Sites likely to have received intense radiation exposure because of their location close to the pelvis include the small intestine, colon, rectum, corpus uteri, ovary, other genital organs, bladder, bone and connective tissue (Figure 2). Statistically significant excesses of cancers were observed for all these heavily irradiated sites except the colon, uterine corpus and ovary. For cancers of the last two sites overall comparisons with the general population are misleading, since many of the cervical cancer cases had had their uterus and ovaries removed.

(a) Small intestine (152)

A two-fold risk was apparent among the irradiated cervical cancer patients (RR=2.2; 95% CI=1.4-3.4). The relative risk did not vary among women exposed at different ages. Denmark and Ontario contributed most to the reported excess. The excess risk first appeared in years 5-9 after irradiation (Figure 2). Although these data are consistent with an increased risk following large radiation doses, an elevated risk of similar magnitude occurred among non-exposed invasive, but not in-situ, cervical cancer patients. Cell type was not specifically evaluated, and it is possible that the excess might reflect an increase in sarcomas of the small intestine resulting from high dose radiotherapy. The Danish registry, however, which contributed a considerable part of the excess, excludes sarcomas from the small intestine classification as it does from all other sites except connective tissue (Clemmesen, 1965).

Evidence for an increased risk of cancer of the small intestine due to radiation exposure comes mainly from studies of women irradiated for metropathia haemorrhagica (Smith & Doll, 1976; Advisory Committee on the Biological Effects of Ionizing Radiations, 1980).

(b) Colon (153)

No excess of colon cancer was seen in this series (RR=1.0; 95% CI=0.9-1.2), and risk did not increase with time following radiation exposure [χ^2_1(trend)=0.88; p=0.17] (Figure 2). In years 1-9 after exposure, there was a significant excess among those under age 50 at exposure (48 *versus* 30), contrasted with a significant deficit among those over age 70 at exposure (20 *versus* 40). Among those aged 50-69, the observed number of cancers was approximately equal to that expected (98 *versus* 99). For this first nine-year period of follow-up, the trend in the observed:expected ratio with age at exposure is highly significant (p<0.001). Factors that might contribute to this effect are the diagnosis of indolent colon tumours at the time of diagnosis of the cervical cancer, the misdiagnosis of recurrence of the cervical cancer as a new primary cancer of the colon, and misdiagnosis of genuine primary cancers of the colon as recurrences of the primary cervical cancer (perhaps more common in the oldest age group). The second factor would affect the observed:expected ratio more markedly among the young (see section 5.1(c)). Ten years or more after exposure, no appreciable variation by age at exposure was observed.

The absence of an overall excess is somewhat surprising in view of the high dose received by the colon. Significant excess mortality from colon cancer has been observed in patients irradiated for ankylosing spondylitis (Court Brown & Doll, 1965; Smith & Doll, 1982) and in women irradiated for metropathia haemorrhagica (Smith & Doll, 1976). A relationship with radiation also has been recently observed among atomic bomb survivors (Kato & Schull, 1982). General population rates may not be appropriate for predicting second tumours of the colon, since cervical cancer patients, often of low socioeconomic status, may have a lower risk of colon cancer than the population in general. This effect, however, should be small, of the order of 10% or less (see section 5.3(d)), and among non-exposed cervical cancer patients the observed:expected ratio is slightly above one. In addition, the absence of an increasing risk with time since irradiation argues against a radiation effect in this series. An analogy to the findings for leukaemia can perhaps be drawn: cells in the large intestine are rapidly dividing and may be sensitive to the cell killing effects of radiation. The absence of an effect in this series and in other studies of cervical cancer patients (Wagoner, 1970; Dickson, 1972) may be due to radiation-induced cellular inactivation that might occur when high doses of radiation are received by rapidly dividing cells.

(c) Rectum (154)

A significant excess of cancer of the rectum was observed among patients treated with radiotherapy (RR=1.3; 95% CI=1.1-1.4), which was confined to women followed for more than ten years (RR=1.7; 95% CI=1.4-2.0). The risk increased steadily with time since diagnosis of cervical cancer [χ^2_1(trend)=21.9; p<0.001], but only for women given radiotherapy (Figure 2). Among women living for ten or more years after treatment, there was no suggestion that the relative risk changed with age at exposure. No excess of cancer of the rectum was found in patients with in-situ cancer or those not treated with radiotherapy. Although increased rates of rectal cancer have been observed in several groups of women who received radiotherapy for benign gynaecological diseases (Advisory Committee on the Biological Effects of Ionizing Radiations, 1980) and in a small study of cervical cancer patients (Dickson, 1972), no excess of this cancer was found among atomic bomb survivors (Beebe et al., 1978; Kato & Schull, 1982) or ankylosing spondylitis patients (Smith & Doll, 1982).

(d) Uterine corpus (172)

There was a statistically significant deficit of cancer of the uterine corpus among women given radiotherapy (RR=0.6; 95% CI=0.5-0.7), which was observed mainly in the early years after exposure (Figure 2). A great many irradiated women would have had their uterus removed (Storm & Jensen, this monograph). The overall deficit was due mainly to reduced rates in Denmark, Finland and Sweden. Connecticut stands out by reporting a significant excess of uterine cancer. Among women over age 40 at exposure, there is an almost 90% deficit of endometrial cancer in years 1-4 after exposure (7 observed versus 65 expected; RR=0.11), a 45% deficit in years 5-9 after exposure (32 versus 59; RR=0.54) and only a 5% deficit among ten-year survivors (64 versus 66.9; RR=0.96). For women under age 40 at exposure, an excess of endometrial cancer is seen in each time interval after exposure (RR=1.5; 95% CI=0.96-2.1). In both groups of non-exposed women, a substantial deficit of endometrial cancer was seen, but in neither group did the observed:expected ratios increase with time since treatment. The large deficit seen in the first years of follow-up for women over age 40 at exposure, and the increase in the observed:expected ratios with time since exposure, are difficult to interpret since the correct denominator is the number of uteri at risk, at present unknown, rather than the number of women. The planned case-control studies will provide estimates of the proportion of patients on whom a hysterectomy was performed. In the Finnish material (this monograph), all cases of corpus or ovarian cancer among those with invasive cervical cancer and who were treated with radiation occurred in the group treated only by irradiation, that is, without surgery. A relative risk of nearly one in the women followed for more than ten years probably corresponds to a considerable real excess in women with an intact uterus.

Cancer of the uterine corpus is known to occur at higher than expected rates in women irradiated for benign menstrual diseases (Advisory Committee on the Biological Effects of Ionizing Radiations, 1980), but it is not increased among atomic bomb survivors (Kato & Schull, 1982).

(e) Ovary (175)

A significant deficit of ovarian cancer was observed among women treated with radiation (RR=0.7; 95% CI=0.6-0.8). The observed:expected ratios increased with time for women of all ages [χ_1^2(trend)=15.2; p<0.001]. In years 1-9 after diagnosis, there was a 47% deficit, whereas long-term survivors appeared to be at elevated risk (Figure 2). The deficit and the trend with time since exposure varied little with age at exposure, except for those under 30 years of age, who were at significantly increased risk (5 *versus* 1.6) of developing ovarian cancer. Denmark reported a substantial deficit of ovarian cancer, whereas Connecticut reported a significant excess. Patients with invasive cervical cancer not treated with radiotherapy had nearly a 50% deficit of ovarian cancer, which varied little with time since diagnosis. Observed and expected numbers of ovarian cancer were similar among women with in-situ cervical cancer (Table 3). The general population is not a correct comparison group, because many of the women with invasive cervical cancer would also have had their ovaries removed during treatment. A radiation effect is suggested because an increased risk over time is seen only for women treated with radiation, and because of the consistency with other studies of women who received ovarian radiation for castration and who subsequently developed ovarian malignancies (Advisory Committee on the Biological Effects of Ionizing Radiations, 1980).

(f) Other genital (176)

There was a substantial excess of other genital cancers, i.e., vulva, vagina and sites not otherwise specified (RR=2.4; 95% CI=1.9-2.9), but the increase in risk did not change appreciably with time since exposure (Figure 2) [χ_1^2(trend)=0.41; p=0.26]. The risk was also high in patients with invasive and in-situ cervical cancer who did not receive radiation, with no systematic change in risk with time since treatment (Figure 2). Denmark, Finland, Sweden and Connecticut contributed most to the reported excess among radiotherapy patients. The risk was most marked in women under 50 years of age at the time of radiotherapy (48 *versus* 11) and decreased with increasing age at exposure (p=0.02). Among women irradiated under age 50, the risk increased significantly with time (p=0.02). The problem in distinguishing a new primary cancer at these sites from a recurrence of the original cervical cancer makes any conclusion difficult.

(g) Bladder (181)

Among women treated by radiation, a substantial risk of bladder cancer was observed (RR=2.6; 95% CI=2.3-3.0), which increased with time since exposure [χ^2_1(trend)=14.4; p<0.001]. The relative risks varied, however, both with age at diagnosis and with time since exposure. In years 1-9 of follow-up, those aged less than 50 years at exposure had an observed:expected ratio of 5.1 (30 versus 6.3), whereas the ratio for those aged over 60 was 1.1 (25 versus 23.1). By contrast, in the 15-year survivors, the relative risk varied only slightly with age (RR=3.9; 95% CI=3.0-4.9), reflecting an increase during follow-up for older groups and little change for the younger groups. Several factors may have contributed to these results. First, metastases from the primary cervical cancer may have been misdiagnosed as primary bladder cancer. This effect on the relative risk would be greatest among the young (see section 5.1(c)), most marked in the first few years of follow-up and relatively small among 15-year survivors. Second, smoking is more common among both bladder and cervical cancer patients. As discussed in section 5.3(d), however, the confounding effect of smoking should not increase the relative risks by more than 50%. Third, the excess in the first ten years may result in part from the relatively early diagnosis of bladder cancer due to greater medical surveillance of the women, with routine cystoscopy and urography. None of these factors would seem to be responsible for a relative risk of nearly 4 among 15-year survivors, which may thus be related mainly to radiation.

This interpretation is supported by the findings in the two non-exposed groups. Among the invasive cancer patients not treated by radiotherapy, the observed:expected ratio, initially high, decreases with time since treatment (Figure 2). This decline probably represents the decreasing effect of misdiagnosed metastases from the cervical cancer. Among in-situ cancer patients, there is a 50% excess of bladder cancer, consistent with the expected influence of smoking as a confounder (see section 5.3(d)).

Although studies of various irradiated populations have yielded equivocal results as to an association of radiation with bladder cancer (Advisory Committee on the Biological Effects of Ionizing Radiations, 1980), in this series both the increased risk over time and the level of the relative risk among 15-year survivors suggest a radiation effect (Figure 2).

(h) Bone (196)

Excess sarcomas of the bone have arisen after the ingestion of bone-seeking isotopes for medical treatment, after occupational exposures and in populations of cancer patients treated with radiotherapy for certain neoplasms and bone disorders (Fraumeni & Boice, 1982). No excess of bone sarcoma is apparent among atomic bomb survivors. The excess in the exposed cervical cancer patients reported here is two-fold and of marginal statistical significance (RR=1.9; 95% CI=1.0-3.5). No excess was observed in the non-exposed women. The distribution of the excess of bone sarcomas over time since exposure (Figure 2) is similar to that seen in other studies of radiogenic bone tumors following short-term exposure (Advisory Committee on the Biological Effects of Ionizing Radiations, 1980). A radiation effect might be supported further if the site distribution of the bone cancers were known.

(i) Connective tissue (197)

Soft-tissue sarcomas have been associated with radiation therapy (Kim et al., 1978), although the magnitude of the risk has not been quantified. The increased risk among irradiated cervical cancer patients was statistically significant (RR=1.9; 95% CI=1.2-2.6) and was concentrated in women over 50 years of age at time of exposure (19 versus 8.9). The relative risk did not change markedly with time since exposure [χ_1^2(trend)=0.70; p=0.20], although it did increase significantly for women over age 50 (p=0.02). An excess was also observed among invasive cervical cancer patients who had not received radiation therapy (5 observed, 1.82 expected) but not among patients with in-situ cancer (6 observed, 8.39 expected). The numbers are small, however. A distribution of connective tissue cancers by anatomic site would assist in evaluating a radiation association. Since a sarcoma occurring in a specific organ is commonly coded as a malignancy of that site, all sarcomas have probably not been included in this analysis, except by the Danish Cancer Registry which, for this study, classified all sarcomas as connective tissue malignancies.

4.4 Sites at intermediate distance from the cervix

Sites considered to be at intermediate distance from the cervix probably received hundreds of rad from the radiotherapy procedures. The stomach, liver, gallbladder, pancreas and kidney were so designated. Only the pancreas showed a statistically significant excess over expectation.

(a) Stomach (151)

There was no excess of stomach cancer in the women treated either with radiation (RR=1.0; 95% CI=0.8-1.1) or without radiation (RR=0.9). A significant excess of stomach cancer reported in Norway was balanced by a significant deficit in Slovenia. The observed:expected ratios did not vary appreciably with age at exposure. There was no change in relative risk with time since treatment [χ_1^2(trend)=0.27; p=0.30] (Figure 2). The absence of any apparent excess is surprising, as this organ received a large radiation dose, and an effect has been seen with similar doses in the studies of patients treated with radiotherapy for ankylosing spondylitis (Smith & Doll, 1982) and in atomic bomb survivors (Kato & Schull, 1982; Advisory Committee on the Biological Effects of Ionizing Radiations, 1980). Moreover, the risk among atomic bomb survivors was in fact concentrated among women (Beebe et al., 1978), although the high 'natural' incidence of stomach cancer in Japan might be a contributing factor. Furthermore, patients with cancer of the cervix and stomach tend to be of a low social class, and a slight excess of stomach cancer might also be expected for this reason alone. On the basis of currently accepted radiation risk estimates for the stomach (Advisory Committee on the Biological Effects of Ionizing Radiations, 1980), approximately 45 extra cancers would have been predicted in this series (see Table 6). Among women treated by radiation and followed for more than ten years, only 86 cases were observed versus 86.5 expected in the absence of a radiation effect. Thus, these data are not compatible with current BEIR risk estimates for radiogenic stomach cancer.

(b) Liver (155) and gallbladder (155.1)

The liver (23 observed versus 23 expected) and gallbladder (41 versus 52) are not known to be particularly radiosensitive to X- or gamma-radiation (Advisory Committee on the Biological Effects of Ionizing Radiations, 1980), and no increased risk of cancer was observed at these sites among cervical cancer patients treated with radiation therapy.

(c) Pancreas (157)

A significant excess of pancreatic cancer was noted among irradiated women (RR=1.3; 95% CI=1.05-1.5), which was concentrated among patients over age 50 at the time of radiotherapy (94 versus 73). Most registries reported only slight increases. There was a peculiar distribution of risk over time with the increase, which occurred mainly in years 1-4 after exposure (47 *versus* 27), and which decreased with time since exposure, although the decrease was of marginal statistical significance (p=0.06). Nevertheless, a slight increase was observed among the ten-year survivors (52 *versus* 42.8). The early risk might be elevated because of increased cigarette consumption, or it might be a diagnostic artefact associated with the increased medical surveillance afforded cancer patients. Pancreatic cancer was not increased among non-irradiated invasive cervical cancer patients, although it was elevated among women with in-situ cancer. The low rate of histological confirmation seen in this series is common in other cancer registry material (Waterhouse *et al.*, 1976, 1982) and adds uncertainty to the interpretation of these data.

Evidence for an increase in the incidence of cancer of the pancreas following irradiation comes mainly from the study of ankylosing spondylitis patients treated with radiotherapy (Advisory Committee on the Biological Effects of Ionizing Radiations, 1980), where much of the excess is also seen soon after irradiation (Smith & Doll, 1982), and also from a small study of cervical cancer patients (Dickson, 1972). Pancreatic cancer was also increased among US atomic energy workers (Mancuso *et al.*, 1977; Gilbert & Marks, 1979). The atomic bomb data are equivocal (Beebe *et al.*, 1978), and a radiation effect is not established (Kato & Schull, 1982). Although the pancreas received substantial radiation exposure during radiotherapy for cervical cancer, a radiation association is not convincingly demonstrated.

(d) Kidney (180)

There was no overall increase in risk of cancer of the kidney, despite the fact that this organ received a relatively large radiation dose (RR=1.0; 95% CI=0.8-1.3). The distribution of risk over time, however, is erratic (Figure 2). There was an appreciable excess in years 1-4 after irradiation, a deficit in years 10-14, and an excess risk of borderline significance among 20-year survivors (12 *versus* 6.4), which might reflect a radiation component, although seen only in Connecticut. The observed:expected ratios in years 1-4 after exposure fell markedly with age at exposure [χ^2_1(trend)=15.9; p<0.001]. Among the 20-year survivors, the excess was not related to age. Close clinical surveillance, with routine urography, perhaps greatest among the youngest age groups, may have contributed to the variation in risk both with age and with time. A significant elevation was also observed for non-radiotherapy patients with invasive cancer, with no appreciable variation by time since diagnosis. Kidney cancer has not been reported previously to be induced by radiation, except in the study of patients treated with radiotherapy for ankylosing spondylitis (Advisory Committee on the Biological Effects of Ionizing Radiations, 1980; Smith & Doll, 1982).

4.5 Sites remote from the cervix

For those organs that received minimal radiation exposure (average dose, under 50 rad), two observations stand out: the substantial excess of lung cancer and other smoking-related sites and the substantial deficit of breast cancer (Figure 2).

(a) Buccal cavity and nasopharynx (140-148)

Among irradiated women, cancers of the buccal cavity and nasopharynx combined were more common than expected (RR=1.3; 95% CI=1.0-1.7), although the risk did not increase with time since treatment [χ^2_1(trend)=0.30; p=0.29]. Norway and Connecticut accounted for most of the excess. The excess was confined to cancers commonly associated with alcohol and tobacco consumption. Neither the salivary gland nor the nasopharynx showed an increased risk. An excess was also apparent among non-irradiated women with invasive cancer and a significant excess occurred among in-situ cancer patients (RR=1.7; 95% CI=1.1-2.5).

(b) Oesophagus (150)

The pattern for oesophageal cancer was similar to that seen for the alcohol- and tobacco-related sites of the buccal cavity. A significant excess was found (RR=1.5; 95% CI=1.1-2.1), but with no variation of relative risk over time since treatment (Figure 2). Most registries contributed only a small number to the overall excess. This risk is probably related to cigarette smoking and/or, possibly, alcohol consumption. No excess was observed among non-irradiated or in-situ cancer patients, but the numbers are small.

(c) Lung (162-163)

Lung cancer risk was substantially increased among all three groups of women. In the irradiated group the risk was highly significant (RR=3.6; 95% CI=3.3-4.0) and was most prominent 1-10 years after diagnosis of cervical cancer (Figure 2). The risk decreased significantly with time since diagnosis and returned to normal levels within 20 years [χ_1^2(trend)=50; p<0.001]. There was considerable change in the observed: expected ratios with age at exposure in the period 1-9 years after exposure [χ_1^2(trend)=74.0]. Among those under age 40 when irradiated, 40 lung cancers were registered *versus* 3.2 expected (RR=12.5), whereas in those aged 60 or over, 96 were observed and 33.2 expected (RR=2.9). The relative risk of 12.5 seen in the younger women is very much greater than could be attributed to the possible confounding effect of cigarette smoking and probably arises from the misclassification of metastases to the lung. The change of the relative risk with age at exposure and the decline in the relative risk with time since exposure are consistent with this explanation.

Among the patients with invasive cancers not treated by radiotherapy, a similar pattern of risk ratios was seen by age at diagnosis and time since diagnosis of cervical cancer. The patients with in-situ lesions, by contrast, among whom metastatic lesions would not be expected, had an approximately two-fold excess of lung cancer throughout follow-up for all age groups. Cigarette smoking might be expected to produce an excess of this magnitude (see section 5.3(d)). The pattern of risk over time among women with invasive cancer might also reflect a cohort effect, long-term survivors being women who were less likely to be cigarette smokers. Since the radiation dose to the lung was relatively low, any radiation effect would be difficult to detect, given the substantially elevated background risk.

(d) Breast (170)

Cancer of the breast was of special interest since it is the most frequent cancer among females and since breast tissue is particularly susceptible to the carcinogenic effects of radiation (Boice et al., 1979; Land et al., 1980). Nevertheless, the effect of radiotherapy for cervical cancer on ovarian function might be expected to lower the subsequent risk of breast cancer (Smith & Doll, 1976; Boice & Hoover, 1981). The observed and expected numbers of breast cancers are given by time since first treatment in Appendix A and by age at first treatment in Table 4 and Appendix B. Among patients irradiated for invasive cervical cancer, 569 breast cancers occurred more than one year after first treatment whereas 804 were expected on the basis of general population rates (RR=0.7; 95% CI=0.6-0.8). Registries not demonstrating a reduction in breast cancer risk include Birmingham, Finland, New Brunswick, and Nova Scotia. The observed and expected numbers for those with invasive cancer not treated with radiotherapy were 118 *versus* 125 (RR=0.9; 95% CI=0.8-1.1) and for in-situ cancer 409 *versus* 427 (RR=1.0; 95% CI=0.9-1.1).

Table 4. Observed (O) and expected (E) numbers of breast cancers[a] following an initial cancer of the cervix by state of disease, treatment and age at treatment

Stage	Treatment	Age at treatment (years)	O	E	O/E
Invasive	Radiotherapy	< 30	1	7.7	0.13
		30-39	40	108.4	0.37
		40-49	182	249.8	0.73
		50-59	181	230.1	0.79
		60-69	113	147.0	0.77
		70 +	53	62.1	0.85
		All ages	570	805.1	0.71
Invasive	No radiotherapy	< 30	3	2.7	1.11
		30-39	26	28.1	0.93
		40-49	35	48.0	0.73
		50-59	36	28.5	1.26
		60-69	11	13.2	0.83
		70 +	5	5.2	0.96
		All ages	116	125.7	0.92
In-situ	No radiotherapy	< 30	18	16.8	1.07
		30-39	116	125.0	0.93
		40-49	171	193.5	0.88
		50-59	75	64.9	1.16
		60-69	19	20.3	0.94
		70 +	8	6.4	1.25
		All ages	407	427.9	0.95

[a] Excluding the first year after diagnosis of cervical cancer

Among both groups of women not treated by radiotherapy, a slight deficit of breast cancer was seen (527 *versus* 553; RR=0.95, 95% CI=0.8-1.1), which varied little with age at diagnosis of cervical cancer (Table 4). The magnitude of this deficit is of the order predicted from the likely confounding effect of earlier and more numerous pregnancies among cervical cancer patients, and of a possibly lower socioeconomic status (see section 5.3.(*e*). Among the women treated by radiation, the relative deficit of breast cancer varied sharply with age (Table 4). Those aged under 40 at irradiation had 65% fewer breast cancers than expected (41 *versus* 116; RR=0.35), whereas in women over 50 at irradiation the deficit was only 20% (347 *versus* 439; RR=0.79). The deficit of breast cancer in those irradiated under age 40 is very much greater than could be attributed to socioeconomic status or reproductive history, and is consistent with other studies that show a protective effect of surgical removal or radiation sterilization of the ovaries (Trichopoulos *et al.*, 1972; Smith & Doll, 1976). Among women over age 50 at diagnosis of cervical cancer, most of whom are post-menopausal, the risk is slightly, but significantly, lower among the irradiated women than in the two non-irradiated groups. If due to radiation, this difference suggests that a separate mechanism may be operating from the one that lowers risk prior to the menopause. The finding of a lowering of risk among women irradiated after menopause is consistent with some (Smith & Doll, 1976) but not all (Dickson, 1969) studies of women given radiotherapy for benign menstrual disorders. There was little change in the observed:expected ratios with time since irradiation in most groups, except for women over age 70 at irradiation, among whom a significant increase with time since exposure was seen (χ_1^2(trend)=3.4, p=0.03).

On the basis of estimates of the radiogenic risk of breast cancer from other studies and assuming an average dose of approximately 35 rad to the breast, about 37 induced cancers might have been expected among ten-year survivors, in addition to the 305 that were expected from 'natural' causes; a total of only 204 cancers had been observed in this period. Thus, these data indicate no effect on subsequent breast cancer risk from the irradiation to which the breast was exposed; but interpretation is not possible at present.

(e) Brain (193)

Among patients treated with radiotherapy, a marginally statistically significant deficit of brain cancer was observed (RR=0.8; 95% CI=0.6-0.99), reflecting in large part a significant deficit in Denmark. The rate of brain cancer was near expectation among women with in-situ cancer and slightly elevated among women with invasive cancer who did not receive radiotherapy (RR=1.5; 95% CI=0.9-2.5).

(f) Thyroid (194)

A slight excess of thyroid cancer (RR=1.1; 95% CI=0.8-1.6) was observed among women with invasive cervical cancer treated with radiation (36 observed *versus* 31 expected), contrasted with slight deficits among those with invasive cancer not treated with radiation (1 *versus* 4.2) and in-situ cancer patients (19 *versus* 27). The excess occurred mainly in those followed for more than ten years after irradiation (16 *versus* 11.7; RR=1.37, 95% CI=0.8-2.3). The observed:expected ratios did not vary appreciably by age at exposure, although risk appeared to increase over time among women aged 60 or more at exposure (p=0.03). The thyroid is especially sensitive to the carcinogenic action of ionizing radiation, especially in females, and low doses have been associated with an increased cancer risk (Ron & Modan, 1980). Most studies of radiogenic thyroid cancer, however, have involved newborn or young children, and risk coefficients derived from these groups may not be applicable to older women. Because thyroid cancer appears to be associated with high social class (Williams & Horm, 1977), population rates may overestimate the expected number of thyroid cancers in cervical cancer patients; and, because the risk in non-exposed patients was lower than expected, it is possible that radiation exposure caused the small excess among irradiated patients.

5. Cautions in interpretation

The inferences drawn from this large body of combined material must be considered as preliminary, since there is likely to be some variability in the results from the 15 registries in eight different countries. There may be specific differences in cancer registration, diagnostic and therapeutic practices and in environmental factors, as well as differences in the characteristics of cervical cancer patients that confound comparisons of their morbidity with that of the general population. The special value of this study, however, pertains to the large numbers of irradiated women, the long follow-up available in many registries, the existence of comparison populations of cervical cancer patients not known to have been treated by radiation, and the stringent criteria used by cancer registries to record second primary cancers. It should be emphasized that this is a study of cancer incidence, not cancer mortality. In general, death certificates are a less reliable indicator of cancer occurrence than cancer registration (Engel et al., 1980) and are of very little value in studies of second cancers (Hakulinen & Teppo, 1977). The studies of atomic bomb survivors rely mainly on mortality data (Beebe et al., 1978), and the study of British ankylosing spondylitis patients is only of their mortality experience compared with that of the general population (Smith & Doll, 1982). Thus, despite the several cautions discussed below, this programme of studies can potentially yield substantial information on the carcinogenic effects of ionizing radiation.

5.1 Cancer registration

Cancer registries differ with regard to methods of registration, the length of patient follow-up available for study, the methods by which the occurrence of a second malignancy is determined, including the assessment of possibly metastatic lesions, and the accuracy of treatment details in the records. Such factors, coupled with differences in the degree of medical surveillance afforded cancer patients, are likely to affect the results from different registries in different ways.

(a) Methods of registration

Over the years covered by this study the methods used to register cancers are likely to have changed. Such variation could affect the completeness and validity of the data collected. Some registries were initially based on hospital patients only and then expanded to include all cases of cancer diagnosed in their region, with voluntary or mandatory registration. Differences in the completeness of registration would affect the numbers of second cancers available for study. In like manner, the diagnostic criteria varied over the years and between registries, as evidenced by the differences in histological confirmation of the reported second cancers (Appendix A).

Although women who had a prior history of cancer before the diagnosis of cervical cancer were excluded from study, such prior cancer and any accompanying radiation treatment may not have been recorded if it occurred before the cancer registry began. Thus, some 'second' cancers may be related to radiation therapy other than that given for the cervical cancer, although the number must be small.

(b) Follow-up practices

Patients with an initial primary cancer are not followed in the same way in all countries for the development of a second primary cancer. Some registries follow up all patients on a regular basis to determine their vital status, and the evidence for second cancers is scrutinized specifically. In other registries, follow-up is in large part based on information about death, and little attempt is made to evaluate migration or other factors that might influence the ascertainment of second cancers. Some registries carry out follow-up by means of national population registries in which both the live status (active follow-up) and the occurrence of death are recorded. Differences in follow-up practices are of greater importance for the longer-lived subjects, in whom the occurrence of radiation-induced cancers would be expected.

(c) *Assessment of metastases*

Cancers diagnosed after the occurrence of cervical cancer may be wrongly classified as a new primary tumour when they are in fact metastatic lesions, or a new primary cancer might be inappropriately classified as metastatic and excluded simply because it occurred within the pelvic region (near the primary) or in the lungs. There may be substantial differences between registries in this respect. The lung is a frequent metastatic site, and it may be particularly difficult to establish whether such tumours are primary or metastatic (Van Nagell *et al.*, 1979). The excess of lung cancer is in fact particularly striking, with risk ratios greater than ten in the younger age groups.

Apart from the lung, spread of the original cancer is, perhaps, most likely to be a problem for organs close to the uterine cervix where local invasion may occur. For other sites, the problem may be minimal, since most cervical cancers are squamous-cell carcinomas and most other cancers are adenocarcinomas. The frequency of metastatic lesions is likely to decrease with the length of time following the diagnosis of the primary cervical cancer, although an excess risk of death is seen more than 20 years after diagnosis among cervical cancer patients (Hakulinen *et al.*, 1981).

Misclassification of metastases may generate an apparent age effect. If the same proportion of primary cervical cancers is misclassified in each age group - a not unlikely supposition - then the effect on the observed:expected ratio will be greater in the younger age groups, since the expected number of second cancers will be smaller. Such a pattern by age at diagnosis of cervical cancer is seen notably for cancers of the lung and bladder.

(d) *Misclassification of therapy*

Some patients classified as having received only surgery may also have received radiation therapy. In addition, the records in many registries code only treatment received during the first few months after diagnosis of cervical cancer, and subsequent radiation therapy is not noted, although later radiotherapy may sometimes erroneously have been coded as pertaining to the primary treatment. The report from the Danish Cancer Registry is particularly informative in this regard, indicating that as many as 10% of the 'no radiotherapy' patients received radiation treatments that were not recorded in the registry records and that this proportion was even higher in those women who developed a second primary cancer. Similarly, patients with in-situ cancer in Sweden, where the cancer registry does not record treatment, occasionally received radiation therapy. Some 15% of the in-situ patients in Finland received radiation treatment (see this monograph). As in other registries where treatment details are recorded, in-situ patients in Finland for whom radiation treatment was recorded have been excluded from the in-situ group.

(e) *Medical surveillance*

Because cancer patients are under closer medical scrutiny during the first few years after diagnosis, second cancers may be detected sooner than might normally have been the case. The date of diagnosis of the second cancer would thereby be advanced in time. Also, indolent tumours might be detected which otherwise would have remained dormant and not come to medical attention. Thyroid cancer, for example, appears to be a malignancy that is frequently found to be increased following medical screening.

5.2 *Therapeutic procedures*

(a) *Extent of surgery*

Surgical practice is likely to differ between the various countries. Many cervical cancer patients were operated upon and had their uteri and sometimes their ovaries removed. The Danish Cancer Registry report indicated that 10%, 50% and 40% of the radiotherapy, no radiotherapy (invasive) and in-situ cancer patients, respectively, had their uteri removed surgically. In Connecticut, 34% of the cervical cancer patients were known to have had a hysterectomy. Thus, the general population rates used to generate expected numbers of second cancers would not be applicable for some pelvic sites and would not always applicable in the case of breast cancer.

(b) *Radiotherapy practices*

Differences also occur among countries with regard to radiation practices, resulting in different radiation doses to various organs. Differences in the amount of radium implanted and/or external beam therapy could produce differences in the incidence of second tumours in different countries. For example, the kidney is an organ that would receive a high dose of radiation if it were included in the direct radiation field during external beam therapy, and considerably lower doses if not. Organ doses also differ for external beam therapy and for brachytherapy (intracavitary radium), and differences in the combined mode of therapy between clinics and countries, and according to calendar year of treatment, could result in different organ doses. Doses also vary by stage of cervical cancer and by type of external beam used.

5.3 *Host and environmental factors*

Cancers that may have a similar etiology are known to occur together in the same person more frequently than would be expected by chance, e.g., breast and ovary, and cancers related to cigarette consumption. Thus, the occurrence of a second cancer might also reflect host or environmental factors common to both the initial cervical cancer and the second tumour.

(a) *Smoking and drinking*

Several studies have shown that patients with cervical cancer smoke more than people in the general population (Wright *et al.*, 1978). For this reason alone, cancers associated with smoking, such as cancer of the lung, would be expected to be increased irrespective of any effect of radiation therapy. The evidence that cervical cancer patients drink more than the average is equivocal, but this could affect the risk of alcohol-associated cancers.

(b) *Socioeconomic status*

General population rates may not be appropriate for computing expected numbers of second cancers, since cervical cancer patients tend to be of lower socioeconomic status than average (Logan, 1954; Clemmesen, 1965). The extent to which they differ from the general population may vary both between and within countries, although adjusting for urban-rural differences in

Denmark had little effect on the risk of developing a second cancer. Any differences would apply to all sites that show variation by social class, but the cancers for which this bias may be a potential problem are those of the lung, colon, breast and stomach. Cigarette smoking is also strongly correlated with social class in many countries.

(c) Endocrine status and reproductive history

Cervical cancer patients may be at a lower risk of breast cancer than women in the general population, due to their greater average parity and other protective factors associated with their reproductive history. If so, the expected number of breast and other gynaecological cancer cases generated from general population rates would overestimate the true expected number. Surgical removal or radiation inactivation of the ovaries would also be expected to reduce subsequent breast cancer risk, especially among younger women (Trichopoulos et al., 1972).

(d) Magnitude of possible confounding

As discussed above, women with cancer of the cervix differ from the general population with respect to factors other than radiation that might affect their risk of second cancers, and the observed risk ratios of second cancers reflect in part these differences. There is evidence to indicate that women with cervical cancer tend to smoke more, have more children and are of lower socioeconomic status than average. Thus, for some cancer sites the observed:expected ratios will be distorted because of differences in these risk factors. It is possible to compute approximately how large an effect such confounding factors might have on the estimated risk of various second primary cancers.

Cervical cancer patients have been reported to smoke more than average in studies from Canada (Wigle et al., 1980), Sweden (Cederlof et al., 1975), the United Kingdom (Buckley et al., 1981), the United States (Thomas, 1977) and Yugoslavia (Kessler, 1976). In the results reported by Buckley, for example, 71% of cervical cancer patients (including those with in-situ cancer and severe dysplasia) had ever smoked compared with 34% of the controls, who might be assumed to represent the general population. Using these results, the crude relative risk for cervical cancer among women who had ever smoked compared with women who had never smoked is 4.8 [(0.71/0.29)/(0.34/0.66)]. Assuming that the relative risk for lung cancer among women who have ever smoked is ten-fold, then the relative risk for lung cancer among cervical cancer patients compared with women in the general population can be obtained as follows :

		Proportion in population	Relative risk of lung cancer	Average relative risk for lung cancer
Cervical cancer patients	Smokers	71 %	10	$(10 \times 0.71) + (1 \times 0.29) = 7.4$
	Non-smokers	29 %	1	
Women in the general population	Smokers	34 %	10	$(10 \times 0.34) + (1 \times 0.66) = 4.1$
	Non-smokers	66 %	1	

The relative risk of lung cancer among cervical cancer patients can be estimated as 7.4/4.1=1.8, that is about 80% higher than for women in the general population. This estimate would differ somewhat if other assumptions were made regarding the actual proportions of women, with or without cervical cancer, who have ever smoked and the relative risk associated with smoking.

For bladder cancer, the relative risk among those who have ever smoked is about 3, and calculations similar to those above give a value of 1.44 for the likely confounding effect. The higher than average proportion of smokers among cervical cancer patients might therefore lead, for lung cancer, to an observed number of second cancers nearly twice that expected from population rates, and, for other smoking-related cancers such as cancers of the buccal cavity, oesophagus and bladder, to an excess risk of approximately 50%.

Women with cancer of the cervix also tend to have more children and to have had their first pregnancy at an earlier age than women in the general population (Kessler, 1974; Thomas, 1977). Using the results reported by Thomas, 46% of cases (in-situ) compared with 30% of controls had first become pregnant before age 20. For breast cancer, a relative risk of about 2.5 might be expected for women who did not have a pregnancy before age 20 (MacMahon et al., 1973). The confounding effect can be estimated as

$$(0.46+0.54\times2.5)/(0.3+0.7\times2.5) = 0.88.$$

The risk for breast cancer might thus be expected to be about 12% lower among cervical cancer patients than average. The additional effect of parity on breast cancer risk after adjusting for age at first birth is not large (MacMahon et al., 1973; Tulinius et al., 1978) and would not be expected to confound the observations appreciably.

Socioeconomic factors may influence the risk of cervical cancer and are also related to the risk of other cancers. The results from the Third National Cancer Survey in the United States provide data on the effect of socioeconomic status on all major cancer sites (Williams & Horm, 1977). Low socioeconomic status is associated with approximately a three-fold increase in risk for cancer of the cervix. At other sites, no significant risk is greater than two-fold in either direction, the largest being 1.9 for the thyroid (associated with high socioeconomic status). The largest confounding effect one might expect is thus in the order of 15%.

Regional differences in incidence within the area covered by a single cancer registry may also have a confounding effect. Correction for region of residence in Denmark (Storm & Jensen, this monograph), however, made little difference. The regional differences in incidence, at least for cervical cancer, seem as great in Denmark (Clemmesen, 1977) as in other areas (Swedish Cancer Registry, 1971; Norwegian Cancer Society, 1978; Teppo et al., 1980).

The values given in the preceding discussion are based on the results of specific studies in specific populations and may not be applicable exactly to the populations included here. They are indicative, however, of the general level of confounding that might be expected from a range of factors and may help in the interpretation of the results.

5.4 Comparisons

The cancer experience in the radiation treated group has been compared with that of three different groups, namely, the general population, women registered with invasive cancer of the cervix but with no record of radiation treatment, and women registered with an in-situ carcinoma of the cervix, with no record of radiation therapy.

(a) General population

As discussed in the previous section, the distribution of a variety of risk factors for a number of cancers will be different in the general population than in the irradiated cervical cancer group. These differences may lead to underestimation of the number of second cancers attributable to radiation for some sites (e.g., breast, ovary, corpus) and to an overestimation of the numbers for other sites (e.g., lung).

(b) Non-exposed invasive cervical cancer patients

This group should be closest (although not identical) to the radiation-treated group in way of life and socioeconomic level. The comparisons between the two groups are therefore less influenced by confounding factors and are in principle a better reflection of radiation effects. Unfortunately, this group is of much smaller size, especially among ten-year survivors. The reduction in systematic bias in the comparisons is counteracted by a large increase in random variation. In addition, some of this group will have received radiation treatment not recorded in the cancer registry.

(c) In-situ carcinoma patients

The group of in-situ cancer cases provides larger numbers than the previous group, particularly in the first 15 years of follow-up. Rates of second cancers among patients with in-situ cancer must, however, also be viewed cautiously in the light of the variations in registration procedures for this condition. In-situ cancer is not a reportable disease in all registries, and the selection factors associated both with screening for the disease and incomplete reporting could be substantial. Finally, a proportion of 'non-exposed' patients are likely to have received radiotherapy that was not recorded in the registry notes.

6. Heterogeneity of observed:expected ratios among registries

The methods described in section 3 were used, by means of a programme developed by Gail (1978), to compare the observed:expected ratios (O/E) for a particular site or a combination of sites among the cancer registries. The O/E ratio was modelled as the product of a registry effect and a time since irradiation effect. Time since irradiation was categorized into six intervals: <1, 1-4, 5-9, 10-14, 15-19 and 20+ years; these intervals were indexed by $i=1,2,...,6$. According to the programme of Gail (1978), the product model was tested and was found to fit the data well for all registries except Denmark, which exhibited non-increasing ratios (O_i/E_i) of observed cases to expected cases in contrast to the other registries, which experienced increasing ratios with increasing time since exposure. Using the product model, it was possible to detect differences among registries in observed:expected ratios adjusted for time since exposure. Significant variability in these ratios among registries is seen for all sites combined, for close and intermediate sites, and for stomach, lung, corpus uteri, ovary and other genital sites (Table 5). The Connecticut registry tended to give higher ratios than the others, whereas ratios for Saskatchewan and Slovenia tended to be low. Differences among registries could be due to different methods of registering second cancers, international differences in therapy and different distributions of cancer risk factors such as smoking.

Table 5. Analysis of heterogeneity among registries[a] of observed:expected ratios (O/E) for each cancer site in women receiving radiotherapy, after adjustment for the pattern of risk over time since diagnosis

Cancer site (ICD7)	Significance of heterogeneity[b]	Registries omitted[c]	Registries with lowest and highest O/E ratios[d]	
			Lowest	Highest
All (140-205)	****	—	7,11	5,15
Sites at close and intermediate distance[5]	****	—	7,11	1,15
Stomach (151)	***	7	13	1,2
Colon (153)	*	—	—	—
Rectum (154)	*	—	—	—
Pancreas (157)	*	5,11	—	—
Lung (162-3)	****	—	5,7	11,15
Breast (170)	**	—	2,7	4,14
Corpus uteri (172)	****	4,7	—	5,15
Ovary (175)	****	—	8,13	1,15
Other genital (176)	****	13	11	3,5
Kidney (180)	**	5,7,11,13	—	—
Bladder (181)	*	5,7	—	—
Other skin (191)	*	6,10,15	—	—
Lymphoma (200,202)	*	3,5,11,14	—	—
Acute and non-lymphocytic leukaemias (204.1-204.4)	*	5,13	—	—
All leukaemias (204)	*	5,13	—	—

[a] Registry codes:

1 = Alberta	6 = Ontario	11 = Slovenia, Yugoslavia
2= British Columbia	7 = Saskatchewan	12 = Sweden
3 = Manitoba	8 = Denmark	13 = Birmingham, UK
4 = New Brunswick	9 = Finland	14 = South Thames, UK
5 = Nova Scotia	10 = Norway	15 = Connecticut, USA

[b] Based on a chi-square test for heterogeneity (Gail, 1978): *, $p > 0.05$; **, $0.05 > p > 0.01$; ***, $0.01 > p > 0.001$; ****, $p > 0.001$

[c] Registry omitted if no second cancer observed.

[d] The registries with the lowest and highest estimated O/E ratios listed here are based on the Gail procedure (Gail, 1978)

[e] See definition, Table 2

7. Comparisons with current risk estimates

Radiation risks by sex and age at exposure have been estimated by the US National Academy of Sciences (Advisory Committee on the Biological Effects of Ionizing Radiations, 1980), and we have used these to predict the excess of cancers that might be expected among the cervical cancer patients treated with radiation.

Table 6 gives a comparison of the 'predicted' radiogenic excess with that actually observed. The incidence of no second primary cancer except in the lung was elevated to the level predicted on the basis of current radiation risk estimates. Actual excesses came close to those 'predicted' for cancers of the pancreas, bladder, thyroid and lymphoma. Deficits or very small excesses occurred for cancers of the stomach, colon, liver, breast and kidney and for leukaemia. The actual excess of lung cancer stands out as being three times greater than 'predicted' on the basis of radiation exposure alone. The slight excess of leukaemia is not consistent with the very large number 'predicted', and this supports the view that only the active bone marrow outside the pelvic region should be considered as the tissue at risk.

Although the expected numbers of cases have not been modified to account for the influence of confounding factors, the effect of such modification would be small compared with the major differences between observed and expected rates seen in Table 6. These differences may reflect the uncertainty in estimating organ doses to specific organs, the uncertainty in age- and sex-specific radiation risk estimates in the BEIR report, the distribution of organ dose in specific organs, the influence of host and environmental factors, and/or difficulties in using the general population for comparison with cervical cancer patients.

Table 6. Comparison of predicted radiogenic excesses with actual observed excesses

Second primary cancer (ICD7)	BEIR III radiation risk estimate (per 10⁶ PY-rad)[a]	Preliminary estimate of organ dose (rad)	Predicted radiogenic excess	Actual excess[b]
Stomach (151)	1.68	150	45	0
Colon (153)	1.12	500+	100	+13
Liver (155.0)	0.70	250	31	0
Pancreas (157)	0.99	150	25	+8
Lung (162-3)	3.94	35	25	+78
Breast (170)	5.82	35	37	-102
Kidney (180)	0.88	250	40	-6
Bladder (181)	0.88	1000+	150	+33
Thyroid (191)	5.80	10	10	+4
Lymphoma (200-203)	0.27	(500)	25	+12
Acute and non-lymphocytic leukaemias (204.1-204.4)	2.70	750[c]	1000	+20
		250[d]	350	+20
		50[e]	70	+20

[a] Risk estimate for females (age-weighted average) 11-30 years after exposure, except for leukaemia, which is 1-20 years post-exposure

[b] Observed minus expected cancers among women living more than 10 years, except for leukaemia, which is for years 1-20 after irradiation

[c] Approximate dose averaged over entire bone marrow

[d] Approximate dose excluding pelvis contribution

[e] Approximate dose excluding pelvis, lumbar spine and femur contribution

8. Conclusions

The analysis of the combined cancer registry data indicates that, for all sites taken together, the risk of developing second cancers in women treated for cervical cancer, with or without radiation therapy, is only slightly greater than would have been expected by comparison with the general population. Clearly, the large radiation doses experienced by the cervical cancer patients have not substantially altered their risk of developing a second cancer.

However, there are interesting variations by cancer site and time since treatment that suggest radiation associations and areas for further study. For the reasons mentioned in section 5, the following summary statements should be interpreted with caution.

The analysis of the combined registry data suggests that

(1) Heavily and moderately irradiated sites taken together (i.e., those likely to have received over 100 rad of radiation) show a pattern of increased risk with time since exposure that is probably radiation-related.

(2) In particular, cancers of the bladder, rectum, bone, connective tissue, uterine corpus, ovary, small intestine and kidney and multiple myeloma may be associated with radiation in this study.

(3) Substantial doses of radiation to the stomach and colon do not appear to have increased the risk of cancers at those sites beyond normal expectation.

(4) The radiation regimens used to treat cervical cancer are not as effective in inducing leukaemia as are other radiation exposures that have been studied; a slight risk, however, might be associated with the low-dose radiation received by bone marrow outside the pelvis.

(5) Radiation effects on the ovary lower breast cancer risk by over 60% for women under age 40 at exposure. Even among women over 50 years of age at exposure, a reduction in risk of some 20% was seen.

(6) The substantial excess of lung cancer among cervical cancer patients is probably not related to radiation since the organ dose was low; misclassification of metastases from the cervical cancer and the confounding effect of cigarette smoking are more probable explanations.

(7) A small excess of thyroid cancer might be associated with a relatively low exposure.

(8) The rates of cancers at other sites that received relatively low doses of radiation either are not increased beyond expectation or are probably elevated due to exposures to other strong risk factors, such as cigarette or alcohol consumption.

Additional detailed studies of cervical cancer patients should determine to what extent the risk of second cancers is influenced by radiation dose, smoking, reproductive history, social class and other important factors that could not be evaluated in this analysis.

9. References

Advisory Committee on the Biological Effects of Ionizing Radiations (1980) *The Effects on Populations of Exposure to Low Levels of Ionizing Radiation*, National Academy of Sciences - National Research Council, Washington DC, National Academy Press

Baker R.J. & Nelder J.A. (1978) *The GLIM System (Release 3)*, Oxford, Numerical Algorithms Group

Beebe, G.W., Kato, H. & Land, C.E. (1970) *JNIH-ABCC Life Span Study. Report 5. Mortality and Radiation Dose, October 1950-September 1966* (Appendix 3: Methodology of contingency table analyses) (*Atomic Bomb Casualty Commission Technical Report No. 11*), pp. 148-158

Beebe, G.W., Kato, H. & Land, C.E. (1978) Studies of the mortality of A-bomb survivors. 6. Mortality and radiation dose, 1950-1974. *Radiat. Res.*, *75*, 138-201

Boice, J.D., Jr (1981) Cancer following medical irradiation. *Cancer, 47*, 1081-1090

Boice, J.D., Jr & Hutchison, G.B. (1980) Leukemia in women following radiotherapy for cervical cancer. Ten-year follow-up of an international study. *J. natl Cancer Inst.*, *65*, 115-129

Boice, J.D., Jr, Land, C.E., Shore, R.E., Norman, J.E. & Tokunaga, M. (1979) Risk of breast cancer following low-dose radiation exposure. *Radiology, 131*, 589-597

Boice, J.D. & Hoover, R.N. (1981) *Radiogenic breast cancer: age effects and implications for models of human carcinogenesis.* In: Burchenal, J.H. & Oettgen, H.F., eds, *Cancer: Achievements, Challenges, and Pespectives for the 1980's*, Vol. 1, New York, Grune & Stratton, pp. 209-221

Breslow, N.E. & Day, N.E. (1975) Indirect standardization and multiplicative models for rates. *J. chronic Dis.*, *28*, 289-303

Breslow, N.E., Lubin, J.H., Marek, P. & Langholtz, B. (1983) Multiplicative models and the analysis of cohort data. *J. Am. stat. Assoc.* (in press)

Buckley, J.D., Harris, R.W.C., Doll, R., Vessey, M.P. & Williams, P.T. (1981) Case-control study of the husbands of women with dysplasia or carcinoma of the cervix. *Lancet, ii*, 1010-1015

Cederlof, R., Friberg, I., Hrubec, A. & Lorich, U. (1975) *The Relationship of Smoking and Some Social Covariables to Mortality and Cancer Morbidity. A Ten Year Follow-up in a Probability Sample of 55 000 Subjects Aged 18 to 69*, Stockholm, Karolinska Institute

Clemmesen, J. (1965) *Statistical Studies in Malignant Neoplasms, I. Review and Results*, Copenhagen, Munksgaard

Clemmesen, J. (1977) *Statistical Studies in Malignant Neoplasms, V. Trends and Risks, Denmark 1943-77*, Copenhagen, Munksgaard

Court Brown, W.M. & Doll, R. (1965) Mortality from cancer and other causes after radiotherapy for ankylosing spondylitis. *Br. med. J., ii*, 1327-1332

Dickson, R.J. (1969) The late results of radium treatment for benign uterine haemorrhage. *Br. J. Radiol., 42*, 582-594

Dickson, R.J. (1972) Late results of radium treatment of carcinoma of the cervix. *Clin. Radiol., 23*, 528-535

Engel, L.W., Strauchen, J.A., Chiazze, L. & Heid, M. (1980) Accuracy of death certification in an autopsied population with specific attention to malignant neoplasms and vascular diseases. *Am. J. Epidemiol., 111*, 99-112

Fraumeni, J.F., Jr & Boice, J.D., Jr (1982) *Bone*. In: Schottenfeld, D. & Fraumeni, J.F., Jr, eds, *Cancer Epidemiology and Prevention*, Philadelphia, W.B. Saunders Co., pp. 814-826

Gail, M. (1978) The analysis of heterogeneity for indirectly standardized mortality rates. *J. R. stat. Soc. A, 141*, 224-234

Gilbert, E.S. & Marks, S. (1979) An analysis of the mortality of workers in a nuclear facility. *Radiat. Res., 79*, 122-148

Hakulinen, T., Pukkala, E., Hakama, M., Lehtonen, M., Saxen, E. & Teppo, L. (1981) Survival of cancer patients in Finland 1953-1974. *Ann. clin. Res., 13, Suppl. 31*

Hakulinen, T. & Teppo, L. (1977) Causes of death among female patients with cancer of the breast and intestines. *Ann. clin. Res., 9*, 15-24

Hutchison, G.B. (1968) Leukemia in patients with cancer of the cervix uteri treated with radiation. A report covering the first 5 years of an international study. *J. natl Cancer Inst., 40*, 951-982

Kato, H. & Schull, W.J. (1982) Studies of the mortality of A-bomb survivors. 7. Mortality, 1950-1978: Part I. Cancer mortality. *Radiat. Res., 90*, 395-432

Kessler, I.I. (1976) Human cervical cancer as a venereal disease. *Cancer Res., 36*, 783-791

Kim, J.H., Chu, F.C., Woodard, H.Q., Melamed, M.R., Huvos, A. & Cantin, J. (1978) Radiation-induced soft tissue and bone sarcoma. *Radiology, 129*, 501-508

Land, C.E., Boice, J.D., Jr, Shore, R.E., Norman, J.E. & Tokunaga, M. (1980) Breast cancer risk from low-dose exposure to ionizing radiation: results of parallel analysis of three exposed populations of women. *J. natl Cancer Inst., 65*, 353-376

Logan, W.D.P. (1954) Social class variations in mortality. *Br. J. soc. prev. Med., 8*, 124-137

MacMahon, B., Cole, P. & Brown, J. (1973) Etiology of human breast cancer: a review. *J. natl Cancer Inst., 50*, 21-42

Major, I.R. & Mole, R.H. (1978) Myeloid leukemia in X-ray irradiated CBA mice. *Nature, 272*, 455-456

Mancuso, T.F., Stewart, A. & Kneale, G. (1977) Radiation exposure of Hanford workers dying from cancer and other causes. *Health Phys., 33*, 369-385

Mantel, N. (1963) Chi-square tests with one degree of freedom: extensions of the Mantel-Haenszel procedure. *J. Am. stat. Assoc., 58*, 690-700

Norwegian Cancer Society (1978) *Geographical Variations in Cancer Incidence in Norway 1966-1975*, Oslo, Norwegian Cancer Registry

Ron, E. & Modan, B. (1980) Benign and malignant thyroid neoplasms after childhood irradiation for tinea capitis. *J. natl Cancer Inst., 65*, 7-11

Rothman, K.J. & Boice, J.D. Jr. (1979) *Epidemiologic Analysis with a Programmable Calculator (NIH Publication No. 79-1649)*, Washington DC, US Government Printing Office

Smith, P.G. (1977) Leukemia and other cancers following radiation treatment of pelvic disease. *Cancer*, *39*, 1901-1905

Smith, P.G. & Doll, R. (1976) Late effects of irradiation in patients treated for metropathia haemorrhagica. *Br. J. Radiol.*, *49*, 224-232

Smith, P.G. & Doll, R. (1982) Mortality among patients with ankylosing spondylitis after a single treatment course with X rays. *Br. med. J.*, *284*, 449-460

Swedish Cancer Registry (1971) *Cancer Incidence in Sweden 1959-1965*, Stockholm, National Board of Health and Welfare

Teppo, L., Pukkala, E., Hakama, M., Hakulinen, T., Herva, A. & Saxen, E. (1980) *Way of Life and Cancer Incidence in Finland - a Municipality-Based Ecological Analysis*, Helsinki, Finnish Cancer Registry

Thomas, D.B. (1977) An epidemiologic study of carcinoma in situ and squamous dysplasia of the uterine cervix. *Am. J. Epidemiol.*, *98*, 10-28

Trichopoulos, D., MacMahon, B. & Cole, P. (1972) Menopause and breast cancer risk. *J. natl Cancer Inst.*, *48*, 605-613

Tulinius, H., Day, N.E., Johannesson, G., Bjarnason, O. & Gonzalez, M. (1978) Reproductive factors and risk for breast cancer in Iceland. *Int. J. Cancer*, *21*, 724-730

Van Nagell, J.R., Rayburn, W., Donaldson, E.S., Hanson, M., Gay, E.C., Yoneda, J., Marayuma, Y. & Powell, D.F. (1979) Therapeutic implications of patterns of recurrence in cancer of the cervix. *Cancer*, *44*, 2354-2361

Wagoner, J.K. (1970) *Leukemia and Other Malignancies Following Radiation Therapy for Gynecological Diseases* (unpublished doctoral thesis), Boston, Harvard School of Public Health

Waterhouse, J.A.H., Muir, C., Correa, P. & Powell, J. (1976) *Cancer Incidence in Five Continents*, Vol. III (*IARC Scientific Publications No.15*), Lyon, International Agency for Research on Cancer

Waterhouse, J.A.H., Muir, C., Shanmugaratnam, K. & Powell, J. (1982) *Cancer Incidence in Five Continents*, Vol. IV (*IARC Scientific Publications No.42*), Lyon, International Agency for Research on Cancer

Wigle, D.T., Mao, Y. & Grace, M. (1980) Smoking and cancer of the uterine cervix: hypothesis. *Am. J. Epidemiol.*, *111*, 125-127

Williams, R.R. & Horm, J.W. (1977) Association of cancer sites with tobacco and alcohol consumption and socioeconomic status of patients: interview study from the Third National Cancer Survey. *J. natl Cancer Inst.*, *58*, 525-547

Wright, N.H., Vessey, M.P., Kenward, B., McPherson, K. & Doll, R. (1978) Neoplasia and dysplasia of the cervix uteri and contraception: a possible protective effect of the diaphragm. *Br. J. Cancer*, *38*, 273-279

APPENDICES

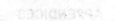

Appendix Table A1. Total number of second cancers by site and time since diagnosis of primary cervical cancer. Invasive cervical cancers treated with radiotherapy

Time since diagnosis of primary cervical cancer (in years)

ICD7	<1 O	<1 O'	<1 E	1-4 O	1-4 O'	1-4 E	5-9 O	5-9 O'	5-9 E	10-14 O	10-14 O'	10-14 E	15-19 O	15-19 O'	15-19 E	20-24 O	20-24 O'	20-24 E	25-29 O	25-29 O'	25-29 E	30+ O	30+ O'	30+ E	Total (excl. <1) O	Total (excl. <1) O'	Total (excl. <1) E
140	0	0	0.58	0	0	1.86	1	1	1.76	1	1	1.35	1	0	0.69	0	0	0.34	0	0	0.11	1	1	0.03	4	3	6.14
141	0	1	0.89	3	3	2.65	3	2	2.46	1	1	1.78	0	0	1.00	0	0	0.45	0	0	0.19	0	0	0.06	9	8	8.59
142	1	1	1.16	1	1	3.34	1	1	2.89	3	3	1.94	1	1	0.98	0	0	0.43	0	0	0.15	0	0	0.05	8	6	9.78
143	3	3	1.13	4	2	3.39	7	6	3.23	6	6	2.33	4	4	1.27	0	0	0.67	0	0	0.30	0	0	0.10	19	15	11.29
145	0	0	1.01	6	5	2.89	5	5	2.63	1	1	1.77	4	4	0.87	0	0	0.38	0	0	0.10	0	0	0.04	17	15	8.68
146	0	0	0.28	1	1	0.82	0	0	0.68	2	2	0.42	0	0	0.18	0	0	0.05	0	0	0.01	0	0	0.01	3	3	2.17
150	3	3	3.03	15	13	8.42	13	7	7.69	9	7	5.67	3	2	3.27	0	0	1.53	0	0	0.55	0	0	0.19	40	29	27.32
151	13	9	23.57	57	29	65.22	57	45	59.10	43	29	42.84	30	25	24.98	8	6	12.65	5	5	4.53	1	1	1.05	200	139	210.37
152	2	2	0.98	3	3	2.91	9	7	2.77	2	2	2.00	5	4	1.03	1	1	0.49	0	0	0.20	0	0	0.06	21	18	9.46
153	15	13	29.85	81	58	86.03	88	71	82.39	70	53	62.43	42	32	37.52	15	12	21.02	16	14	9.12	2	1	3.02	314	241	301.53
154	9	7	16.00	36	25	45.51	43	32	43.28	55	44	32.41	31	26	19.78	18	12	10.77	9	8	4.38	5	1	1.25	197	151	157.38
155.0	0	1	2.01	5	4	5.73	6	4	5.39	11	8	4.02	1	1	2.57	1	0	1.38	2	0	0.63	1	1	0.16	19	14	19.88
155.1	1	1	5.33	12	12	15.31	11	11	15.06	11	8	11.63	5	5	7.40	3	4	4.20	2	2	1.62	1	0	0.47	45	41	55.69
157	4	3	9.22	47	25	26.83	23	11	26.33	24	17	20.02	17	9	12.31	6	6	6.80	2	1	2.77	1	0	0.82	120	67	95.88
160	1	0	0.73	3	2	2.03	3	3	1.85	4	4	1.26	1	1	1.44	1	1	0.36	0	0	0.13	0	0	0.05	13	11	7.12
161	0	0	0.76	4	3	2.20	6	5	2.05	2	2	1.48	3	2	0.82	0	0	0.45	0	0	0.17	0	0	0.04	16	13	7.21
162-3	12	9	13.72	174	122	39.40	183	134	37.71	86	64	27.72	35	25	16.28	7	7	9.12	9	6	3.73	1	1	0.98	491	354	134.94
170	66	45	90.80	176	144	262.05	190	153	237.73	118	100	160.11	53	47	84.75	22	18	40.42	6	6	15.10	4	1	4.25	569	472	804.41
172	18	14	22.02	12	12	64.72	36	30	61.01	41	38	43.18	19	19	23.88	13	13	11.35	5	3	3.94	2	2	1.05	126	117	209.13
173	1	1	2.43	4	4	6.63	3	3	5.63	6	6	3.39	0	0	1.50	1	1	0.65	3	3	0.24	0	0	0.07	15	15	18.11
175	24	21	21.92	35	31	63.83	32	27	58.39	28	24	39.89	20	15	21.49	14	12	10.23	4	3	3.56	3	3	0.92	136	115	198.31
176	8	8	4.69	27	22	13.01	27	24	11.76	23	21	8.44	12	11	5.02	7	7	3.15	4	2	1.21	1	1	0.41	101	90	43.00
180	22	19	6.42	28	22	19.28	18	13	18.81	6	6	13.89	5	5	8.19	7	7	4.27	2	2	1.64	3	3	0.42	69	57	66.50
181	16	11	7.05	46	36	20.47	36	25	20.13	42	35	15.31	36	29	9.41	21	19	5.37	8	8	2.29	5	0	0.76	194	155	73.74
190	5	4	4.96	10	10	14.93	12	11	14.01	10	10	9.56	2	2	5.17	1	1	2.39	5	5	0.80	0	0	0.22	36	34	47.08
191	42	27	22.65	60	44	61.43	58	43	58.68	29	29	45.18	24	21	29.61	16	13	17.50	5	0	6.40	0	0	0.96	206	154	219.76
192	0	0	0.95	2	2	2.73	2	1	2.48	1	1	1.68	1	1	0.93	1	1	0.46	4	4	0.16	0	0	0.03	7	6	8.47
193	3	3	7.80	18	16	22.24	16	16	19.89	7	6	13.34	3	3	7.10	5	5	3.41	1	1	1.25	0	0	0.31	51	46	67.54
194	1	0	3.57	10	10	3.71	10	8	9.43	9	9	6.33	3	3	3.35	3	3	1.47	1	1	0.45	0	0	0.11	36	31	31.47
195	2	0	1.22	4	3	3.71	5	5	3.66	3	3	2.41	1	1	0.84	0	0	0.19	1	1	0.08	0	0	0.02	13	12	10.91
196	0	0	0.69	3	1	2.02	4	4	1.64	1	1	1.09	0	0	0.56	1	1	0.29	0	0	0.10	0	0	0.02	11	9	5.72
197	3	3	1.64	8	8	4.87	7	5	4.11	7	6	2.98	3	3	1.43	1	1	0.63	1	1	0.19	0	0	0.06	27	24	14.57
200	2	1	5.25	17	12	15.78	16	12	14.88	18	13	11.08	9	6	6.56	2	2	3.41	2	2	1.55	0	0	0.06	61	46	53.77
201	1	1	1.96	5	5	5.70	3	3	4.97	2	2	3.28	1	1	1.68	2	1	0.79	1	1	0.31	0	0	0.51	14	13	16.87
203	2	0	3.16	3	1	9.56	8	5	9.52	6	6	7.25	5	5	4.32	3	3	2.16	2	2	0.84	0	0	0.14	33	23	33.92
204.0	2	2	2.35	5	2	6.60	3	2	6.26	2	2	4.63	3	3	2.84	1	1	1.52	1	1	0.63	2	2	0.27	18	12	22.64
204.1-4	3	2	4.43	28	19	12.61	17	14	11.61	10	5	8.26	2	2	4.70	1	1	2.42	0	0	1.01	0	0	0.16	58	41	40.94
204	6	4	7.01	32	21	19.91	23	18	18.55	12	7	13.43	5	5	7.84	2	2	3.97	1	1	1.60	0	0	0.53	77	54	65.83
TOTAL	287	217	326.44	952	712	937.74	971	747	872.85	715	575	622.89	387	316	356.02	183	151	183.20	85	73	70.40	31	27	19.44	3324	2601	3062.54

O : All tumours observed
O': Histologically confirmed tumours observed
E : Expected

Appendix Table A2. Total number of second cancers by site and time since diagnosis of primary cervical cancer. Invasive cervical cancers not registered as having received radiotherapy

Time since diagnosis of primary cervical cancer (in years)

ICD7	<1			1-4			5-9			10-14			15-19			20-24			25-29			30+			Total (excl. <1)		
	O	O'	E	O	O'	E	O	O'	E	O	O'	E	O	O'	E	O	O'	E	O	O'	E	O	O'	E	O	O'	E
140	0	0	0.06	1	1	0.19	0	0	0.19	0	0	0.13	1	1	0.08	0	0	0.03	0	0	0.01	0	0	0.00	2	2	0.63
141	0	0	0.08	0	0	0.23	1	1	0.31	0	0	0.18	0	0	0.12	0	0	0.05	0	0	0.02	0	0	0.01	1	1	0.92
142	0	0	0.14	0	0	0.49	1	0	0.43	0	0	0.23	0	0	0.12	1	1	0.05	0	0	0.02	0	0	0.00	1	0	1.34
143-4	0	0	0.10	0	0	0.33	1	0	0.41	1	1	0.26	0	0	0.17	0	0	0.08	0	0	0.04	0	0	0.01	2	2	1.30
145,7-8	0	0	0.11	0	0	0.29	0	0	0.31	1	1	0.22	0	0	0.10	0	0	0.05	0	0	0.01	0	0	0.00	2	2	0.98
146	0	0	0.00	0	0	0.06	1	0	0.04	0	0	0.02	0	0	0.01	0	0	0.00	0	0	0.00	0	0	0.00	1	0	0.13
150	1	1	0.35	1	1	0.86	2	1	0.85	0	0	0.63	0	0	0.36	0	0	0.15	0	0	0.06	0	0	0.02	3	2	2.93
151	2	2	2.91	5	5	7.28	11	7	7.51	2	2	5.75	3	3	3.51	1	1	1.54	1	1	0.37	0	0	0.15	23	17	26.11
152	0	0	0.09	2	2	0.26	1	1	0.28	1	1	0.19	0	0	0.13	1	0	0.06	1	1	0.02	0	0	0.00	4	4	0.94
153	3	3	3.38	10	9	9.92	9	4	10.83	8	6	8.34	13	13	5.34	1	1	2.75	1	1	0.99	0	0	0.29	42	34	38.46
154	1	1	1.98	5	5	5.64	6	5	6.30	8	8	4.80	2	2	2.97	1	1	1.45	1	1	0.47	0	0	0.15	29	22	21.78
155.0	0	0	0.22	0	0	0.60	1	1	0.65	0	0	0.49	1	1	0.30	0	0	0.16	0	0	0.06	0	0	0.02	2	2	2.28
155.1	0	0	0.55	3	3	1.75	2	2	2.03	2	2	1.65	1	1	1.06	2	2	0.54	0	0	0.15	0	0	0.04	7	7	7.22
157	0	0	1.03	3	3	2.93	2	2	3.35	1	1	2.62	3	3	1.72	0	0	0.71	0	0	0.26	0	0	0.07	10	5	11.66
160	0	0	0.07	0	0	0.21	2	2	0.22	2	2	0.14	2	2	0.09	0	0	0.04	0	0	0.02	0	0	0.00	4	4	0.72
161	0	0	0.09	0	0	0.30	2	2	0.33	2	2	0.24	2	2	0.14	2	2	0.07	0	0	0.02	0	0	0.00	4	4	1.10
162	1	1	1.60	25	23	5.31	14	9	6.12	9	9	4.70	5	4	2.90	2	1	1.33	0	0	0.45	0	0	0.15	60	46	20.96
170	8	5	11.58	40	35	37.42	35	30	39.31	24	20	26.35	9	9	14.14	7	7	5.72	3	3	1.61	0	0	0.36	118	104	124.91
172	2	2	2.49	0	0	8.34	1	1	9.51	1	1	7.11	0	0	4.21	0	0	1.72	0	0	0.44	0	0	0.11	2	2	31.44
173-4	0	0	0.18	0	0	0.61	0	0	0.50	0	0	0.32	2	2	0.13	0	0	0.10	0	0	0.03	0	0	0.03	0	0	1.72
175	5	5	2.70	7	7	9.00	5	3	9.69	1	1	6.67	2	2	3.67	2	1	1.44	1	1	0.34	0	0	0.14	16	13	30.95
176	6	5	0.47	4	4	1.72	3	3	1.72	3	3	1.25	2	2	0.72	1	1	0.27	0	0	0.15	0	0	0.11	17	16	5.94
180	2	2	0.68	6	6	2.13	3	3	2.51	3	3	1.89	2	2	1.20	1	1	0.48	0	0	0.16	0	0	0.04	18	18	8.41
181	3	3	0.80	5	5	2.23	2	2	2.70	2	2	2.10	2	2	1.29	1	1	0.63	0	0	0.24	0	0	0.07	16	12	9.26
190	0	0	0.69	3	3	2.51	2	2	2.63	2	2	1.63	0	0	0.77	1	1	0.34	0	0	0.09	0	0	0.02	8	7	7.99
191	4	3	3.30	9	8	9.15	17	13	10.31	7	7	7.88	5	5	4.63	1	1	2.02	2	1	0.42	0	0	0.07	40	34	34.48
192	0	0	0.10	1	1	0.31	1	1	0.32	1	1	0.23	0	0	0.12	1	1	0.04	0	0	0.02	0	0	0.00	2	2	1.04
193	1	1	0.93	4	4	3.16	3	3	3.25	3	3	2.20	3	3	1.14	0	0	0.45	0	0	0.12	1	1	0.02	16	15	10.34
194	0	0	0.34	0	0	1.33	0	0	1.35	1	1	0.89	0	0	0.45	1	1	0.14	1	1	0.05	0	0	0.00	1	1	4.23
195	1	0	0.04	0	0	0.14	1	1	0.16	0	0	0.09	0	0	0.05	0	0	0.02	0	0	0.00	0	0	0.00	1	1	0.46
196	0	0	0.07	1	1	0.24	2	2	0.21	0	0	0.14	0	0	0.06	0	0	0.03	0	0	0.01	0	0	0.00	0	0	0.69
197	0	0	0.16	1	1	0.60	0	0	0.67	1	1	0.35	1	1	0.16	0	0	0.05	0	0	0.00	0	0	0.00	5	5	1.85
200,202	0	0	0.61	5	4	1.87	2	1	2.13	1	1	1.45	1	1	0.87	0	0	0.37	0	0	0.18	0	0	0.12	8	6	6.99
201	0	0	0.24	2	2	0.83	0	0	0.75	1	1	0.42	0	0	0.26	1	1	0.15	0	0	0.04	0	0	0.01	3	3	2.46
203	0	0	0.27	0	0	0.97	4	4	1.21	0	0	0.92	0	0	0.46	0	0	0.27	0	0	0.15	0	0	0.04	1	1	4.02
204.0	0	0	0.26	2	2	0.89	2	2	0.94	0	0	0.68	0	0	0.29	0	0	0.16	0	0	0.06	0	0	0.02	6	6	3.04
204.1-.4	1	1	0.47	2	2	1.54	4	4	1.66	1	1	1.11	0	0	0.58	0	0	0.34	0	0	0.14	0	0	0.04	6	3	5.41
204	1	1	0.79	4	4	2.51	5	5	2.70	1	1	1.86	0	0	0.91	0	0	0.52	1	0	0.20	0	0	0.06	13	10	8.76
TOTAL	45	38	39.20	149	128	121.72	140	109	131.79	95	79	94.34	61	55	54.36	22	19	23.82	10	7	7.24	2	2	2.13	479	399	435.40

O : All tumours observed
O': Histologically confirmed tumours observed
E : Expected

Appendix Table A3. Total number of second cancers by site and time since diagnosis of primary cervical cancer. In-situ cervical cancers not registered as having received radiotherapy

Time since diagnosis of primary cervical cancer (in years)

ICD7	<1 O	<1 O'	<1 E	1-4 O	1-4 O'	1-4 E	5-9 O	5-9 O'	5-9 E	10-14 O	10-14 O'	10-14 E	15-19 O	15-19 O'	15-19 E	20-24 O	20-24 O'	20-24 E	25-29 O	25-29 O'	25-29 E	30+ O	30+ O'	30+ E	Total O	Total O'	Total E
140	0	0	0.13	6	2	0.61	1	1	0.55	0	0	0.26	0	1	0.05	0	0	0.01	0	0	0.01	0	0	0.00	7	4	1.49
141	1	1	0.21	3	2	1.01	2	2	0.99	0	0	0.52	1	1	0.22	0	0	0.05	0	0	0.01	0	0	0.00	6	5	2.86
142	1	1	0.68	6	2	2.33	1	1	1.61	1	1	0.52	0	0	0.10	0	0	0.03	0	0	0.00	0	0	0.00	9	5	4.59
143-4	0	0	0.33	2	2	1.48	3	3	1.44	0	0	0.71	1	1	0.21	1	1	0.07	0	0	0.01	0	0	0.00	7	7	3.92
145,7-8	1	1	0.28	3	3	1.25	4	4	1.18	2	2	0.50	1	1	0.17	1	1	0.04	0	0	0.00	0	0	0.00	11	11	3.15
146	0	0	0.11	1	0	0.43	0	0	0.36	0	0	0.14	0	0	0.04	0	0	0.01	0	0	0.00	0	0	0.00	2	2	0.98
150	0	0	0.43	6	0	2.05	0	0	2.07	1	1	0.96	1	1	0.33	1	1	0.14	0	0	0.00	0	0	0.00	3	3	5.55
151	8	7	4.43	15	13	17.76	15	9	16.56	10	10	7.61	2	2	2.83	1	1	0.60	0	0	0.00	0	0	0.00	42	34	45.49
152	1	1	0.36	1	1	1.56	2	2	1.41	0	0	0.55	0	0	0.14	0	0	0.03	0	0	0.00	0	0	0.00	3	3	3.76
153	8	7	7.84	43	39	31.76	21	20	29.95	11	11	14.32	9	8	5.68	1	1	1.87	0	0	0.41	0	0	0.10	85	79	84.09
154	4	1	3.96	18	14	16.27	19	19	15.70	8	8	7.33	2	2	2.77	1	1	0.79	0	0	0.12	0	0	0.02	48	44	43.00
155.0	0	0	0.53	0	0	2.31	6	6	2.10	0	0	0.73	0	0	0.27	0	0	0.03	0	0	0.01	0	0	0.00	6	6	5.45
155.1	0	0	1.06	3	2	4.54	6	6	4.55	0	0	2.12	1	1	0.82	0	0	0.18	0	0	0.03	0	0	0.01	10	9	12.25
157	2	0	2.68	14	11	8.85	9	9	9.20	5	5	4.39	3	2	1.71	0	0	0.55	0	0	0.11	0	0	0.06	34	26	24.82
160	0	0	0.22	2	2	0.95	2	2	0.79	7	7	0.35	1	1	0.09	0	0	0.03	0	0	0.00	0	0	0.00	6	5	2.21
161	0	0	0.31	2	2	1.41	2	1	1.21	0	0	0.49	0	0	0.16	0	0	0.04	0	0	0.06	0	0	0.00	4	4	3.33
162	7	6	4.09	33	29	18.58	43	30	18.29	21	19	8.07	6	6	3.02	3	3	0.83	0	0	0.01	0	0	0.01	166	87	48.91
170	25	24	45.66	169	155	182.80	158	140	160.14	59	58	60.45	19	18	18.19	3	3	4.21	1	1	0.79	0	0	0.01	409	375	426.59
172	12	12	7.93	18	18	34.71	20	20	34.89	10	9	15.38	0	0	5.20	0	0	1.42	0	0	0.21	0	0	0.02	48	47	91.83
173-4	1	1	1.41	2	1	5.31	3	3	4.25	1	1	1.42	0	0	0.39	0	0	0.13	0	0	0.02	0	0	0.00	6	6	11.52
175	14	13	11.42	32	31	44.57	45	39	38.38	16	16	14.19	2	2	4.12	1	1	0.86	1	1	0.12	0	0	0.03	91	84	102.25
176	15	12	2.17	32	28	5.08	47	46	4.46	12	12	2.01	4	4	0.69	1	1	0.17	0	0	0.03	0	0	0.00	95	96	12.44
180	3	3	2.57	12	11	10.37	8	8	9.61	3	3	3.91	2	2	1.19	1	2	0.22	0	0	0.04	0	0	0.00	27	26	25.34
181	4	4	1.94	11	10	7.98	9	8	7.57	9	8	3.33	2	2	1.15	1	1	0.39	0	0	0.07	0	0	0.00	31	28	20.49
190	2	2	5.43	23	20	19.32	13	13	14.47	7	7	4.46	0	0	1.23	1	1	0.14	0	0	0.02	0	0	0.00	44	41	39.69
191	4	4	4.83	14	13	18.79	19	18	17.61	9	9	8.88	0	0	3.26	0	0	0.78	0	0	0.15	0	0	0.02	43	41	49.49
192	0	0	0.46	1	1	1.77	1	1	1.41	2	1	0.52	0	0	0.11	0	0	0.03	0	0	0.00	0	0	0.00	4	4	3.84
193	1	1	5.76	22	19	20.82	14	14	15.59	2	2	4.68	2	2	1.04	0	0	0.18	0	0	0.02	0	0	0.00	39	36	42.33
194	3	2	2.91	16	16	10.40	5	5	8.16	3	3	2.65	2	2	0.69	0	0	0.16	0	0	0.01	0	0	0.00	19	18	22.07
195	3	2	1.86	6	6	7.31	6	6	6.24	3	1	1.70	0	0	0.23	0	0	0.06	0	0	0.00	0	0	0.00	12	12	15.54
196	0	0	0.45	0	0	2.18	1	1	1.08	1	1	0.35	0	0	0.06	0	0	0.01	0	0	0.00	0	0	0.00	2	2	3.68
197	3	1	1.08	1	1	1.99	7	7	3.12	6	6	1.65	1	1	0.98	0	0	0.65	0	0	0.02	1	1	0.01	6	6	8.39
200,202	2	1	2.21	14	13	9.25	7	7	7.83	1	1	3.14	1	1	0.37	0	0	0.12	0	0	0.00	0	0	0.00	28	27	20.71
201	0	0	1.87	14	10	5.78	2	2	3.73	1	1	1.22	1	1	0.69	0	0	0.09	0	0	0.02	0	0	0.00	14	13	11.21
203	1	1	0.88	6	5	3.80	3	2	3.92	1	1	1.94	1	1	0.38	0	0	0.17	0	0	0.00	0	0	0.00	12	9	10.56
204.0	1	1	0.55	3	2	2.33	2	2	2.26	1	1	1.61	0	0	0.77	0	0	0.67	0	0	0.02	0	0	0.00	7	5	6.67
204.1-4	1	6	2.32	12	12	8.24	12	7	6.66	3	3	2.38	1	1	1.15	1	1	0.22	0	0	0.03	0	0	0.01	31	24	18.25
204	2	2	2.95	16	17	10.91	16	16	9.08	4	4	3.46	1	1	1.15	1	1	0.29	0	0	0.05	0	0	0.01	39	36	24.95
Total	129	119	136.84	543	489	517.64	513	456	459.56	204	196	184.31	62	59	59.65	18	18	14.72	5	3	2.56	1	1	0.27	1346	1222	1238.05

O : All tumours observed
O': Histologically confirmed tumours observed
E : Expected

Appendix B. Second cancers by age at diagnosis of cervical cancer, time since diagnosis of cervical cancer, stage and treatment

Table B1. Stomach (ICD 151)

TIME SINCE DIAGNOSIS OF PRIMARY CERVICAL CANCER (IN YEARS)

INVASIVE — RADIOTHERAPY

Age	<1 O	<1 E	1–4 O	1–4 E	5–9 O	5–9 E	10–14 O	10–14 E	15–19 O	15–19 E	20–24 O	20–24 E	25–29 O	25–29 E	30+ O	30+ E	Total (excl. <1) O	Total (excl. <1) E
<30		0.00		0.00		0.06		0.07		0.08		0.07		0.03		0.01		0.36
30–39	2	0.30	3	1.37	3	1.91	3	2.10		1.80	2	1.16		0.56		1.52	11	10.42
40–49	1	1.77	7	6.15	10	7.87	6	7.67	8	6.06	6	4.19	2	1.92		0.57	39	34.43
50–59	3	4.17	15	14.30	23	15.98	21	14.20	14	9.71		4.89	3	1.67		0.23	76	60.98
60–69	2	7.41	13	22.43	19	21.09	12	14.31	4	6.40	1	1.83		0.25		0.03	49	66.34
70+	5	9.85	17	21.27	5	12.08	4	4.08		0.84		0.15		0.05		0.01	26	38.48

INVASIVE — NO RADIOTHERAPY

Age	<1 O	<1 E	1–4 O	1–4 E	5–9 O	5–9 E	10–14 O	10–14 E	15–19 O	15–19 E	20–24 O	20–24 E	25–29 O	25–29 E	30+ O	30+ E	Total (excl. <1) O	Total (excl. <1) E
<30		0.00		0.01	1	0.03		0.04		0.04		0.01		0.01		0.00	1	0.14
30–39		0.06		0.33	1	0.54		0.55		0.38		0.17		0.04		0.02	1	2.03
40–49	1	0.25		0.97	4	1.36	1	1.30	1	1.04	1	0.55		0.16		0.06	7	5.44
50–59	1	0.41	2	1.41		1.81	2	1.70	1	1.16		0.48		0.13		0.01	5	6.70
60–69		0.55	2	1.52	2	1.63	1	1.03		0.44		0.17		0.04		0.00	5	4.83
70+	1	1.01	1	1.36		0.83		0.29		0.06		0.02		0.00		0.00	1	2.56

IN SITU

Age	<1 O	<1 E	1–4 O	1–4 E	5–9 O	5–9 E	10–14 O	10–14 E	15–19 O	15–19 E	20–24 O	20–24 E	25–29 O	25–29 E	30+ O	30+ E	Total (excl. <1) O	Total (excl. <1) E
<30		0.10	1	0.44	1	0.41		0.13		0.04		0.01		0.00		0.00	2	1.03
30–39	3	0.57	2	2.39	6	2.40	1	1.10		0.41		0.08		0.01		0.00	9	6.39
40–49	1	1.21	3	4.95	2	4.54	5	1.96		0.71		0.19		0.06		0.01	10	12.42
50–59	2	0.81	5	3.16	1	2.91	1	1.33		0.50		0.12		0.02		0.00	7	8.04
60–69	1	0.58	2	2.18	1	1.75	1	0.59		0.15		0.04		0.00		0.00	4	4.71
70+	1	0.48		1.48	1	0.75		0.15		0.02		0.00		0.00		0.00	1	2.40

O : All tumours observed
E : Expected

Table B2. Small Intestine (ICD 152)

TIME SINCE DIAGNOSIS OF PRIMARY CERVICAL CANCER (IN YEARS)

	<1 O	<1 E	1–4 O	1–4 E	5–9 O	5–9 E	10–14 O	10–14 E	15–19 O	15–19 E	20–24 O	20–24 E	25–29 O	25–29 E	30+ O	30+ E	Total (excl. <1) O	Total (excl. <1) E
<30		0.00		0.00		0.00		0.00		0.00		0.00		0.00		0.00	0.00	0.00
30–39	1	0.02		0.10	1	0.15	1	0.15		0.11		0.08		0.04		0.02	2	0.65
40–49	1	0.09	1	0.35		0.52	1	0.47		0.28	1	0.19		0.09		0.03	4	1.93
50–59	2	0.20	4	0.80	2	0.86	2	0.68	1	0.34		0.16		0.06		0.00	11	2.90
60–69		0.24	3	0.86		0.81	1	0.41		0.16		0.04		0.00		0.00	4	2.28
70+		0.23		0.61		0.27		0.08		0.01		0.00		0.00		0.00		0.97

O : All tumours observed
E : Expected

APPENDIX B

Table B3. Colon (ICD 153)

TIME SINCE DIAGNOSIS OF PRIMARY CERVICAL CANCER (IN YEARS)

INVASIVE — RADIOTHERAPY

Age	<1 O	<1 E	1–4 O	1–4 E	5–9 O	5–9 E	10–14 O	10–14 E	15–19 O	15–19 E	20–24 O	20–24 E	25–29 O	25–29 E	30+ O	30+ E	Total (excl. <1) O	Total (excl. <1) E
<30		0.02		0.09		0.15	1	0.20	1	0.22		0.22	1	0.13		0.04	3	1.05
30–39	1	0.50	5	2.13	2	3.39	5	4.12	1	3.65	1	2.70		1.49	1	0.57	19	18.05
40–49	2	2.73	14	10.22	12	14.27	9	14.12	7	10.46	7	7.47		4.14	2	1.63	73	62.31
50–59	2	6.53	24	21.44	26	23.96	13	20.15	5	12.75	7	7.93		3.00	2	0.54	101	89.77
60–69	5	9.12	27	27.38	23	25.92	13	17.93	1	8.31	1	2.67	1	0.47		0.08	87	82.76
70+	5	11.00	9	24.85	6	14.80	3	5.37	1	1.01		0.18		0.07		0.02	30	46.30

INVASIVE — OTHER

Age	<1 O	<1 E	1–4 O	1–4 E	5–9 O	5–9 E	10–14 O	10–14 E	15–19 O	15–19 E	20–24 O	20–24 E	25–29 O	25–29 E	30+ O	30+ E	Total (excl. <1) O	Total (excl. <1) E
<30		0.00		0.05		0.07		0.07		0.05		0.04		0.02	1	0.01	1	0.31
30–39	1	0.10	1	0.51		0.85	3	0.95	1	0.79	1	0.40		0.15		0.06	4	3.71
40–49	3	0.43	3	1.78	2	2.58	3	2.31	1	1.72	1	1.05		0.48		0.20	13	10.12
50–59	1	0.66	1	2.31	1	2.63	5	2.14	1	1.47		0.71		0.22		0.02	9	9.50
60–69	3	0.70	3	2.04	2	2.08	2	1.30		0.58		0.23		0.08		0.00	7	6.31
70+	1	1.11	1	1.83	1	1.11	1	0.42	1	0.12		0.04		0.00		0.00	3	3.52

IN SITU

Age	<1 O	<1 E	1–4 O	1–4 E	5–9 O	5–9 E	10–14 O	10–14 E	15–19 O	15–19 E	20–24 O	20–24 E	25–29 O	25–29 E	30+ O	30+ E	Total (excl. <1) O	Total (excl. <1) E
<30	1	0.33	1	1.32	1	0.94	1	0.28		0.09		0.04		0.01		0.00	2	2.68
30–39	1	1.12	6	4.46	2	4.62	1	2.28	1	1.00		0.32		0.06		0.01	10	12.75
40–49	3	2.42	12	10.34	4	10.32	4	4.62	1	1.61		0.59		0.22		0.03	22	27.73
50–59	1	1.74	13	6.78	6	5.92	1	2.48		1.04		0.33		0.09		0.02	24	16.66
60–69	2	1.11	7	4.09	2	3.21	2	1.27		0.40		0.12		0.02		0.00	11	9.11
70+	2	0.74	2	2.37	2	1.27		0.32		0.05		0.00		0.00		0.00	4	4.01

O : All tumours observed
E : Expected

Table B4. Rectum (ICD 154)

TIME SINCE DIAGNOSIS OF PRIMARY CERVICAL CANCER (IN YEARS)

INVASIVE — RADIOTHERAPY

Age	<1 O	<1 E	1-4 O	1-4 E	5-9 O	5-9 E	10-14 O	10-14 E	15-19 O	15-19 E	20-24 O	20-24 E	25-29 O	25-29 E	30+ O	30+ E	Total (excl. <1) O	Total (excl. <1) E
<30		0.00		0.00		0.03	1	0.07	1	0.10		0.09	1	0.11	1	0.07	4	0.49
30-39	1	0.28	1	1.15	3	1.90	5	2.38	3	2.29	2	1.66		0.87	2	0.33	16	10.58
40-49	2	1.64	7	5.90	4	8.38	13	8.37	12	6.24	12	4.13	5	1.94	1	0.62	54	35.58
50-59	3	3.78	10	12.34	13	13.76	24	10.99	7	7.02	5	3.63	3	1.26	1	0.20	63	49.20
60-69	3	4.97	9	14.56	14	12.90	8	8.19	7	3.68		1.09		0.16		0.03	38	40.61
70+	1	5.18	9	11.11	8	6.27	5	2.31	1	0.42		0.07		0.03		0.01	23	20.22

INVASIVE — NO OTHER

Age	<1 O	<1 E	1-4 O	1-4 E	5-9 O	5-9 E	10-14 O	10-14 E	15-19 O	15-19 E	20-24 O	20-24 E	25-29 O	25-29 E	30+ O	30+ E	Total (excl. <1) O	Total (excl. <1) E
<30	1	0.00		0.01		0.02		0.02		0.03		0.02		0.01		0.00		0.11
30-39	2	0.05		0.31	1	0.52	2	0.59	1	0.53		0.26	1	0.08		0.02	6	2.31
40-49	1	0.27		1.11	1	1.62	2	1.51	1	1.05	1	0.80	1	0.19		0.07	4	6.10
50-59	2	0.44	2	1.49	2	1.66		1.29	1	0.80		0.32	1	0.09		0.01	5	5.66
60-69	3	0.40	3	1.14	1	1.11	1	0.60		0.27		0.09		0.03		0.00	7	3.24
70+	1	0.54		0.81		0.47		0.17		0.05		0.01		0.00		0.00		1.51

IN SITU — NO TREATMENT

Age	<1 O	<1 E	1-4 O	1-4 E	5-9 O	5-9 E	10-14 O	10-14 E	15-19 O	15-19 E	20-24 O	20-24 E	25-29 O	25-29 E	30+ O	30+ E	Total (excl. <1) O	Total (excl. <1) E
<30	2	0.08		0.35	1	0.35	1	0.14		0.05		0.05		0.00		0.00	2	0.90
30-39	5	0.49	4	2.12	7	2.36	3	1.20	1	0.53	1	0.13		0.02		0.00	9	6.36
40-49	2	1.29	5	4.55	7	5.69	3	2.48	3	0.80	1	0.24	1	0.07		0.01	16	13.84
50-59	2	0.96	2	3.75	3	3.17	3	1.22	1	0.43	1	0.11	1	0.02		0.01	9	8.71
60-69	1	0.58	2	2.03	3	1.43	1	0.46	1	0.13		0.03		0.00		0.00	7	4.08
70+	1	0.32	1	0.98	1	0.51	1	0.12		0.01		0.00		0.00		0.00	2	1.62

O : All tumours observed
E : Expected

Table B5. Pancreas (ICD 157)

TIME SINCE DIAGNOSIS OF PRIMARY CERVICAL CANCER (IN YEARS)

INVASIVE — RADIOTHERAPY

AGE	<1 E	<1 O	1–4 E	1–4 O	5–9 E	5–9 O	10–14 E	10–14 O	15–19 E	15–19 O	20–24 E	20–24 O	25–29 E	25–29 O	30+ E	30+ O	Total (excl. <1) E	Total O
<30	0.00		0.00		0.01		0.02		0.04		0.05		0.03		0.02		0.17	
30–39	0.05	1	0.36	1	0.71	1	0.97	3	1.00	1	0.83	1	0.50		0.21		4.58	7
40–49	0.56	1	2.50	4	4.00	4	4.40	8	3.65	2	2.50		1.27	1	0.43		18.75	20
50–59	1.88	21	6.73	8	8.24	10	7.27		4.80		2.47		0.90		0.14		30.57	44
60–69	3.10	12	9.43	7	8.93	9	5.81	3	2.60	1	0.77	1	0.12	1	0.02		27.68	33
70+	3.65	12	7.85	3	4.52	1	1.62	1	0.29		0.04		0.02		0.01		14.35	17

INVASIVE — NO RADIOTHERAPY

AGE	<1 E	<1 O	1–4 E	1–4 O	5–9 E	5–9 O	10–14 E	10–14 O	15–19 E	15–19 O	20–24 E	20–24 O	25–29 E	25–29 O	30+ E	30+ O	Total (excl. <1) E	Total O
<30	0.00		0.00		0.00		0.01		0.01		0.01		0.01		0.00		0.04	
30–39	0.01		0.08		0.17		0.26	1	0.24		0.12		0.05		0.02		0.94	1
40–49	0.07		0.40		0.71		0.71	2	0.57		0.35		0.13		0.05		2.92	2
50–59	0.18		0.70		0.88		0.75		0.48		0.21		0.07		0.01		3.10	
60–69	0.23	1	0.65		0.67		0.38		0.16		0.06		0.02		0.00		1.94	3
70+	0.32	1	0.52		0.32		0.13		0.03		0.01		0.00		0.00		1.01	1

IN SITU — RADIOTHERAPY

AGE	<1 E	<1 O	1–4 E	1–4 O	5–9 E	5–9 O	10–14 E	10–14 O	15–19 E	15–19 O	20–24 E	20–24 O	25–29 E	25–29 O	30+ E	30+ O	Total (excl. <1) E	Total O
<30	0.03		0.10		0.10		0.04		0.01		0.01		0.00		0.00		0.26	
30–39	0.14	1	0.77	1	1.04	1	0.53		0.26		0.08		0.02		0.00		2.70	5
40–49	0.57	1	2.69		2.99	4	1.44	2	0.51		0.15		0.05		0.01		7.84	13
50–59	0.50	2	2.18		2.12	2	0.87		0.29	1	0.07		0.01		0.00		5.54	5
60–69	0.40	1	1.47		1.09		0.36		0.11		0.03		0.00		0.00		3.06	3
70+	0.26	1	0.82		0.40	1	0.09		0.01		0.00		0.00		0.00		1.32	1

O : All tumours observed
E : Expected

Table B6. Lung (ICD 162-163)

TIME SINCE DIAGNOSIS OF PRIMARY CERVICAL CANCER (IN YEARS)

INVASIVE — RADIOTHERAPY

Age	<1 O	<1 E	1-4 O	1-4 E	5-9 O	5-9 E	10-14 O	10-14 E	15-19 O	15-19 E	20-24 O	20-24 E	25-29 O	25-29 E	30+ O	30+ E	Total (excl. <1) O	Total (excl. <1) E
<30		0.00	4	0.03	2	0.05		0.12		0.19		0.17		0.10		0.03	6	0.69
30-39		0.20	20	0.99	14	2.10	4	2.74	4	2.51	1	1.90	1	1.04		0.39	44	11.67
40-49	3	1.62	49	6.16	58	8.83	28	8.58	11	6.01	2	3.89	2	1.75	1	0.47	151	35.69
50-59	4	3.81	52	12.41	63	13.08	33	9.66	17	5.32	5	2.56	2	0.82		0.11	172	43.96
60-69	2	4.38	37	12.13	36	9.66	15	5.24	3	1.98		0.59		0.10		0.02	91	29.72
70+	2	3.52	14	7.11	9	4.29	6	1.24		0.20		0.04		0.02		0.01	29	12.91

INVASIVE — NO RADIOTHERAPY

Age	<1 O	<1 E	1-4 O	1-4 E	5-9 O	5-9 E	10-14 O	10-14 E	15-19 O	15-19 E	20-24 O	20-24 E	25-29 O	25-29 E	30+ O	30+ E	Total (excl. <1) O	Total (excl. <1) E
<30		0.00		0.00	1	0.01		0.04		0.05		0.04		0.03		0.01	1	0.18
30-39	1	0.05	3	0.32	1	0.65	2	0.74	1	0.68		0.33		0.10		0.03	7	2.85
40-49		0.27	6	1.34	2	1.95	6	1.73	2	1.13		0.59		0.18		0.05	16	6.97
50-59		0.40	10	1.59	6	1.80	3	1.29	1	0.64	2	0.24		0.06		0.00	22	5.62
60-69		0.38	3	1.14	4	0.92	2	0.43		0.13		0.04		0.02		0.00	9	2.68
70+		0.34		0.51		0.25		0.08		0.01		0.01		0.00		0.00		0.86

IN SITU

Age	<1 O	<1 E	1-4 O	1-4 E	5-9 O	5-9 E	10-14 O	10-14 E	15-19 O	15-19 E	20-24 O	20-24 E	25-29 O	25-29 E	30+ O	30+ E	Total (excl. <1) O	Total (excl. <1) E
<30		0.08	1	0.32		0.34	3	0.18		0.08		0.03		0.00		0.00	4	0.95
30-39		0.50	9	2.70	6	3.41	4	1.69	4	0.73		0.23		0.04		0.00	23	8.80
40-49	4	1.75	17	7.62	10	7.88	9	3.25	2	1.08	1	0.27		0.08	1	0.01	40	20.19
50-59	2	1.22	11	4.74	5	3.96	2	1.32	1	0.37		0.08		0.01		0.00	19	10.48
60-69	1	0.56	5	2.03	1	1.34		0.34		0.08		0.01		0.00		0.00	6	3.80
70+		0.24	2	0.72	1	0.31		0.05		0.01		0.00		0.00		0.00	3	1.09

O : All tumours observed
E : Expected

Table B7. Breast (ICD 170)

TIME SINCE DIAGNOSIS OF PRIMARY CERVICAL CANCER (IN YEARS)

O : All tumours observed
E : Expected

INVASIVE — RADIOTHERAPY

Age	<1 O	<1 E	1–4 O	1–4 E	5–9 O	5–9 E	10–14 O	10–14 E	15–19 O	15–19 E	20–24 O	20–24 E	25–29 O	25–29 E	30+ O	30+ E	Total O	Total E
<30		0.10		0.57	1	1.20	1	1.81		1.94		1.43	1	0.61	1	0.18	4	7.74
30–39	2	3.89	9	18.05	14	29.23	8	28.60	5	18.00	2	9.33	1	3.88	1	1.34	40	108.43
40–49	15	22.48	42	71.11	62	73.42	35	52.06	26	29.28	11	15.52	3	6.41	3	1.99	182	249.79
50–59	18	26.25	59	77.04	51	68.80	46	45.42	14	23.74	8	10.92	3	3.58		0.56	181	230.06
60–69	22	21.80	46	60.30	43	46.13	14	26.09	8	10.66	2	3.15		0.56		0.14	113	147.03
70+	9	16.75	20	34.99	25	18.90	8	6.52		1.24		0.31		0.09		0.02	53	62.07

INVASIVE — NO THERAPY

Age	<1 O	<1 E	1–4 O	1–4 E	5–9 O	5–9 E	10–14 O	10–14 E	15–19 O	15–19 E	20–24 O	20–24 E	25–29 O	25–29 E	30+ O	30+ E	Total O	Total E
<30		0.02		0.22	1	0.56	1	0.74		0.65	1	0.40		0.13		0.04	3	2.74
30–39	5	0.86	5	5.20	11	8.61	6	7.59	3	4.52	1	1.59		0.43		0.14	26	28.08
40–49	2	3.75	14	14.27	9	15.36	4	9.71	4	5.17	2	2.42	1	0.75	1	0.27	35	47.95
50–59	3	2.96	12	9.75	12	8.95	8	5.58	2	2.80	1	1.12	1	0.28		0.02	36	28.50
60–69	1	1.94	6	5.17	2	4.49	3	2.21		0.87		0.34		0.09		0.00	11	13.17
70+	2	1.82	3	2.89	2	1.54		0.54		0.15		0.04		0.00		0.00	5	5.16

IN SITU

Age	<1 O	<1 E	1–4 O	1–4 E	5–9 O	5–9 E	10–14 O	10–14 E	15–19 O	15–19 E	20–24 O	20–24 E	25–29 O	25–29 E	30+ O	30+ E	Total O	Total E
<30	1	0.92	6	5.45	6	6.65	4	3.19	2	1.13		0.36		0.04		0.00	18	16.82
30–39	5	9.05	33	43.93	51	50.47	26	21.99	6	7.07		1.41		0.14		0.01	116	125.02
40–49	11	22.44	79	88.45	68	71.72	17	24.61	4	6.83	2	1.71	1	0.18		0.04	171	193.54
50–59	4	8.74	34	30.77	27	22.78	9	8.13	4	2.55	1	0.57		0.12		0.01	75	64.93
60–69	2	3.20	11	10.40	4	6.94	3	2.20	1	0.62		0.15		0.02		0.00	19	20.33
70+	2	1.25	6	3.89	2	1.87		0.53		0.08							8	6.37

Table B8. Corpus uteri (ICD 172)

TIME SINCE DIAGNOSIS OF PRIMARY CERVICAL CANCER (IN YEARS)

INVASIVE — RADIOTHERAPY

Age	<1 O	<1 E	1–4 O	1–4 E	5–9 O	5–9 E	10–14 O	10–14 E	15–19 O	15–19 E	20–24 O	20–24 E	25–29 O	25–29 E	30+ O	30+ E	Total (excl. <1) O	Total (excl. <1) E
<30		0.00	1	0.03	1	0.08	1	0.15		0.24		0.28		0.18		0.05	3	1.01
30–39		0.35	4	1.74	4	3.90	5	5.83	6	5.33	6	3.25	2	1.34		0.43	27	21.82
40–49	4	3.44	3	14.27	11	20.64	16	17.79	12	10.41	4	5.05	3	1.86		0.51	49	70.53
50–59	6	8.67	2	25.79	12	22.85	15	14.01	3	6.53	4	2.57	1	0.73		0.11	37	72.59
60–69	2	6.89		17.73	7	12.03	6	5.68		1.92		0.46		0.07		0.02	13	37.91
70+	7	3.46	2	7.06	2	3.19		0.85		0.14		0.02		0.01		0.00	4	11.27

INVASIVE — NO RADIOTHERAPY

Age	<1 O	<1 E	1–4 O	1–4 E	5–9 O	5–9 E	10–14 O	10–14 E	15–19 O	15–19 E	20–24 O	20–24 E	25–29 O	25–29 E	30+ O	30+ E	Total (excl. <1) O	Total (excl. <1) E
<30		0.00		0.01		0.02		0.04		0.06		0.05		0.03		0.02		0.23
30–39		0.07		0.39		0.90		1.25		1.12		0.50		0.13		0.03		4.32
40–49		0.48		2.19		3.37		2.83		1.71		0.74		0.22		0.07	1	11.13
50–59		0.80		2.64		2.56		1.55		0.73		0.25		0.05		0.00		7.78
60–69		0.51		1.31		0.95		0.39		0.12		0.04		0.02		0.00		2.83
70+	2	0.27		0.43		0.22		0.05		0.02		0.00		0.00		0.00		0.72

IN SITU

Age	<1 O	<1 E	1–4 O	1–4 E	5–9 O	5–9 E	10–14 O	10–14 E	15–19 O	15–19 E	20–24 O	20–24 E	25–29 O	25–29 E	30+ O	30+ E	Total (excl. <1) O	Total (excl. <1) E
<30		0.08	1	0.40		0.48		0.26		0.12		0.05		0.01		0.00	1	1.32
30–39	3	0.71	2	3.68	5	5.65	3	3.55		1.54		0.40		0.05		0.00	10	14.87
40–49	2	3.25	6	15.82	9	16.73	5	6.35		1.68		0.41		0.10		0.01	20	41.10
50–59	5	2.52	7	8.81	4	6.06		1.91		0.53		0.11		0.02		0.00	11	17.44
60–69	1	0.85	1	2.76	1	1.59		0.44		0.09		0.01		0.00		0.00	2	4.89
70+		0.27		0.77		0.30		0.06		0.01		0.00		0.00		0.00		1.14

O : All tumours observed
E : Expected

Table B9. Ovary (ICD 175)

TIME SINCE DIAGNOSIS OF PRIMARY CERVICAL CANCER (IN YEARS)

INVASIVE — RADIOTHERAPY

Age	<1 O	<1 E	1-4 O	1-4 E	5-9 O	5-9 E	10-14 O	10-14 E	15-19 O	15-19 E	20-24 O	20-24 E	25-29 O	25-29 E	30+ O	30+ E	Total (excl. <1) O	Total (excl. <1) E
<30	1	0.05	1	0.20	2	0.26		0.33	2	0.37		0.32		0.13		0.03	5	1.64
30-39	1	0.84	3	3.68	2	5.88	8	6.43	2	4.61	2	2.62	2	1.10	1	0.32	20	24.64
40-49	6	4.53	5	16.02	12	18.87	6	14.35	7	8.32	5	4.36	3	1.68	1	0.43	39	64.03
50-59	7	7.13	14	21.11	11	18.70	12	12.16	5	6.08	3	2.51		0.72		0.09	45	61.37
60-69	5	5.85	11	15.61	6	11.30	5	5.67	2	1.98	1	0.48		0.07		0.02	25	35.13
70+	3	3.35	2	6.92	2	3.30	1	0.95		0.16		0.03		0.01		0.00	5	11.37

INVASIVE

Age	<1 O	<1 E	1-4 O	1-4 E	5-9 O	5-9 E	10-14 O	10-14 E	15-19 O	15-19 E	20-24 O	20-24 E	25-29 O	25-29 E	30+ O	30+ E	Total (excl. <1) O	Total (excl. <1) E
<30		0.01		0.06		0.11		0.12		0.12		0.06		0.02		0.01		0.50
30-39	2	0.19		0.90	1	1.53		1.57		1.04		0.39		0.10		0.02	1	5.55
40-49	1	0.71	1	2.75	1	3.31		2.34	2	1.33		0.59		0.17	1	0.21	5	10.70
50-59		0.71	1	2.26	1	2.10		1.33		0.66		0.23		0.05		0.00	2	6.63
60-69	2	0.45	1	1.16	1	0.92	1	0.39		0.13		0.03		0.01		0.00	3	2.64
70+	1	0.28	1	0.43		0.21		0.06		0.01		0.01		0.00		0.00	1	0.72

IN SITU — SURGERY

Age	<1 O	<1 E	1-4 O	1-4 E	5-9 O	5-9 E	10-14 O	10-14 E	15-19 O	15-19 E	20-24 O	20-24 E	25-29 O	25-29 E	30+ O	30+ E	Total (excl. <1) O	Total (excl. <1) E
<30	3	0.66	4	2.45	2	1.69		0.48		0.17		0.04		0.01		0.00	6	4.84
30-39	1	2.09	7	8.68	7	8.94	3	3.56	1	1.06		0.17		0.03		0.00	18	22.44
40-49	4	4.39	23	18.51	11	15.40	3	4.71		1.05		0.25		0.06		0.01	37	39.99
50-59	1	2.27	3	7.79	5	5.24	2	1.52		0.40		0.07		0.01		0.00	10	15.03
60-69	2	0.81	1	2.57		1.52		0.37		0.07		0.01		0.00		0.00	1	4.54
70+	1	0.26	1	0.76		0.31		0.05		0.00		0.00		0.00		0.00	1	1.12

O : All tumours observed
E : Expected

Table B10. Other female genital (ICD 176)

TIME SINCE DIAGNOSIS OF PRIMARY CERVICAL CANCER (IN YEARS)

O : All tumours observed
E : Expected

INVASIVE — RADIOTHERAPY

Age	<1 O	<1 E	1-4 O	1-4 E	5-9 O	5-9 E	10-14 O	10-14 E	15-19 O	15-19 E	20-24 O	20-24 E	25-29 O	25-29 E	30+ O	30+ E	Total (excl. <1) O	Total (excl. <1) E
<30			1	0.00		0.02		0.03	1	0.03	1	0.03		0.02		0.01	3	0.14
30-39			2	0.11	2	0.42	5	0.61	2	0.68	2	0.52		0.34		0.14	14	2.76
40-49	2		5	0.45	7	1.72	10	2.06	4	1.78	3	1.31	2	0.76	1	0.35	31	8.10
50-59	3		5	0.93	7	2.92	3	3.00	2	2.51	1	1.50	2	0.77		0.25	20	10.99
60-69	1		13	1.11	9	3.42	4	3.08	3	1.98	1	0.90		0.28		0.02	30	9.68
70+	2		4	1.27	4	2.72	1	1.56		0.55		0.13		0.01		0.01	9	4.98

INVASIVE — (no data shown)

Age	<1	1-4	5-9	10-14	15-19	20-24	25-29	30+	Total (excl. <1)
<30									
30-39									
40-49									
50-59									
60-69									
70+									

IN SITU — RADIOTHERAPY

Age	<1 O	<1 E	1-4 O	1-4 E	5-9 O	5-9 E	10-14 O	10-14 E	15-19 O	15-19 E	20-24 O	20-24 E	25-29 O	25-29 E	30+ O	30+ E	Total (excl. <1) O	Total (excl. <1) E
<30	1		3	0.02	2	0.27		0.15	2	0.07		0.02		0.01		0.00	7	0.52
30-39	2		5	0.18	11	0.99	1	0.96	1	0.53		0.21		0.04		0.01	18	2.74
40-49	8		10	0.62	15	1.48	4	1.55	1	0.60		0.16		0.04		0.01	30	3.84
50-59	1		1	0.29	10	0.80	2	0.65		0.27		0.08		0.02		0.00	13	1.82
60-69	2		10	0.16	4	0.41		0.32		0.10		0.02		0.01		0.00	14	0.86
70+	1		1	0.07	2	0.21		0.12		0.01		0.00		0.00		0.00	3	0.34

Table B11. Kidney (ICD 180)

TIME SINCE DIAGNOSIS OF PRIMARY CERVICAL CANCER (IN YEARS)

INVASIVE — RADIOTHERAPY

AGE	<1 O	<1 E	1-4 O	1-4 E	5-9 O	5-9 E	10-14 O	10-14 E	15-19 O	15-19 E	20-24 O	20-24 E	25-29 O	25-29 E	30+ O	30+ E	Total (excl. <1) O	Total E
<30		0.00		0.02		0.03		0.03	1	0.05		0.06		0.04		0.01	1	0.24
30-39	2	0.10	3	0.55	2	1.02	2	1.28	1	1.14	1	0.76	3	0.40		0.13	11	5.28
40-49	7	0.80	10	2.92	5	4.17	2	3.97	2	2.90	1	1.79	1	0.79		0.23	22	16.77
50-59	1	1.78	10	5.75	8	6.31	1	4.97	2	2.85	1	1.38	1	0.42		0.06	23	21.74
60-69	9	2.11	3	6.22	4	5.38		3.04	2	1.22		0.29		0.04		0.01	9	16.20
70+	3	1.86	2	3.85	2	2.04		0.66		0.12		0.00		0.01		0.00	4	6.68

INVASIVE — NO RADIOTHERAPY

AGE	<1 O	<1 E	1-4 O	1-4 E	5-9 O	5-9 E	10-14 O	10-14 E	15-19 O	15-19 E	20-24 O	20-24 E	25-29 O	25-29 E	30+ O	30+ E	Total (excl. <1) O	Total E
<30		0.00		0.00		0.01		0.01	1	0.02		0.01		0.01		0.00	1	0.06
30-39		0.01	1	0.12		0.23	1	0.29		0.23		0.10		0.04		0.02	2	1.03
40-49	1	0.12		0.49	1	0.68	2	0.59		0.40		0.19		0.08		0.02	4	2.45
50-59		0.15	2	0.56	2	0.64	1	0.49		0.29		0.11		0.04		0.00	6	2.13
60-69		0.14	2	0.40	2	0.39	1	0.20		0.07		0.03		0.01		0.00	3	1.10
70+	1	0.14		0.22	1	0.12		0.02		0.01		0.00		0.00		0.00	1	0.37

IN SITU

AGE	<1 O	<1 E	1-4 O	1-4 E	5-9 O	5-9 E	10-14 O	10-14 E	15-19 O	15-19 E	20-24 O	20-24 E	25-29 O	25-29 E	30+ O	30+ E	Total (excl. <1) O	Total E
<30		0.07		0.28		0.24		0.08		0.02		0.01		0.00		0.00		0.63
30-39	1	0.32	1	1.47		1.54		0.65		0.22		0.05	1	0.01		0.00	3	3.94
40-49		0.88	3	3.78	3	3.71	1	1.38		0.36		0.09		0.02		0.00	11	9.34
50-59	2	0.63	4	2.35	4	1.86	1	0.64		0.17		0.02		0.01		0.00	8	5.05
60-69		0.33	3	1.12	1	0.72		0.19		0.03		0.01		0.00		0.00	4	2.07
70+		0.15		0.47		0.20		0.03		0.00		0.00		0.00		0.00		0.70

O : All tumours observed
E : Expected

Table B12. Bladder (ICD 181)

TIME SINCE DIAGNOSIS OF PRIMARY CERVICAL CANCER (IN YEARS)

INVASIVE

Age	<1 O	<1 E	1-4 O	1-4 E	5-9 O	5-9 E	10-14 O	10-14 E	15-19 O	15-19 E	20-24 O	20-24 E	25-29 O	25-29 E	30+ O	30+ E	Total O	Total E
<30	1	0.00	1	0.01		0.01		0.02		0.04		0.04		0.04		0.01	1	0.17
30-39	3	0.09	3	0.36	7	0.68	4	0.89	7	0.91	2	0.72	1	0.41		0.18	27	4.15
40-49	12	0.47	11	2.10	13	3.18	10	3.50	4	2.62	4	2.03	3	1.08		0.38	57	14.89
50-59	13	1.52	13	4.98	13	5.92	17	5.27	6	3.57	3	2.04	2	0.74		0.12	67	22.64
60-69	10	2.20	7	6.85	8	6.66	5	4.42	4	2.03		0.62		0.10		0.02	34	20.70
70+	6	2.74	2	6.12	2	3.48		1.24		0.20		0.03		0.01		0.00	10	11.08

IN SITU

Age	<1 O	<1 E	1-4 O	1-4 E	5-9 O	5-9 E	10-14 O	10-14 E	15-19 O	15-19 E	20-24 O	20-24 E	25-29 O	25-29 E	30+ O	30+ E	Total O	Total E
<30		0.00		0.00		0.01		0.01		0.01		0.01		0.01		0.00		0.05
30-39		0.01		0.11		0.19		0.24		0.24		0.11		0.03		0.02		0.94
40-49	3	0.09	3	0.44	3	0.65		0.59	1	0.42		0.24		0.11		0.04	4	2.49
50-59	2	0.13	2	0.58	1	0.66	3	0.53	1	0.36		0.18		0.05		0.00	7	2.36
60-69	1	0.13	1	0.51	2	0.55		0.32		0.12		0.04		0.02		0.00	3	1.56
70+	2	0.25	2	0.43		0.24		0.10		0.02		0.01		0.00		0.00		0.80

UNKNOWN

Age	<1 O	<1 E	1-4 O	1-4 E	5-9 O	5-9 E	10-14 O	10-14 E	15-19 O	15-19 E	20-24 O	20-24 E	25-29 O	25-29 E	30+ O	30+ E	Total O	Total E
<30		0.09	1	0.30		0.19		0.06		0.02		0.01		0.00		0.00	1	0.58
30-39	2	0.22	2	0.97	1	1.08		0.52		0.21		0.06		0.01		0.00	3	2.85
40-49		0.56	3	2.60	2	2.77	5	1.15	2	0.37		0.11		0.03		0.01	12	7.04
50-59	1	0.48	3	1.92	3	1.69	3	0.61		0.22		0.06		0.01		0.00	9	4.51
60-69	1	0.31	2	1.11	1	0.82	1	0.27		0.08		0.02		0.00		0.00	4	2.30
70+		0.19	1	0.58	1	0.28		0.08		0.01		0.00		0.00		0.00	1	0.95

O : All tumours observed
E : Expected

Table B13. Thyroid (ICD 194)

TIME SINCE DIAGNOSIS OF PRIMARY CERVICAL CANCER (IN YEARS)

INVASIVE

AGE	<1 O	<1 E	1–4 O	1–4 E	5–9 O	5–9 E	10–14 O	10–14 E	15–19 O	15–19 E	20–24 O	20–24 E	25–29 O	25–29 E	30+ O	30+ E	Total (excl. <1) O	Total (excl. <1) E
<30		0.02		0.12		0.12		0.11		0.06		0.03		0.01		0.00	0.00	0.45
30–39	2	0.29	3	1.10	3	1.25	2	1.04	1	0.60		0.26		0.09		0.04	8	4.38
40–49	3	0.78	1	2.44	4	2.61	?	1.83	2	1.08	2	0.65		0.21		0.07	7	8.89
50–59	2	0.86	4	2.63	4	2.58	2	1.96	2	1.03	1	0.44	1	0.13		0.02	11	8.79
60–69	1	0.85	3	2.43	4	2.01	1	1.15		0.51		0.10		0.02		0.00	7	6.22
70+		0.74	2	1.58	2	0.90	1	0.26		0.06		0.01		0.00		0.00	3	2.81

INVASIVE

AGE	<1 O	<1 E	1–4 O	1–4 E	5–9 O	5–9 E	10–14 O	10–14 E	15–19 O	15–19 E	20–24 O	20–24 E	25–29 O	25–29 E	30+ O	30+ E	Total (excl. <1) O	Total (excl. <1) E
<30																		
30–39																		
40–49																		
50–59																		
60–69																		
70+																		

IN SITU

AGE	<1 O	<1 E	1–4 O	1–4 E	5–9 O	5–9 E	10–14 O	10–14 E	15–19 O	15–19 E	20–24 O	20–24 E	25–29 O	25–29 E	30+ O	30+ E	Total (excl. <1) O	Total (excl. <1) E
<30	1	0.59	2	1.96	1	1.03		0.20	1	0.04		0.01		0.00		0.00	3	3.24
30–39	2	0.93	3	3.17		2.43	1	0.71		0.17		0.02		0.00		0.00	4	6.50
40–49		0.83	1	3.02	1	2.24		0.68		0.17		0.02		0.01		0.00	2	6.14
50–59		0.29	3	1.00		0.73		0.25		0.08		0.01		0.00		0.00	3	2.07
60–69		0.10		0.36		0.25		0.05		0.01		0.00		0.00		0.00		0.67
70+		0.05		0.14		0.05		0.01		0.00		0.00		0.00		0.00		0.20

O : All tumours observed
E : Expected

Table B14. Connective tissue (ICD 197)

TIME SINCE DIAGNOSIS OF PRIMARY CERVICAL CANCER (IN YEARS)

INVASIVE — RADIOTHERAPY

AGE	<1 O	<1 E	1-4 O	1-4 E	5-9 O	5-9 E	10-14 O	10-14 E	15-19 O	15-19 E	20-24 O	20-24 E	25-29 O	25-29 E	30+ O	30+ E	Total (excl. <1) O	Total (excl. <1) E
<30		0.00		0.04		0.02		0.02		0.02		0.01	1	0.00		0.00	1	0.11
30-39		0.10		0.40		0.42		0.38		0.26		0.11		0.05	1	0.02	1	1.64
40-49	1	0.31	3	1.04	1	1.10	1	0.88	1	0.57		0.33		0.08		0.03	6	4.03
50-59	1	0.38	4	1.29	6	1.35	1	0.95	1	0.51		0.19		0.05		0.01	12	4.35
60-69	1	0.48	2	1.23		1.05	1	0.65	1	0.21		0.07		0.01		0.00	4	3.22
70+	1	0.32	1	0.85	1	0.39		0.13	1	0.00		0.00		0.00		0.00	3	1.37

INVASIVE — SURGERY

AGE	<1 O	<1 E	1-4 O	1-4 E	5-9 O	5-9 E	10-14 O	10-14 E	15-19 O	15-19 E	20-24 O	20-24 E	25-29 O	25-29 E	30+ O	30+ E	Total (excl. <1) O	Total (excl. <1) E
<30																		
30-39																		
40-49																		
50-59																		
60-69																		
70+																		

IN SITU — SURGERY

AGE	<1 O	<1 E	1-4 O	1-4 E	5-9 O	5-9 E	10-14 O	10-14 E	15-19 O	15-19 E	20-24 O	20-24 E	25-29 O	25-29 E	30+ O	30+ E	Total (excl. <1) O	Total (excl. <1) E
<30																		
30-39																		
40-49																		
50-59																		
60-69																		
70+																		

O : All tumours observed
E : Expected

Table B15. Lymphoma (ICD 200)

TIME SINCE DIAGNOSIS OF PRIMARY CERVICAL CANCER (IN YEARS)

INVASIVE — RADIOTHERAPY

AGE	<1 E	<1 O	1–4 E	1–4 O	5–9 E	5–9 O	10–14 E	10–14 O	15–19 E	15–19 O	20–24 E	20–24 O	25–29 E	25–29 O	30+ E	30+ O	Total (excl. <1) E	Total (excl. <1) O
<30	0.00		0.04		0.06		0.06		0.04		0.03		0.02		0.00		0.25	
30–39	0.19	1	0.71	1	1.08	1	1.08		0.88		0.55		0.26		0.11	2	4.67	2
40–49	0.68	5	2.61	2	3.23	3	2.92	1	2.21	1	1.37		0.58		0.19	12	13.11	12
50–59	1.32	5	4.47	5	4.93	8	3.98	2	2.31	1	1.17	2	0.37		0.06	23	17.29	23
60–69	1.72	4	4.96	6	4.38	7	2.67	2	1.09	2	0.26		0.04		0.01	21	13.41	21
70+	1.48	3	3.41	3	1.81	1	0.58	1	0.12		0.02		0.01		0.00	4	5.95	4

INVASIVE — NO RADIOTHERAPY

AGE	<1 E	<1 O	1–4 E	1–4 O	5–9 E	5–9 O	10–14 E	10–14 O	15–19 E	15–19 O	20–24 E	20–24 O	25–29 E	25–29 O	30+ E	30+ O	Total (excl. <1) E	Total (excl. <1) O
<30																		
30–39																		
40–49																		
50–59																		
60–69																		
70+																		

IN SITU — RADIOTHERAPY

AGE	<1 E	<1 O	1–4 E	1–4 O	5–9 E	5–9 O	10–14 E	10–14 O	15–19 E	15–19 O	20–24 E	20–24 O	25–29 E	25–29 O	30+ E	30+ O	Total (excl. <1) E	Total (excl. <1) O
<30	0.20		0.73		0.62		0.20		0.05		0.01		0.00		0.00		1.61	
30–39	0.54	1	2.11	3	1.94	1	0.77		0.29		0.07		0.01		0.00	5	5.19	5
40–49	0.65	7	2.73	1	2.73		1.20		0.37		0.09		0.03		0.00	8	7.15	8
50–59	0.42	4	1.58	2	1.32	3	0.50		0.17		0.04		0.01		0.00	9	3.62	9
60–69	0.22		0.79	1	0.59	1	0.19		0.04		0.01		0.00		0.00	2	1.62	2
70+	0.10		0.36		0.17		0.03		0.00		0.00		0.00		0.00		0.56	

O : All tumours observed
E : Expected

Table B16. Hodgkin's disease (ICD 201)

TIME SINCE DIAGNOSIS OF PRIMARY CERVICAL CANCER (IN YEARS)

INVASIVE / RADIOTHERAPY

AGE	<1 O	<1 E	1-4 O	1-4 E	5-9 O	5-9 E	10-14 O	10-14 E	15-19 O	15-19 E	20-24 O	20-24 E	25-29 O	25-29 E	30+ O	30+ E	Total (excl. <1) O	Total (excl. <1) E
<30		0.04		0.11		0.09		0.06		0.03		0.01		0.01		0.00		0.31
30-39		0.21	1	0.65		0.61		0.42	1	0.26		0.14		0.07		0.04	3	2.19
40-49		0.40	2	1.22	1	1.21		0.96		0.63		0.34	1	0.18		1.41	5	5.95
50-59	1	0.45		1.47	1	1.35	1	1.01		0.64		0.23	1	0.06		0.00	2	4.76
60-69		0.43	1	1.33	1	1.13	1	0.65		0.17		0.02		0.00		0.00	2	3.30
70+		0.30		0.81		0.32		0.08		0.01		0.00		0.00		0.00	1	1.22

INVASIVE / NON RADIOTHERAPY

AGE	<1 O	<1 E	1-4 O	1-4 E	5-9 O	5-9 E	10-14 O	10-14 E	15-19 O	15-19 E	20-24 O	20-24 E	25-29 O	25-29 E	30+ O	30+ E	Total (excl. <1) O	Total (excl. <1) E
<30																		
30-39																		
40-49																		
50-59																		
60-69																		
70+																		

IN SITU / NON RADIOTHERAPY

AGE	<1 O	<1 E	1-4 O	1-4 E	5-9 O	5-9 E	10-14 O	10-14 E	15-19 O	15-19 E	20-24 O	20-24 E	25-29 O	25-29 E	30+ O	30+ E	Total (excl. <1) O	Total (excl. <1) E
<30																		
30-39																		
40-49																		
50-59																		
60-69																		
70+																		

O : All tumours observed
E : Expected

Table B17. Multiple myeloma (ICD 203)

TIME SINCE DIAGNOSIS OF PRIMARY CERVICAL CANCER (IN YEARS)

INVASIVE — RADIOTHERAPY

AGE AT DIAGNOSIS	<1 E	<1 O	1-4 E	1-4 O	5-9 E	5-9 O	10-14 E	10-14 O	15-19 E	15-19 O	20-24 E	20-24 O	25-29 E	25-29 O	30+ E	30+ O	Total Excl. <1 E	Total Excl. <1 O
<30	0.00		0.00		0.00		0.00		0.02		0.01		0.01		0.00		0.04	
30-39	0.02		0.14		0.28		0.43	2	0.46	2	0.33	1	0.16		0.08		1.88	5
40-49	0.24	1	1.09	1	1.69	1	1.91	2	1.41		0.91		0.44		0.15		7.60	4
50-59	0.79	1	2.71	5	3.20	2	2.79	3	1.81	1	0.80		0.24		0.05		11.60	11
60-69	1.10	2	3.39	1	3.23	2	2.00	2	0.80	2	0.19		0.03	1	0.01		9.65	8
70+	1.04	1	2.30	2	1.23	1	0.37	1	0.06		0.01		0.01	1	0.00		3.98	5

INVASIVE — NO RADIOTHERAPY

AGE AT DIAGNOSIS	<1	1-4	5-9	10-14	15-19	20-24	25-29	30+	Total Excl. <1
<30									
30-39									
40-49									
50-59									
60-69									
70+									

IN SITU — NO THERAPY

AGE AT DIAGNOSIS	<1	1-4	5-9	10-14	15-19	20-24	25-29	30+	Total Excl. <1
<30									
30-39									
40-49									
50-59									
60-69									
70+									

O : All tumours observed
E : Expected

Table B18. Chronic lymphocytic and other leukaemias (ICD 204.1)

TIME SINCE DIAGNOSIS OF PRIMARY CERVICAL CANCER (IN YEARS)

INVASIVE — RADIOTHERAPY

AGE	<1 O	<1 E	1-4 O	1-4 E	5-9 O	5-9 E	10-14 O	10-14 E	15-19 O	15-19 E	20-24 O	20-24 E	25-29 O	25-29 E	30+ O	30+ E	Total (excl. <1) O	Total (excl. <1) E
<30		0.00		0.00		0.00		0.00		0.00		0.00		0.01		0.01	0	0.02
30-39	1	0.01		0.07		0.15		0.19		0.19		0.15		0.11		0.06	2	0.92
40-49		0.11	1	0.47		0.80		0.87		0.76		0.52		0.30		0.12	1	3.84
50-59	2	0.35		1.31	1	1.71	1	1.53		1.02		0.61		0.24		0.04	3	6.46
60-69	1	0.67	3	1.99	3	1.92	2	1.25	1	0.57		0.19		0.03		0.00	10	5.95
70+	1	0.81		1.74		1.01	1	0.35		0.06		0.01		0.01		0.00	2	3.18

INVASIVE — RADIOTHERAPY

AGE	<1	1-4	5-9	10-14	15-19	20-24	25-29	30+	Total (excl. <1)
<30									
30-39									
40-49									
50-59									
60-69									
70+									

IN SITU — NO RADIOTHERAPY

AGE	<1 O	<1 E	1-4 O	1-4 E	5-9 O	5-9 E	10-14 O	10-14 E	15-19 O	15-19 E	20-24 O	20-24 E	25-29 O	25-29 E	30+ O	30+ E	Total (excl. <1) O	Total (excl. <1) E
<30		0.01		0.03		0.03		0.00		0.00		0.00		0.00		0.00		0.06
30-39		0.05		0.17		0.20		0.09		0.03		0.01		0.01		0.01	1	0.51
40-49	1	0.11		0.48		0.50		0.20		0.07		0.03		0.01		0.01	3	1.29
50-59		0.09		0.38		0.36	1	0.14		0.05		0.02		0.01		0.01	1	0.96
60-69		0.09		0.28		0.19		0.06		0.02		0.00		0.00		0.00		0.55
70+		0.05		0.15		0.08		0.01		0.00		0.00		0.00		0.00		0.24

O : All tumours observed
E : Expected

Table B19. Acute and myeloid leukaemia (ICD 205 & 207)

TIME SINCE DIAGNOSIS OF PRIMARY CERVICAL CANCER (IN YEARS)

INVASIVE — RADIOTHERAPY

Age	<1 O	<1 E	1-4 O	1-4 E	5-9 O	5-9 E	10-14 O	10-14 E	15-19 O	15-19 E	20-24 O	20-24 E	25-29 O	25-29 E	30+ O	30+ E	Total (excl. <1) O	Total (excl. <1) E
<30		0.01		0.06		0.09		0.07		0.05		0.02		0.01		0.00	0	0.30
30-39	1	0.22	1	0.85	2	0.96		0.85		0.62		0.37		0.19		0.08	4	3.92
40-49	7	0.67	6	2.16	1	2.46	2	1.98	1	1.32		0.86		0.45		0.17	17	9.40
50-59	2	1.07	7	3.16	7	3.19	1	2.53		1.61		0.77		0.27		0.06	17	11.59
60-69	6	1.01	2	3.25	3	2.88		1.85		0.83		0.26		0.02		0.01	11	9.10
70+	3	1.03		2.39	4	1.39		0.48		0.08		0.00		0.00		0.00	7	4.34

INVASIVE — NO RADIOTHERAPY

Age	<1 O	<1 E	1-4 O	1-4 E	5-9 O	5-9 E	10-14 O	10-14 E	15-19 O	15-19 E	20-24 O	20-24 E	25-29 O	25-29 E	30+ O	30+ E	Total (excl. <1) O	Total (excl. <1) E
<30																		
30-39																		
40-49																		
50-59																		
60-69																		
70+																		

IN SITU

Age	<1 O	<1 E	1-4 O	1-4 E	5-9 O	5-9 E	10-14 O	10-14 E	15-19 O	15-19 E	20-24 O	20-24 E	25-29 O	25-29 E	30+ O	30+ E	Total (excl. <1) O	Total (excl. <1) E
<30	1	0.33	1	1.01		0.53		0.08		0.02		0.01		0.00		0.00	2	1.65
30-39	3	0.55	3	1.91		1.41	1	0.35		0.09		0.02		0.00		0.00	7	3.78
40-49	3	0.60	2	2.20		1.64	1	0.47		0.11		0.04		0.02		0.00	6	4.48
50-59	1	0.25	2	0.93	1	0.70		0.21		0.08		0.03		0.01		0.00	4	1.96
60-69	2	0.15	2	0.46		0.32		0.10		0.04		0.01		0.00		0.00	4	0.93
70+		0.07		0.23		0.10		0.02		0.00		0.00		0.00		0.00	0	0.35

O : All tumours observed
E : Expected

Table B20. All leukaemias (ICD 204-207.9)

TIME SINCE DIAGNOSIS OF PRIMARY CERVICAL CANCER (IN YEARS)

O : All tumours observed
E : Expected

INVASIVE — RADIOTHERAPY

RAD/THERAPY	<1 O	<1 E	1–4 O	1–4 E	5–9 O	5–9 E	10–14 O	10–14 E	15–19 O	15–19 E	20–24 O	20–24 E	25–29 O	25–29 E	30+ O	30+ E	Total (excl. <1) O	Total (excl. <1) E
<30		0.01		0.08		0.09		0.08		0.05		0.04		0.02		0.00	0.00	0.36
30–39	1	0.25	2	1.02	2	1.24	2	1.17	1	0.92	1	0.56		0.30		0.14	8	5.35
40–49		0.93	8	3.12	7	3.70	1	3.24	2	2.33	1	1.62		0.76		0.29	19	15.06
50–59	4	1.61	9	5.17	8	5.53	1	4.50	2	2.84	2	1.60		0.50		0.10	22	20.24
60–69		1.98	9	6.06	4	5.51	6	3.59	1	1.59		0.46		0.06		0.01	20	17.28
70+	1	2.13	4	4.76		2.70	4	1.01		0.18		0.01		0.01		0.00	8	8.67

INVASIVE — NO RADIOTHERAPY

NO RADIOTHERAPY	<1 O	<1 E	1–4 O	1–4 E	5–9 O	5–9 E	10–14 O	10–14 E	15–19 O	15–19 E	20–24 O	20–24 E	25–29 O	25–29 E	30+ O	30+ E	Total (excl. <1) O	Total (excl. <1) E
<30																		
30–39																		
40–49																		
50–59																		
60–69																		
70+																		

IN SITU — NO RADIOTHERAPY

NO RADIOTHERAPY	<1 O	<1 E	1–4 O	1–4 E	5–9 O	5–9 E	10–14 O	10–14 E	15–19 O	15–19 E	20–24 O	20–24 E	25–29 O	25–29 E	30+ O	30+ E	Total (excl. <1) O	Total (excl. <1) E
<30	1	0.36	2	1.19	1	0.66		0.15		0.03		0.01		0.00		0.00	3	2.04
30–39		0.69	5	2.49	4	2.13	1	0.78	1	0.26		0.03		0.01		0.00	10	5.70
40–49		0.83	6	3.31	4	2.84	1	1.03		0.27		0.08		0.03		0.00	11	7.56
50–59	1	0.41	3	1.57	2	1.32	1	0.51		0.18		0.04		0.01		0.00	6	3.63
60–69		0.27	2	0.88	3	0.64		0.22		0.06		0.01		0.00		0.00	5	1.81
70+	1	0.13		0.45		0.23		0.04		0.01		0.00		0.00		0.00		0.73

Liver Cancer — No. 1, 1971; 176 pages US$ 10.000; Sw. fr. 30.—

Oncogenesis and Herpesviruses — No. 2, 1972; 515 pages US$ 25.00; Sw. fr. 100.—

N-Nitroso Compounds, Analysis and Formation — No. 3, 1972; 140 pages US$ 6.25; Sw. fr. 25.—

Transplacental Carcinogenesis — No. 4, 1973; 181 pages US$ 12.00; Sw. fr. 40.—

Pathology of Tumours in Laboratory Animals—Volume I—Tumours of the Rat, Part 1 — No. 5, 1973; 214 pages US$ 15.00; Sw. fr. 50.—

Pathology of Tumours in Laboratory Animals—Volume I—Tumours of the Rat, Part 2 — No. 6, 1976; 319 pages US$ 35.00; Sw. fr. 90.— (OUT OF PRINT)

Host Environment Interactions in the Etiology of Cancer in Man — No. 7, 1973; 464 pages US$ 40.00; Sw. fr. 100.—

Biological Effects of Asbestos — No. 8, 1973; 346 pages US$ 32.00; Sw. fr. 80.—

N-Nitroso Compounds in the Environment — No. 9, 1974; 243 pages US$ 20.00; Sw. fr. 50.—

Chemical Carcinogenesis Essays — No. 10, 1974; 230 pages US$ 20.00; Sw. fr. 50.—

Oncogenesis and Herpesviruses II — No. 11, 1975; Part 1, 511 pages US$ 38.00; Sw. fr. 100.— Part 2, 403 pages US$ 30.00; Sw. fr. 80.—

Screening Tests in Chemical Carcinogenesis — No. 12, 1976; 666 pages US$ 48.00; Sw. fr. 120.—

Environmental Pollution and Carcinogenic Risks — No. 13, 1976; 454 pages US$ 20.00; Sw. fr. 50.—

Environmental N-Nitroso Compounds—Analysis and Formation — No. 14, 1976; 512 pages US$ 45.00; Sw. fr. 110.—

Cancer Incidence in Five Continents—Volume III — No. 15, 1976; 584 pages US$ 40.00; Sw. fr. 100.—

Air Pollution and Cancer in Man — No. 16, 1977; 331 pages US$ 35.00; Sw. fr. 90.—

Directory of On-Going Research in Cancer Epidemiology 1977 — No. 17, 1977; 599 pages US$ 10.00; Sw. fr. 25.— (OUT OF PRINT)

Environmental Carcinogens—Selected Methods of Analysis, Vol. 1: Analysis of Volatile Nitrosamines in Food — No. 18, 1978; 212 pages US$ 45.00; Sw. fr. 90.—

Environmental Aspects of N-Nitroso Compounds — No. 19, 1978; 566 pages US$ 50.00; Sw. fr. 100.—

Nasopharyngeal Carcinoma: Etiology and Control — No. 20, 1978; 610 pages US$ 60.00; Sw. fr. 100.—

Cancer Registration and Its Techniques — No. 21, 1978; 235 pages US$ 25.00; Sw. fr. 40.—

Environmental Carcinogens—Selected Methods of Analysis, Vol. 2: Methods for the Measurement of Vinyl Chloride in Poly(vinyl chloride), Air, Water and Foodstuffs — No. 22, 1978; 142 pages US$ 45.00; Sw. fr. 75.—

Pathology of Tumours in Laboratory Animals—Volume II—Tumours of the Mouse — No. 23, 1979; 669 pages US$ 60.00; Sw. fr. 100.—

Oncogenesis and Herpesviruses III — No. 24, 1978; Part 1, 580 pages US$ 30.00; Sw. fr. 50.— Part 2, 522 pages US$ 30.00; Sw. fr. 50.—

Carcinogenic Risks—Strategies for Intervention — No. 25, 1979; 283 pages US$ 30.00; Sw. fr. 50.—

Directory of On-Going Research in Cancer Epidemiology 1978 — No. 26, 1978; 550 pages Sw. fr. 30.—

Molecular and Cellular Aspects of Carcinogen Screening Tests — No. 27, 1980; 371 pages US$ 40.00; Sw. fr. 60.—

Directory of On-Going Research in Cancer Epidemiology 1979 — No. 28, 1979; 672 pages Sw. fr. 30.— (OUT OF PRINT)

Environmental Carcinogens—Selected Methods of Analysis, Vol. 3: Analysis of Polycyclic Aromatic Hydrocarbons in Environmental Samples — No. 29, 1979; 240 pages US$ 30.00; Sw. fr. 50.—

Biological Effects of Mineral Fibres — No. 30, 1980; Volume 1, 494 pages US$ 35.00; Sw. fr. 60.— Volume 2, 513 pages US$ 35.00; Sw. fr. 60.—

N-Nitroso Compounds: Analysis, Formation and Occurrence — No. 31, 1980; 841 pages US$ 40.00; Sw. fr. 70.—

Statistical Methods in Cancer Research, Vol. 1: The Analysis of Case-Control Studies — No. 32, 1980; 338 pages US$ 30.00; Sw. fr. 50.—

Handling Chemical Carcinogens in the Laboratory—Problems of Safety — No. 33, 1979; 32 pages US$ 8.00; Sw. fr. 12.—

Pathology of Tumours in Laboratory Animals—Volume III—Tumours of the Hamster — No. 34, 1982; 461 pages US$ 40.00; Sw. fr. 80.—

Directory of On-Going Research in Cancer Epidemiology 1980 — No. 35, 1980; 660 pages Sw. fr. 35.—

Cancer Mortality by Occupation and Social Class 1851-1971 — No. 36, 1982; 253 pages US$ 30.00; Sw. fr. 60.—

Laboratory Decontamination and Destruction of Aflatoxins B_1, B_2, G_1, G_2 in Laboratory Wastes — No. 37, 1980; 59 pages US$ 10.00; Sw. fr. 18.—

Directory of On-Going Research in Cancer Epidemiology 1981 — No. 38, 1981; 696 pages Sw. fr. 40.—

Host Factors in Human Carcinogenesis — No. 39, 1982; 583 pages US$ 50.00; Sw. fr. 100.—

Environmental Carcinogens—Selected Methods of Analysis, Vol. 4: Some Aromatic Amines and Azo Dyes in the General and Industrial Environment — No. 40, 1981; 347 pages US$ 30.00; Sw. fr. 60.—

N-Nitroso Compounds: Occurrence and Biological Effects — No. 41, 1982; 755 pages US$ 55.00; Sw. fr. 110.—

Cancer Incidence in Five Continents—Volume IV — No. 42, 1982; 811 pages US$ 50.00; Sw. fr. 100.—

Laboratory Decontamination and Destruction of Carcinogens in Laboratory Wastes: Some N-Nitrosamines — No. 43, 1982; 73 pages US$ 10.00; Sw. fr. 18.—

Environmental Carcinogens—Selected
Methods of Analysis, Vol. 5:
Mycotoxins

No. 44, 1983; 455 pages
US$ 30.00; Sw. fr. 60.—

Environmental Carcinogens—Selected
Methods of Analysis, Vol. 6:
N-Nitroso Compounds

No. 45, 1983 ; 508 pages
US $ 40.00; Sw.fr. 80.—

Directory of On-Going Research in
Cancer Epidemiology 1982

No. 46, 1982; 722 pages
Sw. fr. 40.—

Cancer Incidence in Singapore

No. 47, 1982; 174 pages
US$ 15.00; Sw. fr. 30.—

Cancer Incidence in the USSR
Second Revised Edition

No. 48, 1982; 75 pages
US$ 15.00; Sw. fr. 30.—

Laboratory Decontamination and
Destruction of Carcinogens in
Laboratory Wastes: Some
Polycyclic Aromatic Hydrocarbons

No. 49, 1983; 81 pages
US$ 10.00; Sw. fr. 20.-

Directory of On-Going Research
in Cancer Epidemiology 1983

No. 50, 1983; 740 pages
Sw. fr. 50.-

NON-SERIAL PUBLICATIONS

Alcool et Cancer

1978; 42 pages
Fr. fr. 35-; Sw. fr. 14.-

Information Bulletin on the
Survey of Chemicals Being Tested
for Carcinogenicity No. 8

1979, 604 pages
US$ 20.00; Sw.fr. 40.-

Cancer Morbidity and Causes of
Death Among Danish Brewery Workers

1980, 145 pages
US$ 25.00; Sw.fr. 45.-

Information Bulletin on the
Survey of Chemicals Being Tested
for Carcinogenicity No. 9

1981, 294 pages
US$ 20.00; Sw.fr. 41.-

Information Bulletin on the
Survey of Chemicals Being Tested
for Carcinogenicity No. 10

1982, 326 pages
US$ 20.00; Sw.fr. 42.-

Composition, impression et façonnage
Groupe MCP-Mame
Dépôt légal : Février 1984